全球基金疟疾项目
中国高传播区疟疾控制资料汇编

China Global Fund Malaria Program

Malaria Control in High Transmission Regions of China

主　　编：汤林华
副 主 编：周水森　夏志贵

九州出版社
JIUZHOUPRESS

图书在版编目（CIP）数据

全球基金疟疾项目中国高传播区疟疾控制资料汇编 / 汤林华著 .—北京：九州出版社，2009.11
ISBN 978-7-80195-730-6

Ⅰ.全…　Ⅱ.汤…　Ⅲ.疟疾－防治－资料－汇编－中国－2003～2008　Ⅳ.R531.3

中国版本图书馆 CIP 数据核字（2009）第 201587 号

全球基金疟疾项目中国高传播区疟疾控制资料汇编

作　　者	汤林华　著
出版发行	九州出版社
出 版 人	徐尚定
地　　址	北京市西城区阜外大街甲 35 号（100037）
发行电话	(010)68992190/2/3/5/6
网　　址	www.jiuzhoupress.com
电子信箱	jiuzhou@jiuzhoupress.com
印　　刷	三河市东方印刷厂
开　　本	787×1092 毫米　16 开
印　　张	30　彩插 16P
字　　数	550 千字
版　　次	2009 年 12 月第 1 版
印　　次	2009 年 12 月第 1 次印刷
书　　号	ISBN 978-7-80195-730-6
定　　价	70.00 元

全球基金疟疾项目

中国高传播区疟疾控制资料汇编

主　　编：汤林华

副 主 编：周水森　夏志贵

参编人员：（按姓氏笔画排序）

汤林华　周水森　金　璟　夏志贵

贺　杰　黄　颖　盛慧锋

前　言

疟疾是全球广泛关注的重要公共卫生问题之一。根据世界卫生组织报告，全球大约40%的人口受疟疾威胁，每年有3.5亿～5亿人感染疟疾，110万人因疟疾死亡，每天有3 000个儿童因患疟疾而失去生命。据世界卫生组织估计，全球有59%的疟疾病例分布在非洲，38%分布在亚洲，3%分布在美洲。降低疟疾发病率，减轻疟疾疾病负担已列入《联合国千年发展目标》。疟疾也是严重危害我国人民群众身体健康和生命安全、影响社会经济发展的重要传染病。据不完全统计，新中国成立前全国每年的疟疾发病数达3 000万以上。新中国成立后，党和政府把疟疾作为重点防治的五大寄生虫病之一，组织开展了大规模的防治工作。通过五十多年的积极防治，业已取得了举世瞩目的成绩，全国疟疾病人数已减少到21世纪初的数十万，严重流行区的范围已大幅度缩小，除云南、海南两省外各省已消除了当地原发的恶性疟。2006年，卫生部制订下发《2006—2015年全国疟疾防治规划》，提出“到2015年底，云南边境地区和海南中南部山区的高传播地区各县控制疟疾流行，全国其他流行县（市、区）均要基本消除疟疾；海南省消除恶性疟”。

全球抗击艾滋病、结核病和疟疾基金是由联合国前秘书长科菲·安南先生于2002年倡议的全球性赠款项目，旨在筹集各方捐助资金帮助世界上发展中国家遏制这3种疾病的传播，并防止它们对家庭、社区和全球经济造成的危害。截至目前，我国已成功申请了第一轮、第五轮和第六轮疟疾项目，总资金达6 200多万美元。“中国高传播区疟疾控制项目”是2002年第一批成功获得全球基金资助的国际合作项目，申请资金为640多万美元。项目覆盖云南省25个边境县，海南省有恶性疟传播的10个山区县，以及河南、湖北、安徽、江苏、广东、广西、四川、贵州8个省（区）各1～2个试点县，直接目标人群930万。该项目通过5年的实施（2003—2008年），云南省项目县疟疾调查推算发病率由2002年195/万的基线下降到65.88/万，下降了66.22%；海南省项目县疟疾调查推算发病率和恶性疟调查推算发病率分别由2002年的385/万和9.06/万下降到31.13/万和0.40/万，分别下降了91.91%和95.58%，有力地推动了我国高疟区疟疾的防治工作，为国家疟疾防治规划的实现提供了资金和技术补充。

本汇编全面概括了项目实施5年来的执行结果和经验启示，涵盖项目终期总结报告，项目执行的技术方案，项目管理、财务管理及物资采购供应管理的规范，项目标书等，为以后类似项目的申请与实施提供宝贵的经验和借鉴，同时对其他传染病防治也有重要的参考价值。希望对从事疾病防治工作的管理人员和疟疾相关的从业人员有所裨益。

本书的编写，虽然进行了多次审校修改，但由于时间所限，编写中错误和遗漏之处，尚希读者不吝指正。

汤林华

2008年8月

目　录

第一章

终期总结报告

第一节　中文报告

一、项目背景

2002 年项目成功获得全球抗击艾滋病、结核病和疟疾基金（以下简称“全球基金”）资助，执行期为 5 年（2003 年 4 月 1 日 ~ 2008 年 3 月 31 日），总预算 6 406 659 美元。项目覆盖云南省 25 个边境县，海南省有恶性疟传播的 10 个山区县，以及河南、湖北、安徽、江苏、广东、广西、四川、贵州 8 个省（区）各 1 ~ 2 个试点县（表 1–1），直接目标人群为 930 万。项目旨在通过加强对项目地区疟疾的及时诊断、规范治疗和有效防护、加强云南边境地区流动人口疟疾管理、开展健康教育和健康促进、加强疟疾监测和项目管理能力等，遏制项目省疟疾流行，并有效控制多重抗性恶性疟的传播与扩散，到项目结束时，云南省 25 个项目县疟疾发病率至少下降 50%，海南省恶性疟发病率下降到 1/ 万以下。

表 1–1 第一轮中国全球基金疟疾项目省（区）和县（市）

编号	云南	海南	河南	湖北	安徽	江苏	广东	广西	四川	贵州
1	麻栗坡	万宁	淮滨	枣阳	怀远	泗洪	惠阳区	百色	筠连	榕江
2	马关	陵水	商城	曾都区		盱眙	徐闻			
3	富宁	三亚								
4	绿春	保亭								
5	金平	乐东								
6	河口	五指山								
7	江城	琼中								
8	孟连	东方								
9	澜沧	昌江								
10	西盟	白沙								
11	勐腊									
12	景洪									

续表

13	勐海
14	沧源
15	福贡
16	耿马
17	贡山
18	龙陵
19	陇川
20	泸水
21	潞西
22	瑞丽
23	腾冲
24	盈江
25	镇康

二、项目管理

（一）组织机构与管理制度

1．组织机构

项目建立了包括中央执行机构（Principal Recipient, 以下简称 PR）、10 个省级项目办（Sub-Recipients, 以下简称 SR）、47 个县级项目办（Sub-Sub-Recipients, 以下简称 SSR）的三级项目执行机构。

1.1 PR

由全球基金国家协调委员会（Country Coordinating Mechanism, 以下简称 CCM）提名、经全球基金认可，中国疾病预防控制中心作为项目的 PR，负责中国所得赠款的使用和项目实施。

PR 下设 PR 办公室、国家项目办公室、财务部、审计部、物资采购部、监督与评估部等部门，主要负责与全球基金签署项目拨款协议、向全球基金申请资金拨付、项目活动的管理和执行、项目的监督评价、项目的财务管理与审计、项目资金的拨付、项目物资采购与供应管理、向全球基金中国地方代理机构（Local Fund Agency, 以下简称 LFA）及全球基金递交财务报告、审计报告和项目实施进展报告，以及与卫生部、CCM 和 LFA 等机构部门协调有关工作等。

国家疟疾项目办公室为 PR 下设的项目管理和协调机构，负责项目的组织实施、管理、监督、评价，以及办公室日常事务处理，依托中国疾病预防控制中心寄生虫病预防控制所开展工作。

1.2 SR

在10个项目省，均依托各省疾病预防控制中心或寄生虫病预防控制所建立省级项目办公室。省级项目办公室负责本省项目的管理工作，制定和执行本省项目计划，组织实施项目相关活动，如培训、督导、财务管理以及日常事务工作等，与省卫生厅等机构协调有关工作，并接受PR的领导、监督和指导。

1.3 SSR

在10个项目省的47个项目县，均依托各县疾病预防控制中心建立县级项目办公室，负责本县项目的管理工作，制定和执行本县项目计划，组织实施项目相关活动，如开展财务与物资管理、安排和监督乡镇卫生院以及村卫生室的日常项目活动、开展各种培训以及日常事务工作等，并承担与县卫生局等机构部门协调有关工作，接受省级项目办的领导、监督和指导。

1.4 项目领导小组和技术专家组

各级还成立了由卫生行政机构领导组成的项目领导小组，负责领导项目的执行，将项目纳入当地疟疾防治规划，制定年度疟疾防治计划时将项目工作作为疟疾防治规划的重要部分，使项目在卫生行政部门的支持和领导下顺利开展。

此外，各级项目执行机构邀请疟防战线的有关专家、医师组成技术专家组，为项目工作计划、技术方案的制定出谋划策，承担项目技术培训任务，参与项目督导。

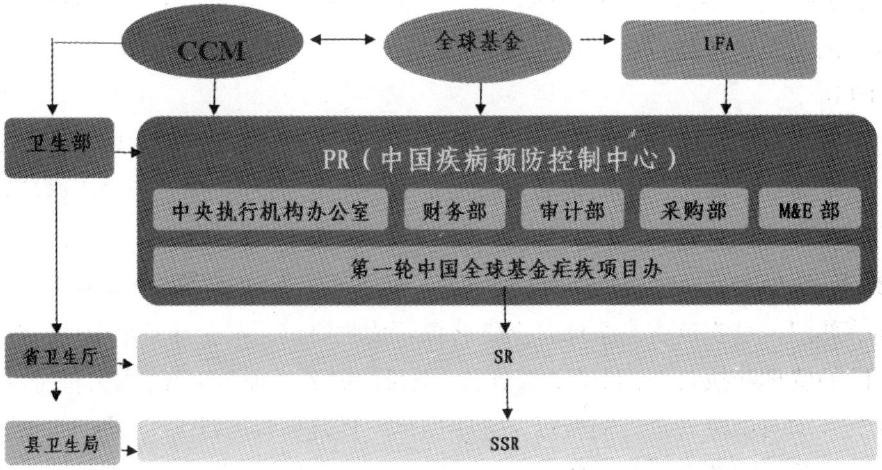

图1–1 第一轮中国全球基金疟疾项目组织机构框架图

2. 管理制度

为加强项目管理，规范项目实施，监督与评价项目进度，保证项目资金物资的安全、有效和专用，以顺利达到项目的预期目标，PR 按照全球基金要求并结合疟疾项目特点，制定了项目管理、监督与评价管理、财务管理以及物资采购与供应管理方面的相关管理手册和指南，主要包括：

（1）中国高传播区疟疾控制项目管理与技术方案；

（2）中国高传播区疟疾控制项目（二期）执行指导手册；

（3）中国高传播区疟疾控制项目监督评价计划与实施指南；

（4）中国全球基金项目财务管理手册；

（5）中国全球基金物资采购与资产管理手册。

各 SR 和 SSR 均依据 PR 下发的管理手册和指南，结合本地区特点，制定并落实了相关的管理制度，确保项目的规范实施。

3. 制定项目工作计划

围绕项目目标，在项目标书和总体计划的基础上，先后制定了项目 6 个月工作计划、两年度工作计划和二期工作计划。

4. 信息管理

为加强对项目进度的监督与管理，在国家、省、县三级建立了项目报表季报制，要求各级项目办由专人负责档案资料、数据报表的管理，及时按计划上报项目季度工作报表、财务报表和年度进展报告，保证报表填写规范，数据准确可靠。

项目实施以来，各级项目办均能及时总结项目进展，及时、规范、准确地上报报表，各项目办还以简讯、简报等形式，加强工作信息交流与反馈。

5. 召开项目年会

为总结项目年度执行进展情况，交流项目执行经验，进一步明确全球基金项目管理、财务管理和审计、采购供应管理、监督与评估管理等方面的要求和规范，国家项目办分别在 2004 年 8 月于河南省郑州市、2006 年 5 月 31 日 ~ 6 月 1 日于海南省三亚市、2007 年 6 月 14 ~ 15 日于云南省昆明市召开年度项目会议，总结年度项目执行进展，进一步明确全球基金管理规范和要求，部署下一年度工作，学习交流管理经验，并就项目存在的问题、困难进行讨论，提出解决方案。

2008 年 11 月 29 日项目终期总结大会在北京召开，会议邀请了卫生部、CCM 疟疾专项工作组成员单位、PR 各部门、各项目省、县主要负责人参加，总结项目 5 年来实施效果、经验，对项目执行过程中的先进集体和个人给予表彰。

（二）监督与评价管理

1. 制定监督评价计划与实施指南

国家项目办组织有关专家总结项目实施经验，不断完善监督评价计划与实施指南，规范各级项目督导活动、实时监控项目进度、客观评价项目实施效果和确保项目实施质量。

2. 按照工作计划开展项目督导

各级项目办均按照要求委派专人负责项目数据的收集、汇总、审核、上报和管理工作，能够按照工作计划开展规范而有成效的督导工作，追踪跟进整改情况。对于项目执行过程中出现的问题，开展有针对性的专项督导。

项目执行5年来，国家项目办共对项目省督导31次（表1–2），重点检查项目管理、财务管理、物资供应管理情况及工作计划和指标完成情况，并核实被督导项目点的上报数据，以及检查上次督导后的整改情况。各省、县项目办也按照工作计划开展了各级督导，并根据需要开展跟踪督导。

表1–2 国家项目办对项目省督导记录

序号	起止日期	被督导项目点
1	2003年6月28～29日	海南省项目办、琼中县、文昌县
2	2004年7月1～5日	海南省项目办、万宁县、陵水县
3	2004年7月5～10日	云南省项目办、景洪市、勐腊县
4	2005年6月28日～7月3日	云南省项目办、海南省项目办
5	2005年11月2～5日	云南省项目办、孟连县、海南省项目办、琼中县
6	2006年6月	云南省项目办、孟连县
7	2006年7月26～31日	云南省项目办
8	2006年9月14～16日	四川省项目办
9	2006年9月4～14日	云南省项目办、腾冲县、盈江县
10	2006年9月21～23日	贵州省项目办
11	2006年10月19～20日	湖北省项目办
12	2006年10月24～26日	广西壮族自治区项目办
13	2006年11月7～9日	河南省项目办
14	2006年11月15～17日	广东省项目办
15	2006年11月14～15日	云南省项目办、孟连县、西盟县
16	2006年12月24～29日	海南省项目办、白沙县、保亭县
17	2007年1月15～20日	云南省项目办、孟连县、西盟县
18	2007年3月14～16日	云南省项目办、勐海县

续表

19	2007 年 3 月 26 ~ 29 日	海南省项目办、保亭县、乐东县
20	2007 年 4 月 17 ~ 21 日	云南省项目办、绿春县
21	2007 年 5 月 20 ~ 24 日	江苏省项目办、盱眙县
22	2007 年 6 月 4 ~ 7 日	安徽省项目办、怀远县
23	2007 年 6 月 26 ~ 30 日	河南省项目办、淮滨县、商城县
24	2007 年 7 月 16 ~ 19 日	广东省项目办、惠州市、惠州市惠阳区
25	2007 年 7 月 23 ~ 27 日	广西壮族自治区项目办、百色市右江区
26	2007 年 8 月 20 ~ 25 日	贵州省项目办、榕江县
27	2007 年 9 月 3 ~ 7 日	湖北省项目办、枣阳市、曾都区
28	2007 年 9 月 17 ~ 21 日	四川省项目办、筠连县
29	2007 年 10 月 22 ~ 26 日	江苏省项目办、盱眙县、泗洪县
30	2007 年 11 月 26 ~ 30 日	海南省项目办、陵水县、三亚市
31	2008 年 3 月 5 ~ 7 日	云南省项目办、景洪市

3. 开展终期评估

为评估项目执行效果，考核项目计划和指标完成情况及工作质量、各级项目办的执行能力以及项目对各级常规疟防的促进作用，按照全球基金提议，由 CCM 组织评估组于 2008 年 5 月 13 ~ 31 日对项目进行了终期评估。

评估组分为云南和海南两个评估组，分别从项目工作计划完成情况、项目考核指标达标情况、项目办执行能力、项目地区疟防投入和受益人群对项目的满意度等方面对项目进行评估。

经过为期 19 天、从省项目办到基层乡村的抽查考核，评估组通过听取项目自评估汇报、查阅项目资料、现场工作人员访谈及目标人群访谈等形式对云南省项目办、景洪市、陇川县、腾冲县以及海南省项目办、白沙县、琼中县进行了全面、综合的现场评估，抽查核实了各级上报的发热病人血检数、疟疾病人治疗数、杀虫剂浸泡蚊帐数和终期专项调查等数据资料，在此基础上给予综合评价。

通过终期评估，评估组充分肯定了项目实施过程中取得的成绩，客观评价了存在的问题，为项目顺利结题做好了准备。

（三）财务管理

项目财务实行分级管理原则，PR 财务工作在中国疾病预防控制中心规划财务处指导下，由中国疾病预防控制中心寄生虫病预防控制所财务处负责会计核算和财务管理工作。各项目点财务设在各省 CDC 或项目办依托单位的财务部门，由其负责会计核算和财务管理工作。

项目财务报表从2003年4月1日到2006年6月30日采用季报形式，从2006年7月1日到2008年6月30日采用半年报形式。国家项目办在每季度、半年结束45天内完成汇总、审核和上报财务报表，根据预算计划和工作进度申请下一周期项目经费，并严格执行基于绩效的拨款机制。

为促进项目工作的深入开展，保证资金安全、有效、专款专用，以顺利完成项目目标，根据工作计划，国家项目办对10省项目点（每个省抽查两个项目县）每年至少进行1次财务督导，对各省项目管理人员及项目财务人员每年举行1次财务培训，并将财务督导报告、财务培训情况上报有关部门。

国家项目办财务督导组以全球基金项目财务管理手册和项目财务督导方案为依据，对各省项目点进行财务督导考评，在充分肯定各省项目进展的同时，指出了项目实施中存在的问题，提出了改进建议。财务督导考评的主要内容包括：预算制订与预算执行情况；银行账号设置情况；财务管理情况；财务核算及资金管理使用情况；固定资产管理；报表及审计情况；培训及督导情况；其他需要检查的内容等。督导组在督导结束15天后完成现场督导报告，并将督导报告报被督导地区单位和上级主管部门。督导报告的内容包括：督导时间、地点、参加督导的人员、督导内容、整改意见与建议等。各省项目办每年对下属县、乡项目点进行了大量的财务督导工作。

（四）物资采购管理

根据项目财务管理手册，使用项目资金购置的使用年限在一年以上，办公设备单位价值在500元以上、专用设备单位价值在800元以上，并在使用过程中基本保持原有物质形态的资产，或单位价值虽不足规定标准，但耐用时间在一年以上，批量（5件以上，含5件）购置的同类物资，使用过程中基本保持原有物质形态的资产为项目固定资产。根据项目财务管理手册，使用项目资金购置的材料、药品、试剂等需要入库保管的物品为项目存货。

项目物资由PR采购部负责进行采购，再调往各项目点使用。为保证采购工作的合法、合规、公开、透明，财务工作有项目依托单位（中国疾病预防控制中心）纪检监察部门或审计部门参与，一次性购置固定资产在50万元人民币（含50万元人民币）以上的大宗采购，均进行招投标。

为保证资产安全，PR采购部在接到售货方的发货通知时，填制项目物资下拨通知单，通知相关项目点接收物资。各项目点按季度对库存项目物品材料进行实地盘点，并编制项目物品材料核查表，进行账实核对。对于盘点出现的盘盈、盘亏和毁损的项目物品材料，及时查明原因，写出详细的书面报告及处理意见。

项目的执行提高了各级项目单位的物资管理水平。项目人员对于物资验收、入库、领用以及登记入账的管理能力较之项目执行前有了大幅度提高。物资管理账目清晰、账物相符、分配及时。项目单位物资的库存条件亦得到改善：绝大部分的项目单位建立了条件良好的库房；药品、非药品、有毒物资分开存放；库房通风条件良好；有温度、湿度的控制；库存管理人员通过项目执行，在入库、出库登记、定期核对、盘点等方面进一步加强了管理。

2003 年 4 月 1 日至 2008 年 6 月 30 日，项目采购了价值 14 628 334.97 元（折合约 180 万美元）的车辆、电脑、显微镜、抗疟药、杀虫剂、蚊帐等物资，并已全部投入项目地区使用。各类办公设备、交通工具和显微镜的配备，提高了基层疾控人员、项目人员的办公自动化、信息化水平，加强了基层单位实验室检测能力，增强了药品、物资运送效率，改善了出差、下乡工作条件，为提高疟疾防治能力，提供了更好的物资保障。

三、项目指标及工作计划完成情况

（一）项目指标完成情况

项目的实施取得了明显的疟疾防治效果，项目各项指标基本达到了预期目标。通过项目的实施，项目地区居民防疟、抗疟知识以及个人自我防护、主动就诊意识显著提高，项目地区拥有杀虫剂浸泡蚊帐的家庭比例也有了很大提高，项目地区疟疾疫情、多重抗性恶性疟的传播与扩散得到了有效的控制。2008 年 1 月开展的项目终期专项调查结果显示：云南省项目县疟疾发病率由 2002 年 195/ 万的基线下降到 65.88/ 万，下降了 66.22%；海南省项目县疟疾发病率和恶性疟发病率分别由 2002 年的 385/ 万和 9.06/ 万下降到 31.13/ 万和 0.40/ 万，分别下降了 91.91% 和 95.58%。实现了云南省 25 个项目县疟疾发病率至少下降 50%，海南省恶性疟发病率下降到 1/ 万以下的项目目标（表 1–3）

表 1–3 项目指标完成情况

项目目标	考核指标	累计目标	累计结果	更新时间
总目标：遏制项目省疟疾流行，控制多重抗性恶性疟扩散。	云南25个项目县和海南10个项目县的疟疾发病率	Y:97/10 000 H: 192/10 000	Y: 65.88/10 000 H: 31.13/10 000	2008-3-31
	海南10个项目县恶性疟发病率	≤ 1/10 000	0.40/10 000	2008-3-31
	云南和海南疟疾报告死亡人数	≤ 17	5	2008-3-31
	拥有杀虫剂浸泡蚊帐的家庭比例	30.00%	37.60%	2008-3-31
	目标地区中小学生能够正确回答至少3个与疟疾相关问题的比例	85.00%	93.18%	2008-3-31
	发热病人在症状出现2天内求诊的比例	90.00%	89.95%	2008-3-31
目标1：使云南省边境地区流动人口更好地获得疟疾诊断和合理治疗。	就诊的流动人口发热病人中得到镜检的人数和比例	118 000/208 300 56.65%	164 433/232 427 70.75%	2008-3-31
	就诊的流动人口疟疾病人得到规范治疗的人数和比例	56 600/144 700 39.12%	57 729/62 604 92.21%	2008-3-31
目标2：使云南和海南流行区居民得到更好的早期诊断和个人防护。	目标地区乡、村医生和镜检员接受早期诊断和规范治疗（EDAT）培训的人数和比例	10 000/10 000 100.00%	11 048/11 048 100.00%	2008-3-31
	云南和海南当地居民疟疾病人中接受规范治疗的人数和比例	261 360/469 200 55.70%	246 885/269 363 91.66%	2008-3-31
	接受规范治疗的疟疾病人中通过镜检确诊的人数和比例	127 422/261 360 48.75%	28 109/246 885 11.39%	2008-3-31
	杀虫剂浸泡蚊帐（ITNs）的数量	333 000	365 039	2008-3-31

续表

目标3：使云南和海南目标地区居民更有效地采取疟疾预防措施，及时治疗。	目标地区家庭收到"信息、教育和交流（IEC）"和健康教育（HE）材料的户数和比例	673 500/2 000 000 33.68%	1 044 055/1 936 021 53.93%	2008-3-31
目标4：优化云南、海南及其他八个项目省疟疾控制项目管理。	疟疾病例通过信息网络报告的比例	40.00%	38.92%	2008-3-31

项目执行5年来，项目主要指标除了"接受规范治疗的疟疾病人中通过镜检确诊的人数和比例"一项由于项目地区多为地处边远的少数民族地区，绝大多数的疟疾病人都在村级就诊，由于村级不具备镜检条件，所以镜检确诊的疟疾病人比例较低的原因导致指标完成率偏低外，其他指标累计结果都已经基本达到项目累计目标。

（二）项目执行进展

各项目单位开展了大量的疟疾诊断、治疗、预防、培训、督导、药品和设备采购分发和管理、健康促进等工作，有力地推动了全国的疟疾防治。截止2008年3月31日，项目累计完成发热病人血检2 530 245例，完成疟疾病人规范治疗517 220例，完成乡、村医生和镜检员早期诊断和规范治疗培训14 745人次，分发杀虫剂浸泡蚊帐365 039顶，在公共场所张贴疟疾防治宣传画259 640份，开展中小学生疟疾知识培训12 644班次，经广播、电视进行疟防知识专题宣传532县次，基本完成了项目工作计划。（表1–4）

表1–4　关键项目活动完成情况

关键项目活动	累计计划数	累计实际数	完成率（%）	更新时间
发热病人血检（人次）	1 929 200	2 530 245	131.16	2008-3-31
疟疾病人治疗（人次）	533 120	517 220	97.02	2008-3-31
乡村/个体医生和镜检员培训（人数）	10 860	14 745	135.77	2008-3-31
杀虫剂浸泡蚊帐（顶数）	333 000	365 039	109.62	2008-3-31
张贴疟疾宣传海报（张数）	241 000	259 640	107.73	2008-3-31
中小学生疟疾知识培训（班数）	9 500	12 644	133.09	2008-3-31
疟防广播电视宣传（县次）	251	532	211.95	2008-3-31

各项关键项目活动分年度计划任务和实际完成数如下（表 1–5）。

表 1–5 各项关键项目活动分年度完成情况

关键项目活动		发热病人血检(人次)	疟疾病人治疗(人次)	乡村 / 个体医生和镜检员培训(人数)	杀虫剂浸泡蚊帐（顶数）	张贴疟疾宣传海报(张数)	中小学生疟疾知识培训（班数）	疟防广播电视宣传(县次)
合计	计划开展	1 929 200	533 120	10 860	333 000	241 000	9 500	251
	实际完成	2 530 245	517 220	14 745	365 039	259 640	12 644	532
2003	计划开展	138 000	22 860	3 050	66 000	4 000	0	0
	实际完成	207 947	28 340	5 208	17 190	4 990	0	0
2004	计划开展	438 200	141 200	3 060	160 750	96 000	3 500	86
	实际完成	523 173	126 498	3 547	69 855	129 860	4 518	172
2005	计划开展	456 000	133 510	1 520	43 000	51 000	2 500	60
	实际完成	580 565	132 591	2 073	62 376	26 082	3 445	205
2006	计划开展	442 000	133 450	2 070	53 250	45 000	2 500	85
	实际完成	616 578	129 208	2 490	205 232	59 349	3 143	135
2007	计划开展	428 000	97 750	1 160	10 000	45 000	1 000	20
	实际完成	556 167	94 401	1 427	10 386	39 349	1 538	20
2008	计划开展	27 000	4 350	0	0	0	0	0
	实际完成	45 815	6 182	0	0	10	0	0

各省分年度计划完成情况详见“终期总结报告附表”。

四、项目资金使用情况

2003 年 4 月 1 日至 2008 年 3 月 31 日为项目执行期，2008 年 4 月 1 日至 2008 年 6 月 30 日经全球基金批准为项目关账期。从 2003 年 4 月 1 日至 2008 年 6 月 30 日，项目累计取得全球基金资助款 6 347 405.31 美元，实际结汇人民币 49 713 251.36 元，累计取得银行存款利息收入人民币 101 181.59 元，项目资金收入累计为人民币 49 814 432.95 元，其中：采购经费人民币 15 013 798.77 元，活动经费人民币 34 800 634.18 元。各项目点经费收入情况如下（表 1–6）。

表 1–6 项目经费收入情况

单位：人民币（元）

项目点	目标 1	目标 2	目标 3	目标 4	合计
中央	0.00	0.00	371 994.30	7 638 535.34	8 010 529.64
采购	0.00	0.00	0.00	15 013 798.77	15 013 798.77
云南	1 479 589.65	4 387 032.76	1 870 875.26	5 873 114.50	13 610 612.17
海南	0.00	2 341 522.89	1 454 659.61	2 107 314.84	5 903 497.34
安徽	0.00	329 214.68	0.00	658 028.45	987 243.13
河南	0.00	552 054.44	0.00	431 135.65	983 190.09
湖北	0.00	458 903.05	0.00	575 161.28	1 034 064.33
江苏	0.00	580 101.04	0.00	411 695.91	991 796.95
广东	0.00	466 082.46	0.00	340 345.27	806 427.73
广西	0.00	356 745.70	0.00	427 299.30	784 045.00
四川	0.00	288 862.73	0.00	514 558.37	803 421.10
贵州	0.00	506 786.55	0.00	277 838.54	784 625.09
合计	1 479 589.65	10 267 306.33	3 697 529.17	34 268 826.21	49 713 251.36

2008 年 6 月 30 日美元对人民币的国家外汇管理局发布的汇率中间价为：USD:RMB = 1:6.8591，按此汇率计算，项目累计发生汇兑损失人民币 6 175 763.60 元。

2003 年 4 月 1 日至 2008 年 6 月 30 日，项目累计经费支出人民币 49 095 615.46 元，累计支出中包括：中央活动经费支出人民币 7 720 347.62 元；设备物资采购经费支出人民币 14 662 815.46 元，十省（SR）活动经费支出人民币 26 712 452.38 元。项目经费总预算 6 406 659.00 美元，累计资金使用率为 99%，累计预算执行率为 96%。

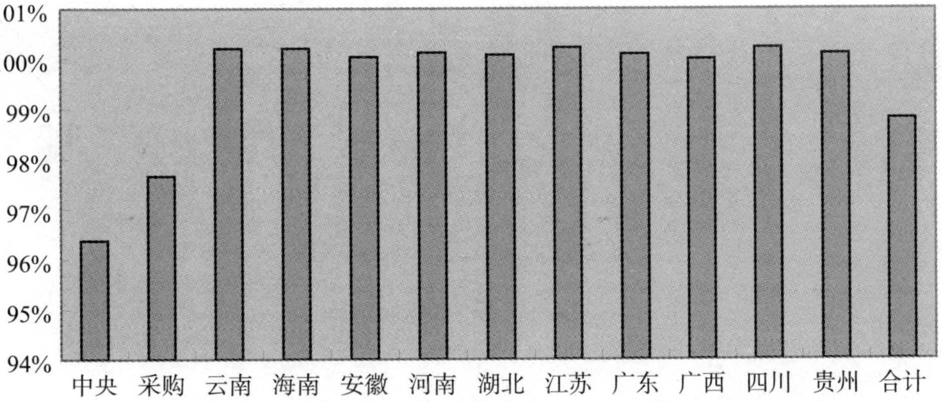

图 1–2 各项目点资金使用率情况分析

截至 2008 年 6 月 30 日，项目经费结余人民币 718 817.49 元，其中：采购经费结余人民币 350 983.31 元，中央活动经费结余人民币 341 848.30 元，10 省活动经费结余人民币 25 985.88 元，其中：云南省经费结余 25 968.88 元，湖北省经费结余 10.09 元，四川省经费结余 6.91 元。

中央及各省的终期审计工作计划已于 2008 年 8 月 4 日完成，终期审计工作根据项目审计工作指南的规定，结合项目的特点和实际情况，公开招标选择了北京兴华会计师事务所有限责任公司对国家项目办进行了审计，各省根据指南规定在本省招标会计师事务所完成了其本省的终期审计。

五、项目设备物资盘点情况

2003 年 4 月 1 日至 2008 年 6 月 30 日，项目采购了价值 14 628 334.97 元（折合约 180 万美元）的车辆、电脑、显微镜、抗疟药、杀虫剂、蚊帐等物资，并已全部投入项目地区使用。项目累计采购固定资产金额为人民币 9 352 909.97 元，其中：显微镜 520 台，电脑 169 台，汽车 22 辆，摩托车 185 辆，数码相机 29 台，打印机 33 台，传真机 3 台，投影仪 3 台等；累计采购抗疟药品及卫生产品金额为人民币 5 275 425.00 元，其中：磷酸氯 / 伯喹片剂 378 500 人份，双氢青蒿素片剂 30 000 人份，蒿甲醚针剂 24 200 人份，复方磷酸哌喹片剂 304 000 人份，青蒿琥酯片剂 26 500 人份，蚊帐 54 000 顶，一次性注射器 23 700 只，氟氯氰菊酯 300 升，溴氰菊酯 8 500 升等。

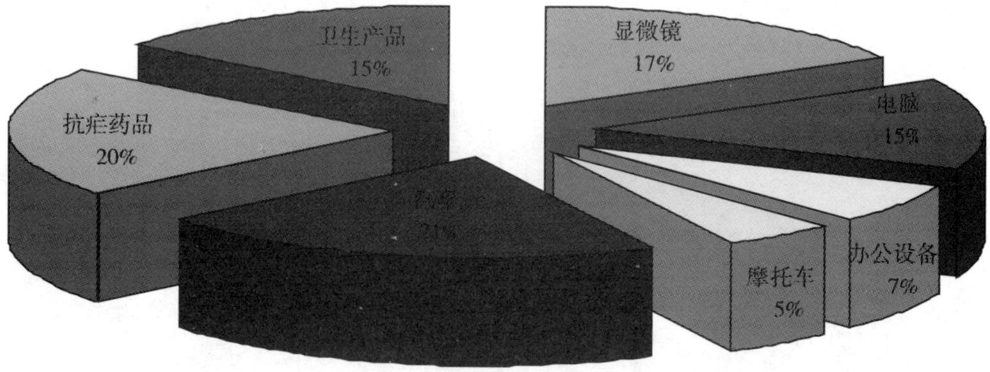

图 1–3 采购物资构成比

经过 PR 采购部物资清查，截至 2008 年 6 月 30 日，各级项目办的抗疟药品和卫生产品均已全部投入项目地区使用，项目固定资产运行良好，项目物资在执行期结束后，移交给项目依托单位（省、县疾病预防控制中心或寄生虫病防治所）使用。

依托单位继续承担其他轮次中国全球基金疟疾项目的，原一轮项目物资用于支持全球基金项目工作。依托单位未承担其他轮次中国全球基金疟疾项目的，原一轮项目物资用于支持国家常规疟疾的防治工作。

六、项目对疟疾防治工作的影响

（一）项目地区疟疾疫情现状

项目执行5年来，有效遏制了云南省、海南省疟疾的流行，并控制了海南省多重抗性恶性疟的传播与扩散，控制了其他八个项目省项目地区疟疾的局部暴发流行。

1. 云南省

根据2008年终期专项调查结果，云南省项目县疟疾发病率已下降到65.88/万，达到项目预期目标。

2. 海南省

根据2008年终期专项调查结果，海南省项目县疟疾发病率已下降到31.13/万，恶性疟发病率已下降到0.40/万。

3. 其他8省项目地区

3.1 河南省每年第4季度开展疟疾病例的主动侦查，深入了解疟疾疫情，及时发现疟疾暴发点，对可能出现的疟疾暴发点及时采取预防措施，避免了疫情的扩大，使项目县的疟疾发病比项目启动前的2002年有大幅降低，2007年估计疟疾病人为210人，疟疾漏报率为37.61%，估计发病人数比2002年估计疟疾病人6 829人下降96.92%。

3.2 湖北省项目县枣阳市2007年度报告疟疾病例441例较2003年（3 052例）下降了85.55%，但局部地区仍有疟疾暴发点发生；曾都区2007年疫情报告病例为77例，目前无暴发点出现。

3.3 安徽省项目县2006—2007年未出现暴发点，有效控制了疟疾的局部暴发流行，2007年推算实际发病数率为6.02/万。

3.4 江苏省项目县在2007年全省网络直报疟疾病人回升的情况下，网报病人数仍呈下降态势，盱眙县和泗洪县2007年网络直报数疟疾发病数分别为42例和106例，较2002年（84例和275例）下降50%以上。

3.5 广东省项目县连续五年均没有暴发流行点出现，且疟疾年发病率均控制在1/10万以下。

3.6 广西区项目县（百色市右江区）5年来当地感染疟疾发病率均控制在1/10

万以下，未发现输入性疟疾继发病例。

3.7 四川省项目县 2007 年报告疟疾病例 5 例，其中本地发病 4 例，输入性疟疾 1 例，发病率 0.12/ 万，5 例疟疾病人均为血检诊断确诊。

3.8 贵州省项目县项目实施以来，疟防工作得到了县政府及卫生局等有关部门高度重视，使疟防措施落到实处。较大程度遏制疟疾发病，5 年来项目地区未发生疟疾暴发流行。

（二）对项目地区疟疾防治工作的促进作用

1. 项目资金投入弥补了项目地区疟疾防治经费的缺口

项目资金、药品和相关器材的投入极大地缓解了项目地区疟防资金、药品和相关器材的不足，同时促使各级政府和卫生主管部门更加重视疟疾防治并给予多方面支持，从而有力地推动了项目地区的疟疾防治工作，提高了抗疟措施的执行力度，有效遏制项目地区疟疾暴发流行，降低了疟疾发病率。

2. 项目的实施和有关培训的开展，提高了项目地区的管理能力和防治水平

开展项目管理、疟防知识和镜检技术、早期诊断和规范治疗等相关培训，提高了项目执行人员管理能力，提高了项目县、乡疟防专业人员的防治水平和镜检员的镜检能力，提高了乡村医生对疟疾的诊断水平和现症病人的根治率，使疟疾的暴发流行得到初步控制，疟疾发病明显下降。

3. 项目的疟防知识宣传活动，提高了居民的自我保护意识

项目覆盖地区广泛开展了疟防知识的宣传，全面提高了广大居民和学生的疟防知识知晓率，增强了居民和学生的自我防护意识，群众对疟疾防治活动的依从性增强，患病后能及时主动就医。

（三）5 年项目执行评价

各级卫生行政部门将项目列入疟疾防治规划的重要组成部分，为项目实施提供了行政保证。项目的实施，对当地的疟疾防治工作起到了积极的促进作用。

项目较好地完成了工作计划各项工作任务，基本达到了项目预期目标；虽然在执行过程中还存在一些问题，但各级项目办的项目执行能力都得到较大提高；项目地区居民防疟、抗疟知识以及个人自我防护、主动就诊意识显著提高，项目地区拥有杀虫剂浸泡蚊帐的家庭比例也都有了很大提高，疟疾漏报率有所降低；项目地区疟疾疫情、多重抗性恶性疟的传播与扩散得到了有效控制。项目的实施还为各级疾控部门培养了疟防人员和项目管理人员，丰富了各级项目依托单位的管理理念和经验，提高了乡、村一级卫生人员的抗疟水平，增强了疟防力量，为国家疟疾防治规

划的实现提供了重要的补充。

七、项目执行经验总结

（一）全球基金项目项目管理理念值得推广

全球基金以财务为基础的项目管理理念、基于绩效的财务管理和贯彻始终的监督与评价机制对于常规疟疾防治工作有很大的参考价值，将先进的管理经验应用于疟防工作，能促进和更新观念，提高管理水平，建立起科学合理的管理体制，推动疟防工作有序开展。

（二）积极开展疟疾防治知识宣传，提高居民疟防知识水平，是遏制疟疾流行的基础

项目 5 年的实践表明：以多种形式开展的全民疟防知识宣传教育，提高了项目地区广大群众的疟疾防治知识水平，增强了自我防病能力，群众对防治活动的依从性大大提高，降低了项目地区疟疾防治措施展开的难度，保证了疟防目标的实现。

（三）坚持不懈地开展各类培训，提高疟疾防治人员技术水平，是推动疟疾防治工作的必要手段

项目执行过程中的经验表明：只有在疟疾防治过程中，不断地开展各类疟防知识和镜检技术的培训，全面提高县、乡、村疟防人员的防治水平和镜检员的镜检能力，才能保证各项防治活动按要求及时开展，保证工作质量。疟防知识和镜检技术的培训应该贯彻疟疾防治的始终，各类强化培训是非常必要的。

（四）针对项目地区目前的疟疾流行特点采取以控制传染源为主的综合性防治措施，能有效控制疟疾的暴发流行

疟疾患者是主要传染源之一，通过对广大群众进行疟防知识宣传教育，加强镜检站建设，反复开展镜检人员培训，并对临床医生进行疟疾诊治技能培训，一方面使疟疾患者能及时主动就医，接受规范治疗，参加休止期根治，从而使患者得到根治，另一方面随着疟防专业技术人员队伍的壮大，血检覆盖范围的扩大使疟疾病人能早发现、早诊断，减少漏诊、误诊，这些举措均对控制疟疾的暴发流行起重要作用。

（五）加强项目执行机构间以及与卫生行政部门间的信息交流，有利于提高项目实施质量

项目5年的实践证明：与省、市、县政府和卫生行政部门加强沟通，密切合作，对确保项目工作顺利开展十分重要。各级项目执行机构间的经验交流，及时发现与解决各种问题，使项目活动不断规范与完善，实施质量不断提高。

（六）加强项目人员与财务人员的及时有效沟通，能提高资金的合理有效利用率

终期评估结果表明：项目实施中项目人员与财务人员及时、有效的沟通非常必要，能做到项目与财务及时有效沟通的项目县，其财务行为出现误操作的现象相对较少，项目活动支出也更加规范，资金使用效率更高。

八、项目省、县执行情况简述

（一）云南省

云南省项目累计完成发热病人血检1 136 911例，完成疟疾病人规范治疗260 367例，完成乡、村医生和镜检员早期诊断和规范治疗培训11 750人次，分发杀虫剂浸泡蚊帐251 070顶，在公共场所张贴疟疾防治宣传画102 906份，开展中小学生疟疾知识培训6 448班次，经广播、电视进行疟防知识专题宣传320县次，基本完成了项目工作计划。

云南省25个县项目办项目执行能力存在着差异，大部分项目县能较好的按照全球基金的要求完成工作任务，部分项目县项目执行能力有待加强，其项目执行过程中的部分血检、治疗等活动数据与原始记录不一致，在后续项目的实施过程中需要督促这些县项目办注意做好报表的审核工作，确保上报数据的准确性。

（二）海南省

海南省疟疾项目累计完成发热病人血检655 175例，完成疟疾病人规范治疗100 785例，完成乡、村医生和镜检员早期诊断和规范治疗培训2 995人次，分发杀虫剂浸泡蚊帐116 611顶，在公共场所张贴疟疾防治宣传画61 126份，开展中小学生疟疾知识培训2 679班次，经广播、电视进行疟防知识专题宣传57县次，基本完成了项目工作计划。

海南省10个县项目办项目执行能力普遍较高，基本上都能按照全球基金的有

关要求，认真开展项目活动，培训乡村医生和镜检员、完成工作任务，保留痕迹资料。

（三）河南省

河南省项目累计完成发热病人血检 58 315 例，完成疟疾病人规范治疗 3 470 例。

（四）湖北省

湖北省项目累计完成发热病人血检 69 907 例，完成疟疾病人规范治疗 22 407 例。

（五）安徽省

安徽省项目累计完成发热病人血检 146 954 例，完成疟疾病人规范治疗 39 358 例。

（六）江苏省

江苏省项目累计完成发热病人血检 53 490 例，完成疟疾病人规范治疗 14 628 例。

（七）广东省

广东省项目累计完成发热病人血检 148 609 例，完成疟疾病人规范治疗 7 615 例。

（八）广西区

广西区项目累计完成发热病人血检 82 178 例，完成疟疾病人规范治疗 2 208 例。

（九）四川省

四川省项目累计完成发热病人血检 33 177 例，完成疟疾病人规范治疗 7 020 例。

（十）贵州省

贵州省项目累计完成发热病人血检 63 773 例，完成疟疾病人规范治疗 5 424 例。

中国全球基金疟疾项目办公室

第二节　英文报告

Malaria Control in High Transmission Regions of China Final Report

1. Introduction

China Global Fund Malaria Program Round 1, which covers 47 target counties in 10 provinces—Yunnan, Hainan, Henan, Hubei, Anhui, Jiangsu, Guangdong, Guangxi, Sichuan, and Guizhou, has been running for five years (April 1, 2003 – March 31, 2008) with the budget of US$ 6 406 659.00, and 9.3 million people have been directly benefited from the program. This program aims to roll back malaria in target provinces of China and limit the spread of multi-drug resistant strains through the following measures: strengthening early diagnosis, appropriate treatment and effective protection; reinforcing malaria management among mobile population in bordering areas of Yunnan Province; holding malaria related health education and promotion; strengthening malaria surveillance, program management capability, etc. The total objective is that malaria incidence in Yunnan decrease by 50%, falciparum malaria incidence in Hainan decrease blow 1/10 000 while closure.

Table 1. Target provinces and counties of China Global Fund Malaria Program Round 1 Phase 2

No.	Yunnan	Hainan	Henan	Hubei	Anhui	Jiangsu	Guang-dong	Guang-xi	Sichuan	Guizhou
1	Malipo	Wanning	Huaibin	Zaoyang	Huai-yuan	Sihong	Huiyang	Baise	Junlian	Rongjiang
2	Maguan	Lingshui	Shang-cheng	Zengdu		Xuyi	Xuwen			
3	Funing	Sanya								
4	Lvchun	Baoting								
5	Jinping	Ledong								
6	Hekou	Wuzhi-shan								
7	Jiang-cheng	Qiong-zhong								
8	Menglian	Dong-fang								
9	Lancang	Chang-jiang								
10	Ximeng	Baisha								
11	Mengla									
12	Jinghong									
13	Menghai									
14	Cangyuan									
15	Fugong									
16	Gengma									
17	Gongshan									
18	Longling									

19	Long-chuan
20	Lushui
21	Luxi
22	Ruili
23	Teng-chong
24	Yingjiang
25	Zhenkang

2 General Information of Program Management

2.1 Program Management

2.1.1 Perfecting the Construction Organization

In order to guarantee smooth implement of the program, China Global Fund Malaria Program Round 1 set up three levels program implement units — PR（including NPO）, 10 PPOs and 47 CPOs:

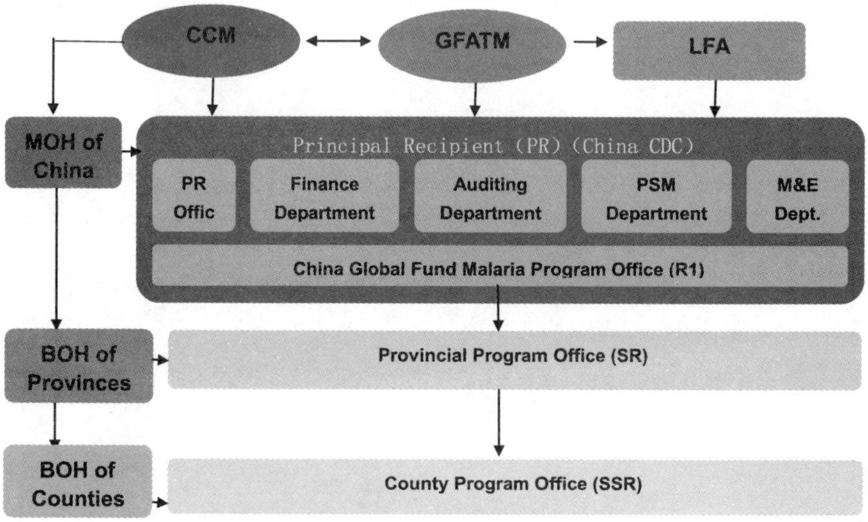

Figure 1. The framework of the organizations of China Global Fund Malaria Program R1

2.1.1.1 Principal Recipient（PR）

Nominated by CCM and recognized by Global Fund, China CDC served as PR for China Global Fund Malaria Program Round 1, and it was responsible for the usage of grants and the program implement.

PR sets PR offices, China Global Fund Malaria National Program Office（Round 1）, finance department, auditing department, PSM department and M&E department and etc. PR was mainly responsible for the following assignments: signing agreement of grant; applying for disbursement of funds from GF; managing and implementing the program, providing M&E for the program; providing finance management and audit; disbursing program grants; procuring and supplying the fixed assets; submitting finance reports; auditing reports and progress reports to LFA and GF; and coordinating with Ministry of Health, CCM and LFA.

China Global Fund Malaria National Program Office（Round 1）is an administered and coordinated unit, it is responsible for organization, implement, monitor, evaluation and regular management of the program and it depends on China CDC National Institutes of Parasitic Diseases to carry out the tasks.

2.1.1.2 Global Fund Malaria Provincial Program Office（SR）

All the Global Fund Malaria Provincial Program Office（SR）in ten target provinces depended on provincial CDC or provincial Institutes of Parasitic Diseases. All SRs are responsible for management of program, formulation and implement of work plan, organizing and conducting program related activities, e.g. trainings, supervisions, finance management, regular work and etc. All SRs coordinate with provincial Bureau of Health, and they are supervised and guided by PR.

2.1.1.3. Global Fund Malaria County Program Office（SSR）

All the Global Fund Malaria County Program Office（SSR）in 47 target counties depended on county CDC. These 47 SSRs are grassroots of program implement units, and they are responsible for management of program, formulation and implement of work plan, organizing and conducting program related activities, e.g. finance and material management, arrangement and evaluation of regular activities in township hospitals, carrying out various trainings, taking regular work and etc.; besides, SSRs coordinate with County Bureau of Health, and accept guidance and evaluation from PPO.

2.1.1.4 Programm leading group and Technical working group

The executing agencies in all levels have established Global Fund Malaria Program leading group made up of major health administration department leaders who lead and paid attention to program implementation and progress all the time, brought Global Fund Malaria Program into local malaria control, always considering program as important part of malaria prevention and control when drawing up annual malaria control plan in order to obtain support and guide from health system. In addition, executing agencies in all levels have invited national malaria control experts, doctors composed of technical working group to advice for wok plan, activities and technical proposals, acting as teacher for progranm technology training, taking part in monitor and evaluation. Smooth implementation of program can not do without the constant guidance of technical experts.

2.1.2 Improvement of Management System

The requirements in the implementation of the program are as follows: to strengthen program management, to standardize implement of program activities, to monitor and evaluate progress of program, to enhance utilization rate of grants, to ensure safe, effective and exclusive use of grants, and to achieve expected goals smoothly. According to these requirements and considering malaria program features, China PR formulated corresponding manuals and guidelines concerning program management, M&E management, finance management and procurement & supply management, the following items are mainly included in:

1) Program Management and Technology Proposal of Malaria Control in High Transmission Regions of China;

2) Program Implementation Guideline of Malaria Control in High Transmission Regions of China (Phase 2);

3) M&E Plan and Guidelines of Malaria Control in High Transmission Regions of China (Year 4 and 5);

4) Manual of Finance Management of China Global Fund;

5) Manual of Procurement and Supply Management of China Global Fund.

According to these manuals and guidelines, and concerning local situations, all SRs and SSRs have formulated and carried out corresponding management system to ensure standardized implement of the program.

2.1.3 Formulation of Work Plan

According to the requirements of GF, concerning the objective of program, based on the program proposal and overall work plan, NPO drew up work plan for the first six months and work plan for the first two years.

As continuity of Phase 1 program (the first two years) , Phase 2 program maintained the designing ideas for the overall program. In order to make use of health resources fully and rationally, combine with National Malaria Control Program better and guarantee smooth implement of program, NPO amended program designing to form Work Plan for China Global Fund Malaria Program Round 1 (Phase 2) based on the experience in the previous two years and communicated with SRs

2.1.4 Information Management

In order to strengthen monitor and evaluation to the program progress, China Global Fund Malaria Program Round 1 set up a system of reporting program progress quarterly, required special staff to be responsible for management of documents and data reports, so as to report program progress every quarter, and send M&E report, finance report and annual progress report in time, ensure that the reports would be filled out standardized, and the data would be accurate and reliable.

Since the implement of the program, program offices at all levels have summarized program progress, and reported the forms to upper levels timely and accurately. These program offices at all levels also strengthened Information exchange and feedback in the form of bulletins and briefings.

2.1.5 Holding Program Annual Meetings

NPO have held three annual meetings: in Zhengzhou, Henan Province in August, 2005; in Sanya, Hainan Province, from May 31-June 1, 2006, in order to summarize progress of program implement, communicate experience in program implement, further specify requirements and standards about Global Fund program management, finance management, audit, procurement and supply management, monitor and evaluation management, and etc.; in Kunming, Yunnan Province, from June 14 ~ 15, 2007, respectively. In these annual meetings, NPO summarized the progress in carrying out the program each year, further specified the requirements and standards of Global Fund program management, disposed work requirement for the next year, communicated experience, talked over current difficulties, and proposed solutions.

The program final summing-up meeting was held in Beijing, on Nov 29, 2008. MOH. CCM Malaria Special Working Group membership units, PR departments, directors in target provinces and counties were invited to join in. NPO summarized working experience during the five years, fully revealed effects of the program, feedback the results of final evaluation, communicated experience in implementing the program and commended the advanced units and individuals during the five years.

2.2 M&E Management

2.2.1 Formulation of M&E Work Plan and Guidelines

NPO organized experts to summarize experience obtained in implementing the program. NPO improved guidelines of M&E and implement manual in order to standardize supervising activities, monitor progress of program in time, objectively evaluate the effectiveness of the program implement and ensure the smooth program implement.

2.2.2 Conducting Supervision according to Work Plan

There are full-time staffs in charge of collection, verification, combination and reporting of progress and finance reports in Program offices at all levels. They conducted effective supervision according to work plan, and inspected rectification of program according to the previous supervision suggestion. For the problems revealed in implementing the program, the program offices at all levels would carry out special supervision as well.

NPO have carried out 31 supervisions to 10 target provinces during the five years, mainly focused on completion of budgeted work-plans, results of M&E indicators, capabilities of program management, finance management, procurement and supply management, verifying reported data, checking whether they rectify according to previous supervisions by upper levels. All PPO and CPO also have carried out supervision and track-supervision according to the work plan.

Table 2 The supervisions conducted by NPO in program provinces

No.	Beginning date	End date	Target sites chosen for supervisions
1	June 28, 2003	June 29, 2003	Hainan PPO, Qiongzhong, Wenchang
2	July 1, 2004	July 5, 2004	Hainan PPO, Wanning, Lingshui
3	July 5, 2004	July 10, 2004	Yunnan PPO, Jinghong, Mengla
4	June 28, 2005	July 3, 2005	Yunnan PPO, Hainan PPO
5	November 2, 2005	November 5, 2005	Yunnan PPO, Menglian, Hainan PPO, Qiongzhong
6	June 2006	June 2006	Yunnan PPO, Menglian
7	July 26, 2006	July 31, 2006	Yunnan PPO
8	September 14, 2006	September 16, 2006	Sichuan PPO
9	September 4, 2006	September 14, 2006	Yunnan PPO, Tengchong, Yingjiang
10	September 21, 2006	September 23, 2006	Guizhou PPO
11	October 19, 2006	October 20, 2006	Hubei PPO

12	October 24, 2006	October 26, 2006	Guangxi PPO
13	November 7, 2006	November 9, 2006	Henan PPO
14	November 15, 2006	November 17, 2006	Guangdong PPO
15	November 14, 2006	November 15, 2006	Yunnan PPO, Menglian, Ximeng
16	December 24, 2006	December 29, 2006	Hainan PPO, Baisha, Baoting
17	January 15, 2007	January 20, 2007	Yunnan PPO, Menglian, Ximeng
18	March 14, 2007	March 16, 2007	Yunnan PPO, Menghai
19	March 26, 2007	March 29, 2007	Hainan PPO, Ledong, Baoting
20	April 17, 2007	April 21, 2007	Yunnan PPO, Luchun
21	May 20, 2007	May 24, 2007	Jiangsu PPO, Xuyi
22	June 4, 2007	June 7, 2007	Anhui PPO, Huaiyuan
23	June 26, 2007	June 30, 2007	Henan PPO, Huaibin, Shangcheng
24	July 16, 2007	July 19, 2007	Guangdong PPO, Huizhou, Huiyang
25	July 23, 2007	July 27, 2007	Guangxi PPO, Youjiang
26	August 20, 2007	August 25, 2007	Guizhou PPO, Rongjiang
27	September 3, 2007	September 7, 2007	Hubei PPO, Zhaoyang, Zengdu
28	September 17, 2007	September 21, 2007	Sichuan PPO, Junlian
29	October 22, 2006	October 26, 2007	Jiangsu PPO, Xuyi, Sihong
30	November 26, 2007	November 30, 2007	Hainan PPO, Lingshui, Sanya
31	March 5, 2008	March 7, 2008	Yunnan PPO, Jinghong

2.2.3 Overall Evaluation

In order to evaluate the effects of the program, NPO organized experts from Chinese Association of Preventive Medicine, Sunshine Doctors Programme, China Association of Ethnic Economy, LFA, Chinese CDC（Audit Department, Finance Department, Procurement Department and National Institute of Parasitic Diseases）and Zhejiang CDC to evaluate five-year program implementation of Yunnan Province and Hainan Province respectively. These experts mainly focused on the completion of budgeted work-plans, results of M&E indicators, program implementation capabilities, investment in malaria control and prevention, and degree of satisfaction for people who were benefit from the program and so on. According to the evaluation proposal, National Evaluation Group checked Yunnan PPO and spot-checked three CPO — Jinghong, Longchuan and Tengchong CPO on May 13 ～ 24, 2008. It also checked Hainan PPO and spot-checked

Baisha & Qiongzhong CPO on May 26-31, 2008. These experts verified the quantities of blood tests, malaria treatment, ITNs Distributed and data of final special surveys. The effects were concluded from the evaluation: in general, the planned activities and key indicators were achieved well, local residents' self protection and treatment-seeking behavior were significantly improved, the program implementation capabilities have been enhanced, however, the malaria control services at village levels need to be given more attention.

National evaluation group assessed the achievement and difficulties during the five-year program implement to make full preparation for closure of China Global Fund Malaria Program R1.

2.3 Financial Management

By principle of graded management, and under the guidance of China CDC Financial Department, the capital audit and financial management of China Global Fund Malaria Program（R1）have been undertaken by Financial Department in the National Institute of Parasitic Diseases, China CDC. The financial sections for each targeted site have been set in the financial department in the targeted provincial CDC or other financial department which the program office relied on

From April 1, 2003 to June 30, 2006, the PUDR reported to GFATM once a quarter. From July 1, 2006 to June 30, 2008, the PUDR reported to GFATM once half a year. Not later than 45 days after the close of each period, did NPO complete the collection, verification, summarization, and reporting of the financial M&E data. According to the performance-based principle, the funds requested from GFATM were forecasted, moreover, the funds were disbursed to SRs and SSRs based on their work-plans and program progress.

According to the work plans, NPO has taken the following measures: supervising the financial state of these ten targeted PPOs（two program counties in each PPO）at least once a year, training the program management officers and financial staffs in the targeted provinces once a year, and delivering report about the financial supervision as well as the financial training circumstances to the corresponding department. Thus, NPO would promote the development of GF Malaria Program, and ensure safe, effective and exclusive use of capital, so as to accomplish the predicted targets of the program successfully.

In accordance with the Financial Management Handbook of GFATM and the supervision projects of China Global Fund Malaria Program（Phase 2, Round1）, the financial supervision section in NPO carried on the financial supervision and evaluation. The financial supervision section confirmed the progress for implementing GF Malaria Program in the targeted provinces, and it also pointed out the problems existed in carrying out the program, then it proposed suggestions for improvement.

The main contents of financial supervision and evaluation are as follows: budgeteering and performance of the budgeted work-plans, bank account, financial management mechanism, budget performance, supervision of fixed assets, financial trainings, financial supervisions and audits, and etc. Not later than 15 days did the supervision group complete the locale supervision report, and submit the reports to the branches which have been supervised and to the upper directing department PR. The content of supervision report includes the following items: time and spots of supervision, the staffs who took part in the supervision, the items for supervising, the suggestions for improvement, and so on. Every PPO also carried out a lot of supervisions to the program sites in its subordinate counties and villages every year.

2.4 PSM Management

According to China Global Fund Program Financial Management Handbook, the definition of fixed asset is as follows: purchased by the program fund and the service lifetime of which is above one year; the cost of office equipment is beyond 500 RMB for each, the cost of special equipment is beyond 800 RMB for each and it keeps its original form basically while it has been put into use; or the cost of each equipment is less than the regulated standard, but it has been bought by wholesale (five or more than five) , the service lifetime is above one year and the original form would be remained.

China PR Procurement Department took charge of purchasing program materials in the process of implementing China GF Malarial Program R1, and then the materials were sent to the targeted areas. To guarantee the legality, regularity, publicity and transparency of purchasing activities, department of discipline inspection & supervision and department of audit (in China CDC, the program-relied institution) took part in the financial affairs. The purchase of fixed assets which cost more than 500 000 RMB (including 500 000RMB) should be conducted by inviting public bidding.

To guarantee the safety of assets, PR Procurement Department filled in China GF Requisition for Assets Allocation to inform the targeted sites to receive the assets. Each program site made a field inventory to the repertory assets every season, and then the program site compiled China GF Assets Checking Table to audit and check. The inventory profit and loss, as well as damage in making an inventory needs to be found out immediately, and then be written down in detail.

The implement of China GF Malaria Program R1 improved the assets management standard of the PR department at all levels. The program managers' capacities about checking-material, material storage, material receiving and using, as well as the material recording and registration were improved greatly than before. The accounts of material managing were clear, the material and account matching with each other, and the materials were distributed in time. The present storage conditions were better than before: the storerooms which were in good condition have been set up in most parts of the program department; medicine, non-medicine and toxicant were disposed separately; the ventilation of the storeroom was good, and temperature & humidity in the storeroom could be controlled; the storage staffs' management capacities have been further improved through the program implementation, their capacities about material storage, material recording & registration, and material checking have been improved.

From April 1, 2003 to March 31, 2008, the total procurement expenditure was 14 628 334.97 RMB (about 1.8 million USD), the materials including vehicles, computers, microscopes, anti-malaria drugs, insecticides, bed nets, and etc., all of these materials have been distributed to the program areas. The outfit of official equipment, vehicles and microscopes provided better material guarantee for the following matters: improving the office automation and information-based capacities of grass-roots disease-controlling staffs and program officers; reinforcing the diagnosis conditions for the laboratories in the grass-roots department; improving the medicine and assets freighting efficiency; meliorating work conditions of business trip and going to villages; and improving malaria professionals' capacities about malaria control and prevention.

3 Fulfillment of Key Indicators and Work Plan

3.1 Fulfillment of key indicators

Generally, through the implementation of the program, significant effects for malaria control in China's high transmission regions were achieved: awareness of prevention and anti-malaria were improved; local residents' self protection and treatment-seeking behavior were significantly promoted; the program implementation capabilities were enhanced; the proportion of families possessing ITNs were increased greatly; transmission and spread of multi-drug resistance falciparum malaria were controlled effectively.

In general, the key indicators were achieved well, and significant effects for malaria control in China's high transmission regions were achieved. The results of the special survey in January 2008 showed that: malaria incidence in target counties of Yunnan Province has been decreased by 66.22%, from 195/10 000 in 2002 to 65.88/10 000 in 2007. Besides, Malaria morbidity and falciparum malaria morbidity in target counties of Hainan Province have been decreased by 91.91% and 95.58% respectively, from 385/10 000 and 9.06/10 000 in 2002 to 31.13/10 000 and 0.40/10 000 in 2007.（See Table 2）

Table 3 update of M&E indicators

Program Objectives	Indicators	Cumulative Targets	Cumulative Results	Update Time
Total objectives: Malaria in target provinces of China is rolled back and the spread of multi-drug resistant strains is limited	Malaria incidence (confirmed and probable) in 25 target counties of Yunnan province and 10 of Hainan province	Y: 97/10 000 H: 192/10 000	Y: 65.88/10 000 H: 31.13/10 000	2008-3-31
	Incidence of confirmed falciparum malaria in 10 target counties of Hainan province	≤ 1/10 000	0.40/10000	2008-3-31
	Number of malaria-associated deaths of Yunnan and Hainan provinces	≤ 17	5	2008-3-31
	Percentage of households owning at least one ITN	30.00%	37.60%	2008-3-31
	Proportion of school children in target areas able to recall at least 3 key messages relating to malaria	85.00%	93.18%	2008-3-31
	Proportion of people with fever seeking treatment within 2 days of the onset of symptoms	90.00%	89.95%	2008-3-31

Objectives1: Mobile populations in border areas of Yunnan Province have better access to diagnosis and appropriate treatment for malaria	Number/proportion of out patients with fever among mobile populations examined by microscope	118 000/208 300 56.65%	164 433/232 427 70.75%	2008-3-31
	Number and percentage of fever cases among mobile populations (in Yunnan province) receiving anti-malaria treatment as per national guidelines (non-ACT)	56 600/144 700 39.12%	57 729/62 604 92.21%	2008-3-31
	Number and proportion of village doctors and township microscopists trained in early detection and treatment of malaria	10 000/10 000 100.00%	11 048/11 048 100.00%	2008-3-31
Objectives2: People living in endemic areas of Yunnan and Hainan Provinces have better access to early diagnosis and personal protection measures	Number and percentage of fever cases among local populations in Yunnan and Hainan provinces receiving anti-malaria treatment as per national guidelines (non-ACT)	261 360/469 200 55.70%	246 885/269 363 91.66%	2008-3-31
	Number and percentage of fever cases examines by microscopy out of all fever cases treated	127 422/261 360 48.75%	28 109/246 885 11.39%	2008-3-31
	Number of ITNs distributed	333 000	365 039	2008-3-31

Objectives3: People living in target areas of Yunnan and Hainan Provinces practice malaria prevention more effectively and access treatment facilities more promptly on getting fever	Number and proportion of targeted families receiving IEC and Health Education Materials	673 500/2 000 000 33.68%	1 044 055/ 1 936 021 53.93%	2008-3-31
Objectives4: Management of malaria control programme optimized in Yunnan Hainan and eight other program supported provinces	Proportion of cases reported by the malaria surveillance network	40.00%	38.92%	2008-3-31

Since the implementation of program, all indicators are achieved well but one indicator Number and percentage of fever cases examines by microscopy out of all fever cases treated is somewhat low because all of the 25 project counties in Yunnan Province are the border counties with inconvenient transportation, slow economic development and large amount of mobile population. Therefore, there are indeed some difficulties existing objectively in the implementation and management of the program. Because most of the target counties are in the minority areas, and the majority of the malaria patients were diagnosed at village clinics which possess no microscopes, the confirmed malaria cases is somewhat low.

3.2 Program Progress

Since the program start in April 2003, it has been implemented for five years and ended on June 30, 2008. During in the five years, China global fund malaria office has held various management activities, and these activities promoted the implement of the whole program effectively. The executive Institutions in all levels held a lot of work, such as malaria diagnosis, treatment, prevention, training, supervision, as well as the distribution and management of medicine and equipment, thus the planned activities and indicators were achieved well, and the malaria control in local areas has been promoted. The cumulative number of blood tests done through this program was 2 530 245 cases; the cumulative number of malaria cases which have been treated was 517 220 cases; 14 745 village doctors and township microscopists have been trained; the cumulative number of ITNs distributed was 365 039; 259 640 anti-malaria posters were exhibited in public areas; about 12 644 classes of anti-malaria IEC courses were held for primary and secondary school students; and malaria programs over radio or TV were broadcasted 532 times for target counties. The objectives of the program have been basically achieved. (See Table 4)

Table 4 Update of key activities (Until June 30, 2008)

Key Activities	Planned	Actual	Rate	Update Time
Blood Tests	1 929 200	2 530 245	131.16%	2008-3-31
Malaria Treatment	533 120	517 220	97.02%	2008-3-31
Village/Private Doctors and Microscopists Trained	10 860	14 745	135.77%	2008-3-31
ITNs Distributed	333 000	365 039	109.62%	2008-3-31
Anti-malaria Posters Put-up	241 000	259 640	107.73%	2008-3-31
IEC Courses for Schoolchildren	9 500	12 644	133.09%	2008-3-31
Anti-malaria Broadcasting	251	532	211.95%	2008-3-31

Work Plan and Actual Completion of Key Activities (See Table 5)

Table 5 Update of key activities in years

Key Activities		Blood Tests	Malaria Treatment	Village/Private Doctors and Microscopists Trained	ITNs Distributed	Anti-malaria Posters Put-up	IEC Courses for School-children	Anti-malaria Broad-casting
Total	Planned	1 929 200	533 120	10 860	333 000	241 000	9 500	251
	Finished	2 530 245	517 220	14 745	365 039	259 640	12 644	532
2003	Planned	138 000	22 860	3 050	66 000	4 000	0	0
	Finished	207 947	28 340	5 208	17 190	4 990	0	0
2004	Planned	438 200	141 200	3 060	160 750	96 000	3 500	86
	Finished	523 173	126 498	3 547	69 855	129 860	4 518	172

2005	Planned	456 000	133 510	1 520	43 000	51 000	2 500	60
	Finished	580 565	132 591	2 073	62 376	26 082	3 445	205
2006	Planned	442 000	133 450	2 070	53 250	45 000	2 500	85
	Finished	616 578	129 208	2 490	205 232	59 349	3 143	135
2007	Planned	428 000	97 750	1160	10 000	45 000	1 000	20
	Finished	556 167	94 401	1427	10 386	39 349	1 538	20
2008	Planned	27 000	4 350	0	0	0	0	0
	Finished	45 815	6 182	0	0	10	0	0

4. Program Fund Performance

The phase from April 1, 2003 to June 30, 2008 is the program implementation period and the phase from April 1 to June 30, 2008 is the program closure period. from April 1, 2003 to June 30, 2008, the program has received all together $ 6 347 405.31,（the actual settlement was RMB 49 713 251.36）, cumulatively receiving bank interest RMB 101 181.59; so the cumulative capital of the program is RMB 49 814.432.95, including RMB 15 013 798.77 for procurement and RMB 34 800 634.18 for activities. The detailed incoming of each target provinces is as follows:

Table 6 Cumulative funding of target province

Currency: RMB（Yuan）

Target site	Objective 1	Objective 2	Objective 3	Objective 4	Total
PR	0.00	0.00	371 994.30	7 638 535.34	8 010 529.64
Procurement	0.00	0.00	0.00	15 013 798.77	15 013 798.77
Yunnan	1 479 589.65	4 387 032.76	1 870 875.26	5 873 114.50	13 610 612.17
Hainan	0.00	2 341 522.89	1 454 659.61	2 107 314.84	5 903 497.34
Anhui	0.00	329 214.68	0.00	658 028.45	987 243.13
Henan	0.00	552 054.44	0.00	431 135.65	983 190.09
Hubei	0.00	458 903.05	0.00	575 161.28	1 034 064.33
Jiangsu	0.00	580 101.04	0.00	411 695.91	991 796.95
Guangdong	0.00	466 082.46	0.00	340 345.27	806 427.73
Guangxi	0.00	356 745.70	0.00	427 299.30	784 045.00
Sichuan	0.00	288 862.73	0.00	514 558.37	803 421.10
Guizhou	0.00	506 786.55	0.00	277 838.54	784 625.09
Total	1 479 589.65	10 267 306.33	3 697 529.17	34 268 826.21	49 713 251.36

According to the exchange rate on June 30, 2008 released by State Administration of Foreign Exchange, the RMB against the dollar is 1:6.8591; the program funds cumulative exchange loss is RMB 6 175 763.60.

From April 1, 2003 to June 30, 2008, the cumulative program expenditure was RMB 49 095 615.46, including RMB 7 720 347.62 at central level, RMB 26 712 452.38 in targeted provinces and RMB 14 662 815.46 for procurement. The total budget is US$6 406 659.00, and the cumulative utilization rate of funds was 99%, the cumulative performance rate was 96 %, (Details in Figure 2).

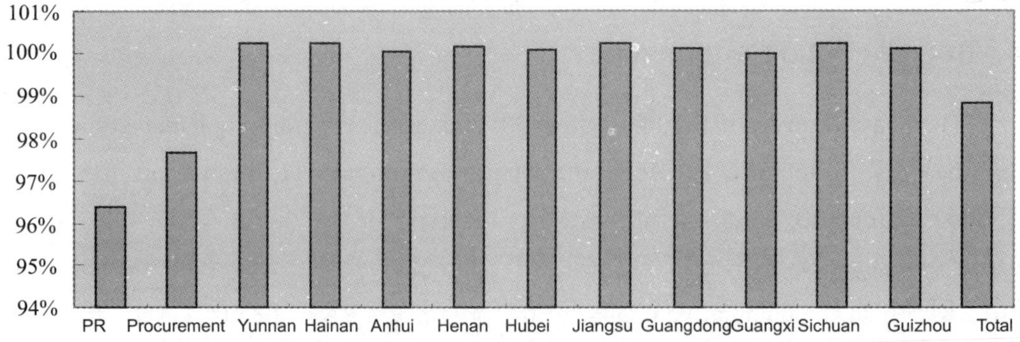

Figure 2. The budget utilization rate in each target sites

Up to June 30, 2008, the cash balance is RMB 718 817.49, including RMB 350 983.31 for procurement activities, RMB 341 848.30 at central level and RMB 25 985.88 in targeted provinces: the savings of RMB 25 968.88 for Yunnan, the savings of RMB 10.09 for Hubei and RMB 6.91 for Sichuan.

External financial auditing to national and provincial levels has been finished by Aug. 4, 2008. According to China Global Fund Program Audit Guideline, considering program features and realities, an invite public bidding was conducted to select XingHua Certified Public Accountants Ltd. Company of Beijing to audit national program office, and ten provinces have finished their audit by the means of an invite public bidding according to China Global Fund Program Audit Guideline.

5. Liquidate and Dispose of Grant Assets and Inventory

From April 1, 2003 to June 30, 2008, RMB 14 628 334.97 (equal to USD 1.8 million) was used to purchase computers, vehicles, microscopes, anti-malaria drugs, insecticides, bed nets, etc., and all procurement has been distributed to the targeted areas. The cumulative fixed assets procurement expenditure was RMB 9 352 909.97. The procured materials included 520 microscopes, 169 computers, 22 vehicles, 185 motorbikes, 29 digital cameras, 33 printers, 3 fax machines, 3 projectors and etc.; the cumulative procured anti-malaria drugs and health products are worth of RMB 5 275 425.00, containing 378 500 cases of Chloroquine phosphate and Primaquine phosphate, 30 000 cases of Dihydroartemisinin, 24 200 cases of Artemether injection, 304 000 cases of Piperaquine Phosphate, 26 500 cases of Artesunate, 54 000 bed nets, 23 700 Disposable Syringes, 300 liters of Cyfluthrin, 8 500 liters of Deltamethrin and etc..（Details in Table 15: List of Products Procured and Distributed）

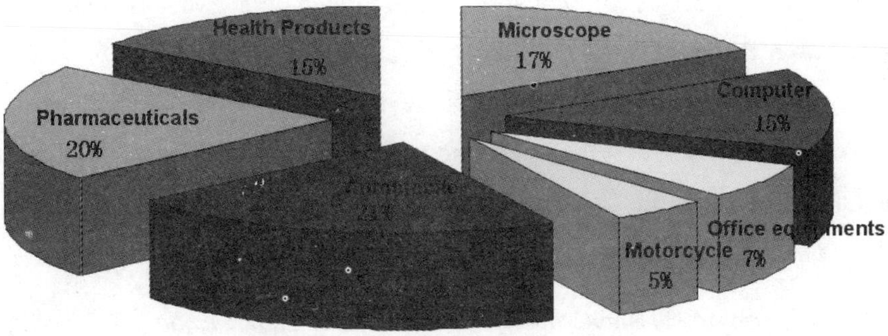

Figure 3. Percentage of procurement

China Global fund PR PSM Department has finished Liquidate and dispose of grant assets and inventory. Up to June 30, 2008, anti-malaria drugs and health products at all levels have been put into use in target areas, and the fixed assets are still in good condition. And all program assets and inventory are proposed to be transferred to the corresponding recipients, e.g. provincial and county CDCs or Institutes of Parasitic Diseases. If these corresponding recipients continue to undertake other rounds of GF malaria programs, the original R1 program assets will support GF program as well. If those corresponding recipients don’t undertake other rounds GF malaria programs any longer, the fixed assets in R1 program would support National Malaria Control Programme as well.

6. The Influence of GF Malaria Program (R1) on the Malaria Control and Prevention in the Targeted Areas

6.1 The Malaria epidemic situation in Target Areas

The Global Fund Program was started 5 years ago, since then, the malaria prevalence has been restrained effectively, and the spreading and transmission of multi-drug resistance Plasmodiom falciparum has been kept within limits; besides, the local break-out and transmission of malaria has been controlled in other 8 targeted provinces.

6.1.1 Yunnan Province

According to the results from special surveys in 2008, malaria incidence in Yunnan Province decreased to 65.88/10 000 in 2007, the predicted objective was achieved.

6.1.2 Hainan Province

According to the results from special surveys in 2008, malaria incidence in Yunnan Province decreased to 31.13/10 000, and falciparum malaria incidence in target counties of Hainan have decreased to 0.40/10 000 in 2007, the resistance of *P falciparum* to chloroquine did not changed significantly. (See Table 7 and Table 8)

Table 7 The susceptibility Surveillance *in vitro* of *Plasmodium falciparum* to chloroquine, pyronaridine in Hainan Province (2005)

Monitoring Points	Drugs	The number of cases	The number of resistant cases	Resistant rates (%)	CIMC* (ρ mol/ μl)	LD_{50} (95 % fiducial interval) (ρ mol/μl)
Baoyou Township of Ledong County	chloroquine	31	19	61.26	3.72	2.07 (1.75-2.45)
	pyronaridine	31	5	16.13	1.39	0.35 (0.27-0.46)
Jiangbian Township of Dongfang County	chloroquine	34	25	73.53	5.41	2.86 (2.39-3.42)
	pyronaridine	34	4	11.76	1.10	0.53 (0.43-0.65)

Note:* The average concentration to completely inhibit the merozoite formation

Table 8 The susceptibility surveillance *in vitro* of *Plasmodium falciparum* to Antimalarials in Hainan Province (2007)

Drugs	The number of cases	The number of resistant cases	Resistant rates (%)	LD_{50} (95% fiducial interval) (ρmol/μl)	CIMC* (ρmol/μl)
Chloroquine	32	23	71.88	2.34 (1.85—2.94)	5.60±5.64
Piperaquine Phosphate	32	13	40.63	1.96 (1.44—2.68)	9.26±13.67
Pyronaridine	32	4	12.50	0.16 (0.13—0.20)	0.55±1.02
Artesunate	32	0	0	0.04 (0.03—0.05)	0.07±0.04

Note:* The average concentration to completely inhibit the merozoite formation

6.1.3 Target Areas in Other 8 Provinces

6.1.3.1 Henan Province: In the purpose of reducing malaria incidence, the program office in Henan Province took active measures to investigate malaria cases in the forth quarter every year, such as to know the malaria epidemic situation deeply, to detect malaria spots in due course, and to take timely preventing measures for possible malaria spots. These measures obtained good results: the spreading of epidemic was prohibited; in 2007, the malaria cases in the targeted counties were decreased to a large extent compared with 2002 (before implementing the program). There were 210 estimated malaria patients in 2007, the missing report rate was 37.61%, it could be seen that the estimated number of malarial patients decreased by 96.92 % compared with 2002 (6 829 patients).

6.1.3.2 Hubei Province: In 2007, there were 441 malaria patients in the malaria-controlling Zaoyang County according to the report, the number of patients decreased by 85.55% compared with 2003 (3052 patients) ; however, the outbreaks of malaria epidemic still occurred in some local places. There were 77 patients in the malaria-supervising Zengdu County, and there were no outbreaks of malaria epidemic at present.

6.1.3.3 Anhui Province: There were no outbreaks of malaria epidemic in the targeted Huaiyuan County in 2006 and 2007, and the transmission of malaria epidemic has been effectively controlled. In 2007, it is estimated that the exact malaria incidence was 6.02/10 000.

6.1.3.4 Jiangsu Province: Although the number of malaria patients reported by the malaria surveillance network throughout Jiangsu Province increased, the number of patients in the targeted program counties in Jiangsu Province still decreased. In 2007, there were 42 and 106 malaria patients reported by the malaria surveillance network in Xuyi County and Sihong County respectively, compared with 2002（Xuyi, 84; Sihong, 275）, the incidence decreased more than 50%.

6.1.3.5 Guangdong Province: There were no malaria outbreaks in Guangdong Province since the program has been carried out, and the malaria incidence has been restricted below 1 /100 000.

6.1.3.6 Guangxi Province: In Baise County, Baise County, the local infected malaria incidence has been restricted below 1/100 000 in the past five years. There were no secondary infection malaria case originated from imported cases, and the malaria incidence was still controlled below 1/10 000.

6.1.3.7 Sichuan Province: There were 5 malaria patients reported in the program county Junlian, from which 4 patients were infected in the local county, 1 patient was infected outside. The total incidence was 0.12/10 000, and all of these cases were diagnosed by examining the blood smear.

6.1.3.8 Guizhou Province: Rongjiang County Rongjiang, the local government and the board of health laid emphasis on malaria control and prevention since the global malaria program has been implemented, thus the anti-malaria measures have been put into effect. Benefiting from the implement of the program, malaria incidence was restrained to a great extent, and there were no malaria outbreaks in targeted areas over the past five years.

6.2 Promotion role of program in program areas

6.2.1 Financial support from the GF program filled the gap of the capital insufficiency for carrying out anti-malaria activities in the targeted areas.

With the implement of China GF Malaria Program（R1）, the investment of capital, medicine and corresponding equipment supplied the gap of anti-malaria capital, medicine and equipment insufficiency. Meanwhile, the implement of the program urged the governments at all levels and the health administrate department to pay more attention to control and prevent malaria, and also urged them to support the anti-malaria activities in many aspects. Therefore, malaria control and prevention has been improved greatly, the outbreaks of malaria in targeted areas were kept within limits, and the malaria incidence was restrained.

6.2.2 The management and anti-malaria capabilities have been enhanced by implementing the global fund program and conducting related trainings.

Since the program has been carried out, a lot of trainings have been conducted, such as the project management trainings, trainings about anti-malaria knowledge and the capability of using microscope, trainings about early diagnoses, and trainings about appropriate treatment. The effects of these trainings were as follows: improving the project executive staffs' management abilities, improving the anti-malaria capabilities of the professionals in the targeted counties and villages, improving the microscopists' capacities of using microscope, improving the village doctors' treatment capacities, and increasing the cure rate of malaria patients.

6.2.3 Residents' self-protection consciousness was improved by conducting propaganda activities about malaria control and prevention.

The propaganda activities about malaria control and prevention were widely conducted in the target areas. The benefits from these propaganda activities are as follows: the local residents and the students had got a better understanding about malaria control and prevention; the residents' self-protection has been improved; people tended to be more reliable to the activities directed at malaria control and prevention, so they would seek treatment immediately after being infected.

6.3 Evaluation about the program implementation

The capital invested by the global fund accounted for 52.70% of the total capital in the targeted areas. As an important supply of China regular malaria control and prevention, the health services at all levels regarded China GF Malaria Program R1 as a main component for the long-term anti-malaria project. These health services considered executing and implementing the program to be an important anti-malaria task, what's more, they took part in the program directly, and also actively support the program, so the implement of the program got necessary and enough executive guarantees. In general, the implement of the global fund program has positive effects on malaria control and prevention in the targeted areas.

According to the results gained from the final evaluation conducted by malarial special working group of CCM in May, 2008, the planned activities and key indicators were achieved well. Although there were some problems existing in the process of the program execution, the program implementation capabilities of the program offices at all levels were enhanced greatly.

The effects of carrying out the program could still be seen as follows: the local residents have got a better understanding about anti-malaria knowledge, besides, local residents' self-protection and treatment-seeking behaviors have significantly improved; the percentage of household ITNs has been improved in a great extent, and the malaria missing report rate has been decreased; the malaria epidemic has been controlled effectively in the targeted areas, and the spreading and transmission of multi-drug resistance P falciparum has been kept within limits; through the implementation of the program, a group of anti-malaria professionals in disease control department at each level have been trained, and a group of program officers have also been trained. Thus, the management concept and experience about program depending on government department have been enriched; the health officers who were in townships and villages have improved their capacities of malaria control and prevention; the precious experience has been gained, the anti-malaria force has been strengthened, then the realization of national malarial control plan gained important supplies.

7. Effects and experience

7.1 The management concept of GF program is worth of being popularized.

In the process of implementing GF, the finance-based management concept, performance-based principle and M&E mechanisms are valuable to the regular malaria control and prevention. Practicing these advanced management experience in malaria control and prevention, the concept could be promoted and renovated, the management standard could be enhanced, the scientific management system could be set up, and anti-malaria tasks could be carried out properly.

7.2 Propagandizing anti-malaria knowledge and making residents have a better understanding about malaria controlling and prevention served as basis for restricting malaria transmission.

In the implement of the program, it could be seen that anti-malaria propaganda served as basis for restricting malaria transmission, the exact effects are as follows: the local residents have got a better understanding about malaria control and prevention; the residents' self-protection consciousness has been improved, and they tended to be more reliable to anti-malaria activities. Thus, the difficulties to conduct anti-malaria activities were reduced, and the realization of the targets got guarantee.

7.3 The trainings which were intended to improve the anti-malaria professionals' technology served as necessary means to facilitate malaria controlling and prevention.

Much experience was gained in carrying out the program, in general, the experience remind us that work quality and conducting of anti-malaria activities could be guaranteed under these circumstances: conducting various trainings about anti-malaria knowledge and microscope technology; improving malaria professionals' anti-malaria capacities and microscopists' technology to use microscope. Thus, the trainings about anti-malaria knowledge and technology to use microscope were very important, so these trainings should be conducted throughout the whole process of the GF malaria control program.

7.4 The outbreaks of malaria have been effectively controlled by adopting comprehensive preventing measures. Aimed at the characteristics of the current malaria propaganda, these measures mainly directed at cutting off infection sources.

Malaria patients are one of the main infection sources. A lot of measures have been taken to control malaria outbreaks: propagandizing malaria control and prevention among people, strengthening the establishment of microscope station, holding trainings repeatedly for the microscopist, and conducting trainings for clinicians' treatment capacities. Thus, on the one hand, the malaria patients would seek timely treatment after they were infected, then they would receive proper treatment and took part in effecting radical cure, so the patients would be cured, and they would not be the source of infection; on the other hand, along with the number of anti-malaria professionals increased and the extending of blood-test areas, the malaria patients could be detected and diagnosed earlier, the missing and improper diagnoses decreased. Thus, these measures are effective in controlling malaria out-breaks.

7.5 The quality of program implement would be improved by strengthening the information exchange between program executive institutions and health services.

It is approved in the five-year program practicing that the information exchange among provinces, cities, county governments and health services helped the program implement gain administrative support and the cooperation from other departments, thus the program could be carried out successfully. The effects of information exchange among the program executive institutions are as follows: various problems were detected and solved early; the program activities were standardized and optimized and the quality for implementing program was enhanced.

7.6 The fund could be more effectively used by strengthening communication between program officers and the financial staffs.

The results from the overall evaluation showed that the effective communication between program officers and financial staffs are very important. For example, there were fewer mistakes in the financial affairs, the program investment tended to be more regular, and the efficiency of using capital tended to be higher in the counties where there were harmonious information exchanging for program condition and financial affairs.

8. Progress in target provinces

China GF Malaria Program Round 1 covered 47 counties in 10 provinces. Yunnan Province and Hainan Province were the key control and prevention provinces in the program, apart from that, other 8 provinces, Henan, Hubei, Anhui, Jiangsu, Guangdong, Guangxi, Sichuan, Guizhou were the monitoring provinces. In the implementation of the program, each program province could examine its own problems existing in the program implementation under the monitoring of NPO, and they could exchange experience with each other. Thus, the program could be carried out well.

Up to Match 31, 2008, all of the targeted provinces completed their planned activities in general:

8.1 Yunnan Province

Basically, all of the planned program activities were completed in Yunnan Province. the cumulative number of blood tests in the program was 1 136 911; the cumulative number of malaria patients who have been treated was 260 367; the cumulative number of distributed ITNs was 251 070; 11 750 village doctors and township microscopists have been trained; 102 906 anti-malaria posters were put-up in public areas; 6 448 classes of IEC course were held for primary and secondary school students; and anti-malaria knowledge was broadcasted 320 times through radio or TV to the target counties.

The planned activities in GF Malaria Program (R1) in Yunnan Province have been implemented well and the targets were reached basically. Although there were some difficulties in implementing the program, the executive capacities of the program office in Yunnan were improved a lot over the 5 years.

The effects of the implementation of the program are as follows: the local residents have got a better understanding about anti-malaria knowledge, besides, local residents' self-protection and treatment-seeking behaviors have significantly improved; the percentage of household ITNs has been increased to a great extent, and the malaria missing report rate was decreased; the malaria epidemic was controlled effectively in the targeted areas; meanwhile, a group of anti-malaria professionals in disease control department at each level have been trained; the management concept and experience about program dependent on the government department have been enriched; the health officers who were in townships and villages have improved their capacities of malaria control and prevention; then the realization of national malarial controlling plan gained important personnel guarantee.

However, there are great differences in program implementation capacities among 25 counties in Yunnan Province. Most of the target counties were able to complete the program tasks well, while some of the counties still need to strengthen their implementation competence, for example, a proportion of the data reported failed to be verified with the original records of blood tests and treatment prescriptions. More strict verifications are in demand in the following program implementation to ensure the accuracy for the reported data.

8.2 Hainan Province

Basically, all the planned program activities were completed in Hainan Province. the cumulative number of blood tests in the program was 655 175; the cumulative number of malaria patients who have been treated was 100 785; 2 995 village doctors and township microscopists have been trained; the cumulative number of ITNs distributed was 116 611; 61 126 anti-malaria posters were put-up in public areas; 2 679 classes of IEC courses were held for primary and secondary school students; and anti-malaria knowledge was broadcasted 57 times through radio or TV to the target counties.

The planned activities in GF Malaria Program (R1) in Yunnan Province were implemented well and the targets were reached basically. The exact effects of the implementation of the program are as follows: the local residents have got a better understanding about anti-malaria knowledge, besides, local residents' self protection and treatment-seeking behaviors have significantly improved; the percentage of household ITNs has been increased to a great extent, and the malaria missing report rate was decreased; the malaria epidemic was controlled effectively in the targeted areas; the spreading and transmission of multi-drug resistance P falciparum was kept within limits; meanwhile, a group of anti-malaria professionals in disease control department at each level have been trained; some anti-malaria equipment were left; the precious experience has been gained, and the anti-malaria force has been strengthened, then the realization of national malarial control plan gained important supplies.

Generally, all of the 10 target counties in Hainan Province possess high program implementation capacities. In accordance with the relevant requirements of Global Fund, program activities have been carried out seriously, village doctors and township microscopists have been trained, the work plan has been completed, and program records were kept in these program counties in Hainan Province.

8.3 Henan Province

The cumulative number of blood tests in Henan GF Malaria Program (R1) was 58 315; the cumulative number of malaria patients who have been treated was 3 470.

8.4 Hubei Province

The cumulative number of blood tests in Hubei GF Malaria Program（R1）was 69 907; the cumulative number of malaria patients who have been treated was 22 407.

8.5 Anhui Province

The cumulative number of blood tests in Anhui GF Malaria Program（R1）was 146 954; the cumulative number of malaria patients who have been treated was 39 358.

8.6 Jiangsu Province

The cumulative number of blood tests in Jiangsu GF Malaria Program（R1）was 53 490; the cumulative number of malaria patients who have been treated was 14 628.

8.7 Guangdong Province

The cumulative number of blood tests in the Guangdong GF Malaria Program（R1）was 148 609; the cumulative number of malaria patients who have been treated was 7 615.

8.8 Guangxi autonomous region

The cumulative number of blood tests in the Guangxi GF Malaria Program（R1）was 82 178; the cumulative number of malaria patients who have been treated was 2 208.

8.9 Sichuan Province

The cumulative number of blood tests in the Sichuan GF Malaria Program（R1）was 33 177; the cumulative number of malaria patients who have been treated was 7 020.

8.10 Guizhou Province

The cumulative number of blood tests in the Guizhou GF Malaria Program（R1）was 63 773; the cumulative number of malaria patients whohave been treated was 5 424.

China Global Fund Malaria National Program Office

第三节 省级报告

一、云南省项目终期总结报告

云南省第一轮全球基金疟疾项目自2003年启动以来，得到了卫生部、国家项目办公室、省卫生厅的支持和帮助。在项目实施的5年中，严格按照项目计划书开展各项活动，完成了既定的任务，达到了预期的目标。现将云南省5年的项目工作执行情况总结如下。

（一）项目概况

第一轮云南省全球基金疟疾项目共实施了5年（2003年4月～2008年3月），覆盖了边境8个市的25个县。项目的总体目标是：通过5年项目的实施，全省的疟疾发病率下降50%，减少多重抗药性恶性疟在项目地区的传播并限制其向中部地区扩散。项目的目标人群和直接受益人群为25个边境县的580万人口以及约1 000万流动人口，间接受益人群为毗邻地区的约2 000万人口和中国中部其他省区已得到控制的原恶性疟流行区的约5 000万人口，共7 000万人口。

（二）项目资金使用情况

截至2008年6月10日，资金结余人民币524 257.96元，其中，目标一结余15 425.94元，目标二结余59 836.60元，目标三结余69 050.71元，目标四结余379 944.71元。

结余的资金部分依照计划，在项目中止前用于完成剩余工作并作相应支出，主要包括：省级、县级总结大会、项目终期审计等。

项目5年总预算为1 015 277美元，折合人民币8 122 216元，实际收到项目经费为人民币13 561 524.60元，共支出经费为人民币12 301 864.20元，预算执行率为151.46%，截止2008年6月30日结余经费为零。各阶段经费收支情况见表1–7。

表 1–7 项目经费执行情况表

单位：人民币（元）

周期序号	年份	科目	目标 1	目标 2	目标 3	目标 4	合计	预算执行率
项目一期	2003—2004	预算		851 336		480 000	1 331 336	384.13%
		到款	1 029 537.10	1 448 809.04	1 083 994.38	2 067 391.31	5 629 731.83	
		支出	985 204.20	1 403 178.77	972 308.99	1 753 369.43	5 114 061.39	
项目二期	2005	预算	122 560	105 8720	320 800	902 000	2 404 080	84.22%
		到款	72 346.20	450 643.30	174 763.45	979 200.12	1 676 953.07	
		支出	137 868.24	510 141.60	211 342.33	1 165 273.46	2 024 625.63	
	2006	预算	180 000	1 061 600	330 000	950 000	2 521 600	137.37%
		到款	259 802.84	1 758 614.55	505 003.30	917 424.48	3 440 845.17	
		支出	200 726.91	1 406 339.59	502 903.61	1 353 882.78	3 463 852.89	
	2007	预算	111 200	748 000	104 000	902 000	1 865 200	91.11%
		到款	117 903.51	728 965.87	107 114.13	1 860 011.02	2 813 994.53	
		支出	108 492.06	714 944.42	109 530.95	766 356.86	1 699 324.29	
累计		预算	413 760	3 719 656	754 800	3 234 000	8 122 216	151.46%
		到款	1 479 589.65	4 387 032.76	1 870 875.26	5 824 026.93	13 561 524.60	
		支出	1 432 291.41	4 034 604.38	1 796 085.88	5 038 882.53	12 301 864.20	
		结余	47 298.24	352 428.38	74 789.38	812 022.54	1 286 538.54	

注：预算数根据工作计划填写（折算汇率 1:8），预算执行率 = 支出数 / 预算数。累计结余含银行利息人民币：26 878.14 元。

（三）项目管理总结

1. 项目管理

1.1 在省内各级成立项目领导小组、项目办公室（以下简称项目办）、项目专家组等管理机构，项目办负责具体的项目执行，鉴于云南省的特殊情况，在市级成立督导组，项目实行分级管理，各级项目办负责管理下级项目办，县级项目办对乡镇卫生院进行管理，乡镇卫生院对村级医疗机构进行管理。

1.2 各级项目管理机构主动与卫生行政部门进行沟通和协调，接受其监督。

1.3 各级项目办由项目办主任、项目主管、财务主管、物资管理、信息管理等人员组成，按照项目管理要求进行分工管理，项目办主任负责整个项目执行管理，其他人员分别按照工作职责和管理要求开展工作，定期组织例会进行内部沟通。

1.4 严格执行项目工作计划和预算，工作计划和预算的调整必须报上级项目办同意后方能改动，项目执行中出现较大问题时必须向上级项目办和卫生行政部门报告。

1.5 积极发挥项目专家组的作用，项目管理和执行中存在技术性问题及时组织专家组进行论证。

1.6 在项目计划的实施过程中，严格按照《全球基金疟疾项目管理与技术方案》、《全球基金疟疾项目执行指导手册》、《监督与评价（M&E）计划与实施指南》、《云南省全球基金疟疾项目实施细则》、《全球基金财务管理手册》等要求进行管理，按要求规范进行 M&E、财务、物资、发热病人血检和治疗、杀虫剂浸泡蚊帐、健康教育、督导等管理工作，确保项目执行的规范性。经逐级检查，未发现违反以上管理要求与规定的事例。

1.7 专人专项负责项目数据、资料信息和原始材料的收集和管理工作，保证数据、信息的完整性、规范性和准确性。

2．监督与评价管理

2.1 严格执行工作计划及其预算，每项工作均有详细的实施方案、工作记录和总结材料。

2.2 省级统一开展 M&E 管理的培训，省级、县级均有专人负责 M&E 数据收集、统计、复核。

2.3 定期逐级进行项目执行情况检查、评价项目执行质量，并及时将结果通报和上报。

2.4 按照季度上报工作报表、M&E 报表和物资库存表，在报表中对任务完成和预算－开支偏差较大的内容详细说明原因并提出改进计划。

2.5 每年均依照 M&E 管理要求组织专项调查，及时上报了调查结果。

2.6 项目人员、财务人员和物资管理人员及时沟通，项目报表统计结束后由项目办负责人签字、项目实施机构盖章后上报。

2.7 县级项目办按月汇总数据形成月报表上报省项目办，在季度结束后 15 日内汇总季度报表上报，省项目办在季度结束后均按时于 30 日内上报全省季度报表。

2.8 各级项目执行机构均执行了原始数据的收集、整理、录入、统计和报告，保证了报表及时上报、填写规范、内容完整、数据准确真实。

2.9 省项目办定期组织了督导评估，对项目数据不实、整改工作不力的县进行通报批评，严重的县予以暂停拨款进行整改直至验收后才拨付经费延续项目实施。

3．财务管理

3.1 财务人员队伍建设

3.1.1 项目办财务人员配置齐全，项目会计、出纳各 1 人。

3.1.2 项目办财务人员不相容职务分人担任。

3.1.3 财务人员和项目人员经常沟通。

3.2 预算制定和预算执行

财务人员参与和了解项目预算，严格按照预算标准进行项目支出并与工作计划相对应。

3.3 项目资金管理

3.3.1 开立全球基金疟疾项目专用银行账户，独立核算。

3.3.2 严格遵守中国人民银行颁布的《现金管理暂行条例》和《银行存款支付结算办法》及《全球基金财务管理手册》中的货币资金管理规定。

3.3.3 现金、银行存款日记账账实相符。

3.3.4 使用"全球基金项目空白票据购置、领用登记簿"，及时登记空白票据的购入、使用和结存。

3.4 会计核算

3.4.1 项目资金支出严格执行授权批准制度，并使用全球基金专用凭证。

3.4.2 合规使用项目资金，不挤占挪用项目资金。

3.4.3 严格按照《全球基金财务管理手册》中规定的科目分轮次建账，并分工作目标进行了财务核算。

3.5 报表及审计

按时上报财务季度报、半年报和年报，并做到账表相符；年报每年进行一次审计，并有审计报告附后一同报出。

3.6 会计档案管理

项目会计资料齐全，财务票据、账簿、报表的装订整齐，每两年的会计资料进行一次归档。

4．物资管理

4.1 项目固定资产管理

4.1.1 自项目启动至今，共收到项目固定资产 3 246 744.08 元（含自购部分 11 730 元），严格按工作计划执行，及时下拨县级项目点，调拨、领用手续健全，固定资产账面余额 870 077.51 元（留用本项目办使用的固定资产总值），其中一般设备 203 449.77 元，专用设备 24 033.88 元，交通工具 642 593.86 元，并按照《全球基金财务管理手册》的要求，建立相应的固定资产辅助账，账账相符，账实相符。

4.1.2 收到和采购的固定资产包括：显微镜 249 台，汽车 13 辆、摩托车 25 辆，台式电脑 27 台，笔记本电脑 5 台，打印机 1 台，传真机 1 台，数码相机 6 台。本轮项目结束后，固定资产转入所在单位进行管理，继续供其他轮次全球基金疟疾项目和常规疟疾防治工作使用。

4.2 项目物品管理

4.2.1 项目物品（用本项目资金购置的材料、药品、试剂等需要入库保管的物品）自项目启动至今，共收到项目物品 2 794 008 元，严格按工作计划执行，及时下拨县级项目点，调拨、领用手续健全。

4.2.2 截至目前，各级结余物资包括：磷酸氯喹、伯氨喹类抗疟药物 19 943 人份，青蒿素类药物 5 126 人份，磷酸哌喹 64 328 片，杀虫剂 4 841 公斤，蚊帐 1 040 顶，一次性注射器 390 支，部分物资的结余主要是由于项目初期物资没有及时到位而各县先期借用本机构常规药物完成项目工作，项目结束后对借用物资予以归还，剩余的少量物资转入其他轮次全球基金疟疾项目进行管理并继续使用。

（四）项目活动执行情况

1. 流动人口血检和规范治疗指标

计划进行流动人口发热病人血检 118 000 人次，实际完成 161 585 人次，完成率 136.94%；计划规范治疗流动人口疟疾病例 58 000 例，实际完成 57 729 例，完成率 99.53%（表 1–8）。

表 1–8 2005—2008 年流动人口血检和规范治疗计划完成情况

内容	年度	计划目标	实际完成	完成率(%)
边境流动人口发热病人血检	2005	38 000	50 092	136.94
	2006	46 000	60 463	
	2007	32 000	44 925	
	2008	2 000	6 105	
	合计	118 000	161 585	
边境流动人口疟疾病人规范治疗	2005	15 400	21 195	99.53
	2006	26 600	20 171	
	2007	15 000	14 952	
	2008	1 000	1 411	
	合计	58 000	57 729	

2. 当地居民发热病人血检及规范治疗指标

计划完成当地居民发热病人血检 432 000 例，实际完成人次 973 175 例，完成率 225.27%；计划完成当地居民疟疾病人规范治疗 226 880 例，实际完成 202 638 例，完成率 898.32%（表 1–9）。

表 1–9　2005—2008 年当地居民血检及规范治疗计划完成情况

内容	年度	计划目标	实际完成	完成率（%）
当地居民发热病人血检	2005	162 000	534 250	225.27
	2006	130 000	208 991	
	2007	130 000	205 864	
	2008	10 000	24 070	
	合计	432 000	973 175	
当地居民疟疾病人规范治疗	2005	90 480	89 211	89.32
	2006	74 400	55 736	
	2007	60 000	53 965	
	2008	2 000	3 726	
	合计	226 880	202 638	

3. 乡村 / 个体医生和基层镜检员培训

计划在 25 个项目县（市）针对疟疾诊断和规范治疗完成培训乡村 / 个体医生 7 025 名，实际完成 11 614 名，完成率 165.32%，通过培训提高了基层疟疾镜检正确诊断的比例，降低漏检率、误检率，使疟疾病人得到及时正确的诊断治疗（表 1–10）。

表 1–10　2003—2007 年乡村 / 个体医生和基层镜检员培训计划完成情况

内容	年度	计划目标	实际完成	完成率（%）
乡、村医生 / 个体医生培训	2003	2 375	4 096	165.32
	2004	1 000	2 565	
	2005	1 000	1 507	
	2006	1 650	2 067	
	2007	1 000	1 379	
	合计	7 025	11 614	

4. 杀虫剂浸泡蚊帐指标

计划杀虫剂浸泡蚊帐 225 000 顶，实际完成 251 070 顶，完成率 111.59%（表 1–11）

表 1–11　2003—2007 年杀虫剂浸泡蚊帐计划完成情况

内容	年度	计划目标	实际完成	完成率(%)
药浸蚊帐	2003	0		111.59
	2004	152 000	22 627	
	2005	33 000	43 845	
	2006	40 000	184 598	
	2007	0	0	
	合计	225 000	251 070	

5. 健康教育

项目目标地区家庭通过广播、电视、各类宣传品接收到“疟疾相关信息、教育和交流以及健康教育材料”的户数计划达到 438 000 户，通过各项目县的努力实际达到 733 378 户，提高了项目地区居民对疟疾防治知识的知晓率，加强了疟疾流行地区居民的疟疾防护能力。其中，使用广播进行疟疾知识宣传共计 320 次，举办中小学生疟防知识课共 6448 个班次，在公共场所张贴疟疾知识宣传画 102 892 张。详见表 1–12。

表 1–12 2005—2007 年健康教育计划完成情况

内容	年度	计划目标	实际完成	完成率(%)
使用广播进行疟疾知识宣传	2005	150	195	142.22
	2006	75	125	
	2007	0	0	
	合计	225	320	
举办中小学生疟防知识课	2005	1 500	1 767	128.96
	2006	2 500	3 143	
	2007	1 000	1 538	
	合计	5 000	6 448	
在公共场所张贴疟疾知识宣传画	2005	41 000	26 082	97.07
	2006	35 000	47 439	
	2007	30 000	29 371	
	合计	106 000	102 892	

（五）项目地区疟疾疫情现状

2007 年云南省共报告疟疾 6 703 例，其中边境 25 县为 5 063 例，占 75.53%，与 2002 年（7553 例）相比，发病数下降 2 490 例，下降率为 32.97%。报告发病数的大幅下降，与终期调查中推算发病率的下降基本吻合（表 1–13）。

表 1–13 2007 年边境 25 市疟疾发病情况表

县名	1 月	2 月	3 月	4 月	5 月	6 月	7 月	8 月	9 月	10 月	11 月	12 月	合计
腾冲	109	78	58	113	273	194	154	111	105	62	50	38	1 345
龙陵	9	6	17	28	35	41	34	20	8	26	22	10	256
江城	0	1	2	1	2	3	3	2	3	0	3	1	21
孟连	5	5	3	5	6	9	12	11	12	14	17	9	108
澜沧	2	1	4	5	2	7	3	4	5	3	2	2	40
西盟	21	3	3	3	6	8	7	16	16	19	14	15	131
镇康	9	1	3	10	7	5	5	7	11	6	9	8	81
耿马	6	4	5	7	7	8	5	11	2	4	8	12	79
沧源	6	3	5	17	11	13	12	9	7	20	12	16	131
金平	6	5	2	14	25	20	27	5	6	12	11	6	139
绿春	4	0	1	0	3	5	5	4	1	4	6	2	35
河口	1	0	2	3	3	5	8	15	6	8	8	1	60
麻栗坡	5	4	6	7	3	3	1	10	3	1	4	1	48
马关	6	4	4	5	7	32	9	9	9	4	0	9	98
富县	0	0	0	1	2	1	0	2	1	1	1	0	9
景洪	10	7	9	14	7	8	16	9	1	3	4	4	92
勐海	4	0	4	1	1	1	5	4	2	2	2	6	32
勐腊	10	9	8	5	7	11	12	8	7	6	7	7	97
瑞丽	39	10	18	20	43	64	54	39	23	49	38	43	440
潞西	27	12	14	23	67	65	62	55	39	47	54	36	501
盈江	46	33	36	54	159	170	101	74	52	80	63	32	900
陇川	9	11	16	11	30	28	40	37	24	28	38	8	280
泸水	0	1	2	7	0	2	0	3	3	0	4	0	22
福贡	1	1	0	2	4	6	5	8	4	2	2	1	36
贡山	0	0	3	5	13	11	30	9	8	2	1	0	82
合计	335	199	225	361	723	720	610	482	358	403	380	267	5 063

（六）项目执行评价

1. 项目目标完成情况

2008 年 1 月，全省组织了项目终期调查，结果与 2003 年基线调查值对比，云南省均顺利完成了项目预定的目标，具体见表 1–14。

表 1–14 第一轮疟疾项目执行情况评价

指标	03 年基线值	目标值	终期调查值	是否实现目标
推算发病率	197.00/ 万	97.00/ 万	65.88/ 万	是
学生知晓率	58.20%	85.00%	94.83%	是
2 天内求诊率	37.95%	90.00%	92.36%	是
ITNs 拥有率	4.30%	30.00%	32.36%	是
病例上报率	8.80%	40.00%	45.30%	是

各指标的完成，得益于多个方面的因素，包括：

1.1 国家、省、县项目办切实加强了项目执行力度，云南省卫生厅高度重视云南省全球基金项目实施情况，并要求项目地区卫生主管部门确实把全球基金疟疾项目作为当地重点疾病防治工作，督促所辖县项目办严格按照要求开展工作。在各级卫生行政主管部门的支持下，各级项目执行机构加强了项目管理，使辖区项目乡、村落实项目工作措施力度得到了有效加强。

1.2 项目地区在第一轮项目启动后，第五轮、第六轮全球基金疟疾项目相继开展，2007 年后，除全球基金疟疾项目以外的国家、省、县等的疟疾及其与蚊媒有关疾病（如登革热和乙型脑炎等）防治项目相继开展，疟疾防治工作的进一步得到了加强。

1.3 云南省新型农村卫生合作医疗工作（新农合）在 25 个边境县得到了较好的开展，使得农村居民就医积极性和规范治疗率较大提高，对当地的疟疾防治工作起到了非常有效的促进作用。

2. 项目终期评估情况

为了较好的总结项目 5 年实施工作情况和实施效果，根据国家项目办要求和云南省项目计划安排，2008 年 3 月 25 日 ~ 4 月 11 日，在云南省项目区域开展了省级项目终期自评估。主要评估内容包括项目计划和指标完成情况及工作质量、评估项目投入产出效果及项目对各级常规疟防的促进作用。

云南省严格按照国家项目办的评估实施方案的要求实施，本着实事求是的原则，对 5 年来的项目工作进行客观评估，抽取了腾冲、龙陵、福贡、陇川、耿马、孟连、西盟、金平、麻栗坡以及全省项目执行情况进行了自评估，得分为 92.64 分，项目执行等级为 A 级。

2008 年 5 月 13 ～ 24 日，国家评估组对云南省进行了项目的评估。

（七）成效与经验

1. 疟疾信息月报表的编制和项目工作信息的及时传递

2003 年下半年云南省项目办编制了《疟疾流行和工作月报表》，并于 2004 年开始执行。内容包括：疟疾发病情况、疟疾发病人群分布、抗疟措施执行情况、疟疾暴发流行、疟疾血检、出入境和到国内高疟区流动人口疟疾监测、疟疾发病人员分类、其他寄生虫病、虫媒病毒性疾病发病情况等。疟疾月报表由村级填报，然后逐级按月汇总上报。大部分乡镇以及所有县均以固定电子邮件定期上传，月报表的成功运转，为全面了解项目动态提供了非常必要、准确、及时的信息内容，有助于项目监控及数据的复核。

2. 建立信息网络

项目启动后，省项目办对 8 个地（市）督导组及 25 个边境项目县项目办技术骨干统一培训了疟疾信息运作流程的使用。建立了县项目办每月及时上报所辖县的乡级疟疾流行及防治情况的制度，为云南省完成全球基金项目的总体目标提供了保障。

3. 采取积极有效措施，改进落后局面

3.1 针对治疗病例痕迹资料丢失严重和漏报的情况，使用个案病例登记卡记录管理病例，对疟疾病例追踪管理、规范治疗回溯起到了良好的作用。

3.2 设计、制作含有免费治疗信息的宣传日历，提高项目宣传力度，提高居民就诊意识，扩大项目人群参与力度。

3.3 定期印发项目简报，对全省项目执行情况作通报，并将简报送达政府和卫生行政部门，加强行政参与力度，提高项目知晓程度。

3.4 利用全省性会议的机会，选取项目执行较好的县交流经验，编制经验交流的材料下发各县，全面提高全省的疟疾项目执行能力和管理水平。

4. 探索适合于云南实际的项目管理模式

4.1 针对云南项目覆盖广、交通不便的情况，省项目办提出分片管理的模式，将全省项目县划片管理，由片区主管直接负责管理，片区主管由项目主管负责管理。

4.2 办公室成员在有分片区管理的同时，还有协作，针对项目工作零碎、临时性的特征，针对临时性的工作给予统一安排，并在项目办内再次分工，分管物资、信息、资料等内容，采取责任落实到人、任务落实到人的管理模式，使项目管理更加灵活和充分。

5．开发项目管理规范材料

针对以往财务活动支出与业务目标活动支出难以核对的情况，云南特别制定了项目用款申请 / 结算单，在单据中明确标明该支出活动应属目标中的活动，避免了因财务人员不熟悉业务活动设置而将活动支出列错目标的问题。2007 年修改完善了第一轮云南省全球基金疟疾项目实施细则。

6．完善了市、县项目管理机制

6.1 提高州市级参与项目管理的程度，加大对县级项目办的管理力度。

在原有省级督导的基础上增加州市级对项目督导、检查的参与程度，逐步加强市级督导组履行监督、检查的能力，利用日常工作到县级进行指导的机会，加强对县级项目办的指导。

6.2 积极与项目实施县卫生主管部门协商，最大限度的提高项目行政干预的力度。

在项目管理中逐步引入行政督导机制，把卫生主管部门参与督导作为项目督导的一个重要组成部分，让卫生主管部门了解项目的进程和实施过程中遇到的困难和阻力，加强对项目执行部门的督导力度，将项目工作纳入卫生责任目标的考核内容，充分的调动基层以及私人 / 个体医疗机构参与项目的积极性，提升项目的运作效果。

7．培养了一批稳定的项目管理人员，使基层疟防网络稳定运转

通过 5 年的项目实施，各级项目机构的培训，培养了一大批较为熟练的项目管理人员，完善了疫情报告、规范了治疗、落实了疟防宣教、健全了疫情处理体系，利用基层卫生网络，形成了一个稳定、灵活、准确的基层疟防工作长效机制。此外，基层的疟防网络的稳定运转，在很大程度上也使其他疾病的防治管理受益，并产生了深远的影响。

尽管项目在云南省实施 5 年中遇到了很多困难和问题，但在卫生部、云南省卫生厅的正确领导下，在国家、省、市、县各级实施机构的共同努力下，不断及时克服和解决各种困难和问题，保障了云南省的项目目标的实现。提高云南省疟疾控制能力，降低了 25 个项目县的疟疾发病率，减少了多重抗药性恶性疟的传播和扩散。项目实施中各级项目执行机构获得的宝贵管理理念和经验，将为后续项目的实施提供重要的参考和帮助。通过第一轮项目的实施，为云南省培养了一大批熟练的项目管理人员，为基层的疟防网络建设提供了重要的人员和物资保证，同时也对基层的防保网络建设起到了积极的促进作用。

云南省全球基金疟疾项目办公室

2008 年 6 月 30 日

二、海南省项目终期总结报告

（一）项目概况

第一轮海南省全球基金疟疾项目（2003 年 4 月 1 日～ 2008 年 3 月 31 日）覆盖海南省万宁市、陵水县、保亭县、五指山市、三亚市、乐东县、琼中县、白沙县、东方市、昌江县等 10 个市县，共 142 个乡镇（场），4860 个自然村（生产队），总人口约 250 万。通过加强对项目地区疟疾的及时诊断、规范治疗和有效防护、开展健康教育和健康促进、加强疟疾监测和项目管理能力等，海南省在遏制疟疾流行、有效控制多重抗性恶性疟的传播与扩散方面有了显著的进展。

项目自 2003 年 4 月启动以来，已执行 5 年，各项目执行单位开展了大量的疟疾诊断、治疗、预防、培训、督导、药品和设备分发和管理、健康促进等工作，项目的顺利实施有力地推动了海南省的疟疾防治。项目的实施为海南省的疟防提供了宝贵的经验，给海南留下一批抗疟设备，同时也为海南培训了大量的疟防人员，增强了海南的疟防力量。项目执行 5 年来，疟疾总发病率从基线的 385/10 000 下降到 31.13/10 000，恶性疟发病率从基线的 9.06/10 000 下降到 0.40/10 000，项目终期调查各项结果显示项目进展良好。

（二）项目剩余资金使用情况

截至结题报告日，第一轮海南省全球基金疟疾项目省本级尚节余 32 917.12 元，用于在 2008 年 6 月底召开项目结题总结大会和项目财务结题审计；10 个项目市县资金节余数为 0。

（三）项目设备物资盘点情况

第一轮海南省全球基金疟疾项目设备盘点情况见表 3–2 第一轮海南省全球基金疟疾项目设备物资一览表。

（四）5 年工作总结

1. 项目管理

1.1 项目办公室建设和运转情况：2003 年 3 月 27 日项目启动后，省级和市县级相继建立和健全项目办公室；省及各市县项目办机构健全，工作正常运行，人员职责清晰，工作规章制度齐全；省、各市县按计划召开或参加项目年会、例会，会议记录齐全。

1.2 项目工作计划和总结：省、各市县制定项目年度和季度工作计划；重要的项目活动都制定具体的实施方案；项目工作记录规范，细致清楚；项目活动结束后都有总结；按规定及时上报项目报表和报告，报表和报告填写规范。

1.3 项目培训：按计划开展培训活动，培训内容针对项目计划的需要，培训的记录、资料齐全；项目管理和执行人员按要求参加了有关的项目培训，培训覆盖率≥90%。

2．项目监督与评估（M&E）管理

各级项目办有专人负责项目数据报表的收集、审核、汇总和上报工作；项目季度报表上报及时、填写规范、数据准确；项目办有 M&E 工作指南和模板；组织开展或参加相关培训，培训记录、资料齐全，内容有针对性；按照工作计划开创性的应用模糊数学综合评价方法开展项目督导，督导规范、有成效，有督导通知、督导报告，督导过程有记录，督导后跟踪整改情况。

3．项目财务及物资管理

3.1 项目财务管理

3.1.1 财务人员队伍建设：各级项目办财务人员配置齐全；各级项目办财务不相容职务分人担任；财务人员与项目人员经常沟通；

3.1.2 预算制订与预算执行：财务人员参与、了解项目预算；项目支出标准符合预算；项目资金的使用与工作计划相对应；预算调整有批准；

3.1.3 项目资金管理：省、市县各级项目办银行账号独立设置；严格遵守中国人民银行颁布的《现金管理暂行条例》和《银行存款支付结算办法》；现金日记账和银行存款日记账账实相符 ；使用“全球基金项目空白票据购置、领用登记簿”，及时登记空白票据的购入、使用和结存；

3.1.4 项目财务管理：各级项目实施单位有项目财务管理相关制度；项目资金支出严格执行授权批准制度，使用全球基金专用凭证；项目资金使用符合规定 ；项目资金按照规定建账管理、分工作目标进行财务核算 ；使用《全球基金财务管理手册》规定的会计科目进行财务核算；

3.1.5 财务报表、审计及会计档案管理：各级项目实施单位账表相符；省市县级项目每年进行财务审计，有审计报告；会计资料，财务票据、账簿、报表装订和保管良好；

3.1.6 财务、物资管理培训及督导：各级项目办按照工作计划对下一级项目点财务人员进行了培训和督导，督导、培训资料记录详细齐全；

3.1.7 内部控制制度：建立项目的内部控制制度、授权批准控制制度、财产保全控制制度、内部报告控制制度、财务电子信息系统的数据输入与输出、文件储存与保管、网络安全等方面的控制制度。

项目累计共收到项目经费（人民币）5 882 497.34 元，累计支出金额为 5 868 476.61 元（详见表 1–15 ）。

表 1–15　第一轮海南省全球基金疟疾项目资金收支情况表

周期序号	年度	科目	目标 2		目标 3		目标 4		合计	
			人民币	百分比（%）	人民币	百分比（%）	人民币	百分比（%）	人民币	百分比（%）
项目一期	2003—2004	预算	2 004 852.00	--	655 320.00	--	473 329.00	--	3 133 501.00	--
		到款	1 223 520.24	61.03	991 390.72	151.28	618 590.56	130.69	2 833 501.52	90.43
		支出	1 226 512.74	61.18	978 490.50	149.31	606 756.74	128.19	2 811 759.98	89.73
项目二期	2005	预算	476 743.00	--	132 000.00	--	373 824.39	--	982 567.39	--
		到款	414 901.84	87.03	287 374.13	217.71	538 142.16	143.96	1 240 418.13	126.24
		支出	405 661.51	85.09	273 708.50	207.35	474 447.07	126.92	1 153 817.08	117.43
	2006	预算	419 232.00	--	42 298.00	--	407 170.73	--	868 700.73	--
		到款	382 594.78	91.26	157 767.76	372.99	357 497.24	87.80	897 859.78	103.36
		支出	403 726.41	96.30	105 464.50	249.34	300 797.38	73.88	809 988.29	93.24
	2007	预算	337 541.00	--	38 959.00	--	359 752.20	--	736 252.20	--
		到款	320 506.04	94.95	18 127.00	46.53	572 084.87	159.02	910 717.91	123.70
		支出	383 397.40	113.59	42 626.00	109.41	344 529.36	95.77	770 552.76	104.66
	2008	预算	28 000.00	--	0.00	--	56 800.00	--	84 800.00	--
		到款	0.00	0.00	0.00		0.00	0.00	0.00	0.00
		支出	25 900.00	92.50	1 450.00		295 008.50	519.38	322 358.50	380.14
累计		预算	3 266 368.00	--	868 577.00	--	1 670 876.32	--	5 805 821.32	--
		到款	2 341 522.90	71.69	1 454 659.61	167.48	2 086 314.83	124.86	5 882 497.34	101.32
		支出	2 445 198.06	74.86	1 401 739.50	161.38	2 021 539.05	120.99	5 868 476.61	101.08
		结余	-17 198.34		48 182.51	3.31	392 125.95	18.80	423 110.12	7.19

3.2 物资供应管理：项目固定资产和各种药品及时下拨给各级项目点；项目固

定资产和药品的调拨、领用手续健全；严格按照《全球基金财务管理手册》的要求，建立相应的固定资产和项目物品辅助账；全球基金项目固定资产和药品账实相符（详见表 1–16 ）。

表 1–16 第一轮海南省全球基金疟疾项目设备物资一览表

设备名称	数量	总金额(元)	获得途径	下拨时间	运行情况	用 途
显微镜	173 台	712 488.09	拨入	2004 ~ 2007	良好	项目专用
电脑	16 台	169 400.00	拨入	2004	良好	项目专用
打印机	12 台	27 600.00	拨入	2004	良好	项目专用
4 轮驱动皮卡车	6 辆	520 800.00	拨入	2005 ~ 2006	良好	项目专用
125C 摩托车	152 辆	576 187.90	拨入	2005 ~ 2006	良好	项目专用
越野车 / 面包车	2 辆	440 649.53	拨入	2005 ~ 2006	良好	项目专用
多媒体投影仪	1 台	17 850.00	拨入	2004	良好	项目专用
数码相机	1 架	7 840.00	拨入	2004	良好	项目专用
数码相机	1 架	4 950.00	自购	2003	良好	项目专用
扫描仪	1 台	990.00	自购	2005	良好	项目专用
文件柜	1 套	1 500.00	自购	2005	良好	项目专用
移动硬盘	1 个	730.00	自购	2006	良好	项目专用
设备小计	–	2 480 985.52	–	–	–	–
磷酸氯 / 伯喹片剂	68786 盒	189 485.20	拨入	2004 ~ 2008		项目专用
双氢青蒿素片剂	20000 盒	330 000.00	拨入	2004		项目专用
蒿甲醚针剂	9200 盒	315 120.00	拨入	2004 ~ 2007		项目专用
复方磷酸哌喹片剂	50 罐	17 000.00	拨入	2007		项目专用
一次性注射器	13500 支	5 900.00	拨入	2004 ~ 2007		项目专用
长效蚊帐	11980 顶	251 960.00	拨入	2004 ~ 2007		项目专用
杀飞克	104 瓶	15 912.00	拨入	2004		项目专用
奋斗呐	2 吨	210 000.00	拨入	2005		项目专用
物资小计	–	1 335 377.20	–	–	–	–
设备物资合计	–	3 816 362.72	–	–	–	–

4. 项目工作计划完成情况

4.1 项目地区居民发热病人血检（人次）：计划血检 628 829 人次，实际血检 655 175 人次，完成率 104.19%（详见表 1–17、图 1–4）。

表 1–17　海南省各项目市县 5 年发热病人血检人次与费用（元）

单　位	计划目标	实际完成	完成率（%）	预算数	实际支出	执行率（%）
万宁市	55 369	56 948	102.85	112 408	115 366	102.63
陵水县	45 600	46 480	101.93	93 348	95 411	102.21
保亭县	66 260	77 269	116.61	138 324	132 788	96.00
五指山市	50 000	51 066	102.13	105 374	108 508	102.97
三亚市	55 400	62 775	113.31	105 558	113 080	107.13
乐东县	86 200	94 172	109.25	146 003	144 765	99.15
琼中县	88 200	80 942	91.77	170 779	159 696	93.51
白沙县	79 700	81 441	102.18	160 413	156 213	97.38
东方市	53 700	55 040	102.50	123 352	122 567	99.36
昌江县	48 400	49 042	101.33	231 228	229 419	99.22
合　计	628 829	655 175	104.19	1 386 787	1 377 814	99.35

* 表内为 2003 年 4 月 1 日至 2008 年 3 月 31 日的数据。

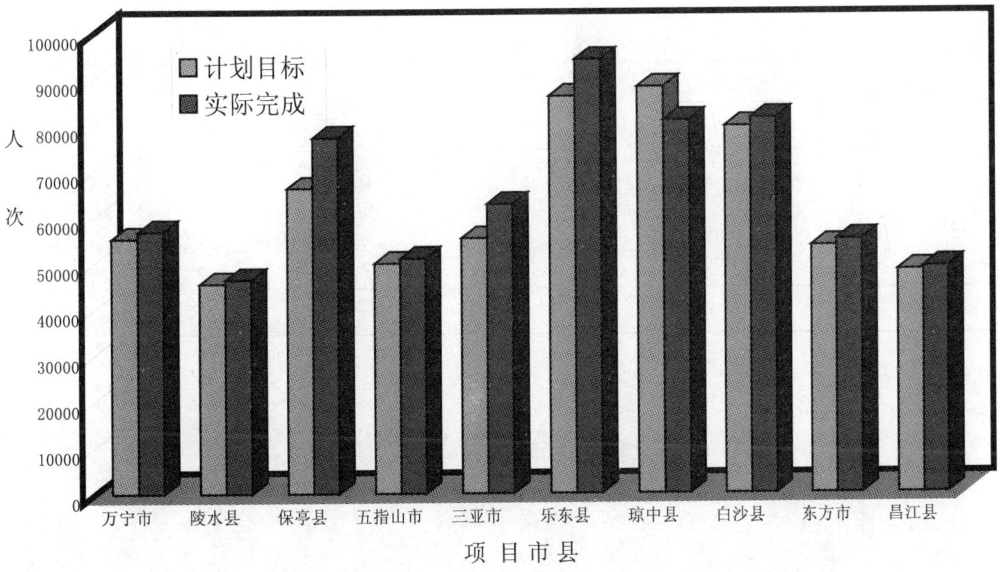

图 1–4　各项目市县 5 年（2003 年 4 月 1 日～ 2008 年 3 月 31 日）发热病人血检完成情况

4.2 项目地区居民疟疾病人规范治疗（例）：计划治疗 101 474 例，实际治疗 100 785 例，完成率 99.32%（详见表 1–18、图 1–5）。

表 1–18　海南省各项目市县 5 年疟疾病人规范治疗例数与费用（元）

单　位	计划目标	实际完成	完成率（%）	预算数	实际支出	执行率（%）
万宁市	7 294	6 865	94.12	45 883	40 846	89.02

续表

陵水县	5 700	5 996	105.19	37 172	38 020	102.28
保亭县	9 210	7 984	86.69	88 098	90 517	102.75
五指山市	12 900	12 199	94.57	57 135	52 077	91.15
三亚市	14 770	18 406	124.62	36 438	35 748	98.11
乐东县	7 340	7 377	100.50	95 891	95 662	99.76
琼中县	15 640	13 050	83.44	80 992	60 291	74.44
白沙县	7 640	7 199	94.23	100 827	101 002	100.17
东方市	6 390	6 653	104.12	55 520	55 515	99.99
昌江县	14 590	15 056	103.19	43 399	41 546	95.73
合 计	101 474	100 785	99.32	641 354	611 223	95.30

*表内为 2003 年 4 月 1 日至 2008 年 3 月 31 日的数据。

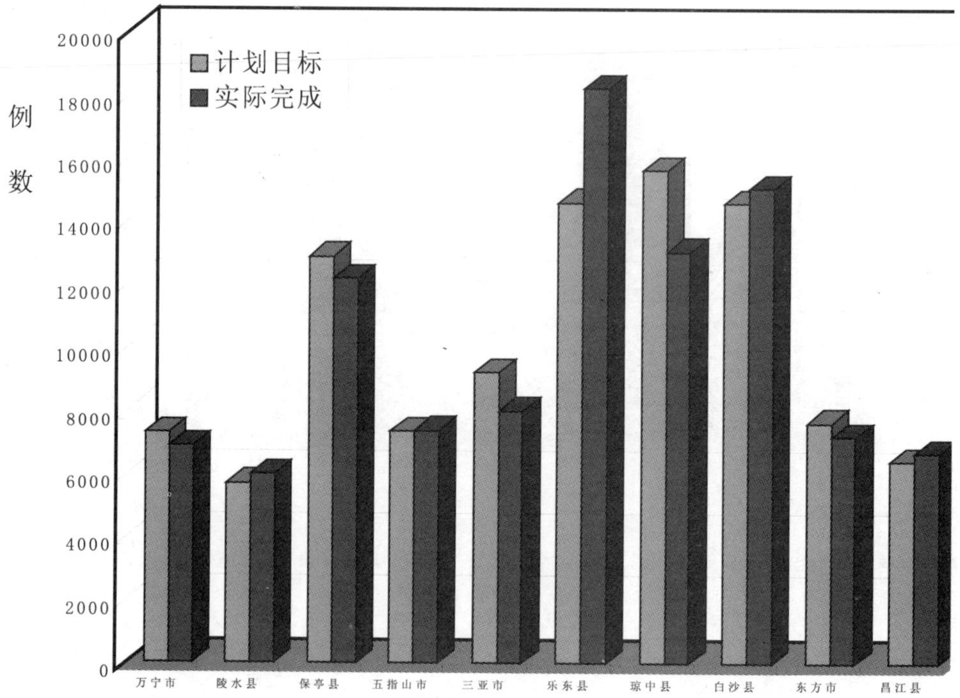

图 1-5 各项目市县 5 年（2003 年 4 月 1 日～ 2008 年 3 月 31 日）疟疾病人规范治疗完成情况

4.3 乡、村医生 / 个体医生及疟原虫镜检员培训：计划培训 2 500 人次，实际培训 2 995 人次，完成率 119.80%（详见表 1-19）。

表 1–19 海南省各项目市县 5 年乡、村医生 / 个体医生培训人次与费用（元）

单　位	计划目标	实际完成	完成率(%)	预算数	实际支出	执行率(%)
省本级	330	427	129.39			
万宁市	200	280	140.00	44 200	44 200	100.00
陵水县	200	186	93.00	56 200	56 200	100.00
保亭县	240	257	107.08	60 600	47 670	78.66
五指山市	240	498	207.50	20 200	19 383	95.95
三亚市	280	281	100.36	82 900	88 139	106.32
乐东县	200	207	103.50	46 731	46 396	99.28
琼中县	160	160	100.00	39 415	40 179	101.94
白沙县	320	333	104.06	60 900	58 250	95.65
东方市	180	197	109.44	34 100	33 601	98.54
昌江县	150	169	112.67	44 200	44 200	100.00
合　计	2 500	2 995	119.80	489 446	478 218	97.71

* 表内为 2003 年 4 月 1 日至 2008 年 3 月 31 日的数据。

4.4 杀虫剂浸泡（处理）蚊帐：计划浸泡（处理）90 375 顶，实际浸泡（处理）116 611 顶，完成率 129.03%（详见表 1–20）。

表 1–20 海南省各项目市县 5 年杀虫剂浸泡（处理）蚊帐顶数与费用（元）

单　位	计划目标	实际完成	完成率(%)	预算数	实际支出	执行率(%)
万宁市	8 050	12 746	158.34	29 476	29 267	99.29
陵水县	7 075	7 105	100.42	23 927	23 911	99.93
保亭县	9 850	12 717	129.11	38 048	32 761	86.10
五指山市	3 100	2 877	92.81	10 838	8 419	77.68
三亚市	8 850	9 560	108.02	21 383	22 530	105.36
乐东县	13 600	14 766	108.57	28 435	28 435	100.00
琼中县	12 800	18 210	142.27	45 048	45 623	101.28
白沙县	13 000	20 964	161.26	45 090	44 240	99.79
东方市	7 100	7 736	108.96	26 888	27 539	102.42
昌江县	6 950	9 930	142.88	26 896	26 896	100.00
合　计	90 375	116 611	129.03	296 029	289 621	97.83

* 表内为 2003 年 4 月 1 日至 2008 年 3 月 31 日的数据。

4.5 高危人群预防服药：计划巡诊 900 次，实际巡诊 714 次，完成率 79.33%。

4.6 健康教育材料印制：计划印制 125 000 份，实际印制 125 000 份，完成率

100.00%。

4.7 健康教育人员培训：计划培训 1 020 人次，实际培训 1 412 人次，完成率 138.43%。

4.8 项目市县用广播电视进行疟疾防治知识宣传：计划进行 60 次，实际进行 60 次，完成率百分百比。

4.9 给项目市县中小学生上疟防知识课：计划上 2 550 班次，实际上了 2 679 班次，完成率 105.06%（详见表 1–21）。

表 1–21 海南省各项目市县 5 年中小学生上疟防知识课的班次与费用（元）

单 位	计划目标	实际完成	完成率(%)	预算数	实际支出	执行率(%)
万宁市	235	235	100.00	19 270	19 270	100.00
陵水县	215	215	100.00	16 630	16 630	100.00
保亭县	285	310	108.77	23 370	21 104	90.31
五指山市	220	225	102.27	17 769	12 500	70.34
三亚市	235	259	110.21	14 600	14 600	100.00
乐东县	300	314	104.67	23 024	22 826	99.14
琼中县	305	311	101.97	24 195	24 795	102.48
白沙县	300	327	109.00	24 600	24 239	98.53
东方市	235	241	102.55	16 200	16 234	100.21
昌江县	220	242	110.00	18 040	18 040	100.00
合 计	2550	2679	105.06	197 698	190 238	96.23

* 表内为 2003 年 4 月 1 日至 2008 年 3 月 31 日的数据。

4.10 在公共场所张贴疟疾知识宣传画：计划张贴 58 000 张，实际张贴 61 126 张，完成率 105.39%（详见表 1–22）。

表 1–22 海南省各项目市县 5 年公共场所张贴疟疾知识宣传画张数与费用（元）

单 位	计划目标	实际完成	完成率(%)	预算数	实际支出	执行率(%)
万宁市	5 600	6 510	116.25	9 761	11 185	114.59
陵水县	4 400	4 736	107.64	7 516	7 513	99.96
保亭县	12 300	12 440	101.14	8 450	8 363	98.97
五指山市	4 600	5 350	116.30	7 711	7 710	99.99
三亚市	4 700	4 704	100.09	7 789	7 778	99.86
乐东县	5 800	5 810	100.17	8 633	8 633	100.00
琼中县	6 000	6 500	108.33	8 856	9 062	102.33
白沙县	5 800	5 781	99.67	8 848	8 830	99.80

续表

东方市	4 400	4 695	106.70	15 500	15 470	99.81
昌江县	4 400	4 600	104.55	9 500	9 460	99.57
合 计	58 000	61 126	105.39	92 564	94 004	101.56

＊表内为 2003 年 4 月 1 日至 2008 年 3 月 31 日的数据。

4.11 项目地区居民疟原虫调查（人次）：计划调查 60 000 人次，实际调查 62 714 人次，完成率 104.52%（详见表 1–23）。

表 1–23　海南省各项目市县 5 年居民疟原虫调查人次与费用（元）

单　位	计划目标	实际完成	完成率(%)	预算数	实际支出	执行率(%)
万宁市	5 400	5 598	103.67	10 359	10 340	99.82
陵水县	4 500	5 298	117.73	5 632	5 625	99.88
保亭县	7 500	8 211	109.48	15 000	49 734	331.57
五指山市	4 500	4 377	97.27	8 707	6 861	78.80
三亚市	4 500	5 216	115.91	8 561	8 704	101.67
乐东县	8 100	8 113	100.16	15 159	15 140	99.88
琼中县	8 400	8 865	115.31	15 858	16 567	104.47
白沙县	8 100	8 169	100.85	15 538	15 379	98.98
东方市	4 500	4 257	94.60	9 000	8 433	93.00
昌江县	4 500	4 610	102.00	9 000	9 000	100.00
合 计	60 000	62 714	104.52	112 814	145 783	129.22

＊表内为 2003 年 4 月 1 日至 2008 年 3 月 31 日的数据。

4.12 目标地区恶性疟原虫对药物抗性的监测：在 2005 及 2007 年分别在乐东县和东方市进行了恶性疟原虫对磷酸氯喹、磷酸哌喹和咯萘啶的敏感性体外测定，显示其对磷酸氯喹和磷酸哌喹的抗性率较高（详见表 1–24、1–25）。

表 1–24　海南省恶性疟原虫对氯喹、咯萘啶的敏感性体外测定（2005）

测定地点	测定药物	测定例数	抗性例数	抗性率 %	CIMC* (ρmol/μl)	LD_{50}（95% 可信限）(ρmol/μl)
乐东县抱由镇	磷酸氯喹	31	19	61.26	3.72	2.07（1.75-2.45）
	咯萘啶	31	5	16.13	1.39	0.35（0.27-0.46）
东方市江边乡	磷酸氯喹	34	25	73.53	5.41	2.86（2.39-3.42）
	咯萘啶	34	4	11.76	1.10	0.53（0.43-0.65）

注：* 完全抑制裂殖体形成的平均浓度

表 1–25 海南省恶性疟原虫对抗疟药敏感性体外测定结果（2007）

药敏	测定例数	抗性例数	抗性率(%)	LD_{50}（95%可信限）（ρmol/μl）	CIMC*（ρmol/μl）
磷酸氯喹	32	23	71.88	2.34（1.85—2.94）	5.60±5.64
磷酸哌喹	32	13	40.63	1.96（1.44—2.68）	9.26±13.67
咯萘啶	32	4	12.5	0.16（0.13—0.20）	0.55±1.02
青蒿琥酯	32	0	0	0.04（0.03—0.05）	0.07±0.04

注：* 完全抑制裂殖体形成的平均浓度

5. 项目考核指标达标情况

5.1 疟疾调查推断发病率：终期目标为 192/10 000，终期调查结果为 31.13/10 000，指标达标率 183.15%（详见表 1–26）。

表 1–26 海南省 10 个项目市县终期专项调查推算的疟疾发病率

县名(1)	被调查县人口数(2)	被调查县上报疟疾病例数(3)	受调查人群中通过网络直报的疟疾病例数(C 值)(4)	走访调查出的疟疾病例数(R 值)(5)	走访调查出的疟疾病例中作为疫情网络直报的病例数(M 值)(6)	推算被调查人群实际疟疾病例数(N 值)(7)	推算被调查县(市)实际发病数(8)=(3)/{(4)/(7)}	推算被调查县(市)实际发病率(1/万)(9)=(8)/(2)×10000
万宁市	565 761	551	138	89	40	304	1 214	21.46
陵水县	343 661	372	171	155	39	670	1 457	42.40
保亭县	160 622	444	59	116	39	175	1 313	81.76
五指山	111 773	98	15	22	10	32	212	18.97
三亚市	533 349	123	24	52	23	54	278	5.21
乐东市	492 114	323	14	68	11	85	1 967	39.97
琼中县	201 321	309	39	90	22	157	1 246	61.89
白沙县	185 727	532	32	59	26	72	1 203	64.75
东方市	403 560	458	194	70	29	461	1 087	26.94
昌江县	253 308	174	26	13	6	53	355	14.00
合 计	3 251 196	3 384	712	734	245	2 129	10 120	31.13

5.2 项目县恶性疟调查推断发病率：终期目标为<1/10 000，终期调查结果为0.40/10 000，指标达标率 107.85%（详见表 1–27、图 1–6）。

表 1–27　海南省 10 个项目市县终期专项调查推算的恶性疟发病率

县名 (1)	被调查县人口数 (2)	被调查县上报恶性疟病例数 (3)	被调查乡镇卫生院恶性疟疫情报告数数(C 值) (4)	被调查乡镇恶性疟病例登记数(R 值) (5)	恶性疟名单相符的病例数 (M 值) (6)	推算被调查乡镇实际恶性疟病例数 (N 值) (7)	推算被调查县(市) 实际恶性疟病例数(8) = (3) / {(4) / (7)}	推算被调查县(市) 恶性疟实际发病率(1/ 万) (9)=(8)/(2) × 10000
万宁市	565 761	1	1	1	1	1	1	0.02
陵水县	343 661	4	3	3	3	3	4	0.12
保亭县	160 622	1	1	1	1	1	1	0.06
五指山	111 773	1	0	0	0	0	1	0.09
三亚市	533 349	42	3	3	3	3	42	0.79
乐东市	492 114	28	5	5	5	5	28	0.57
琼中县	201 321	2	0	0	0	0	2	0.10
白沙县	185 727	10	3	3	3	3	10	0.54
东方市	403 560	29	14	14	14	14	29	0.72
昌江县	253 308	3	2	3	1	5	8	0.30
合 计	3251 196	121	32	33	31	34	129	0.40

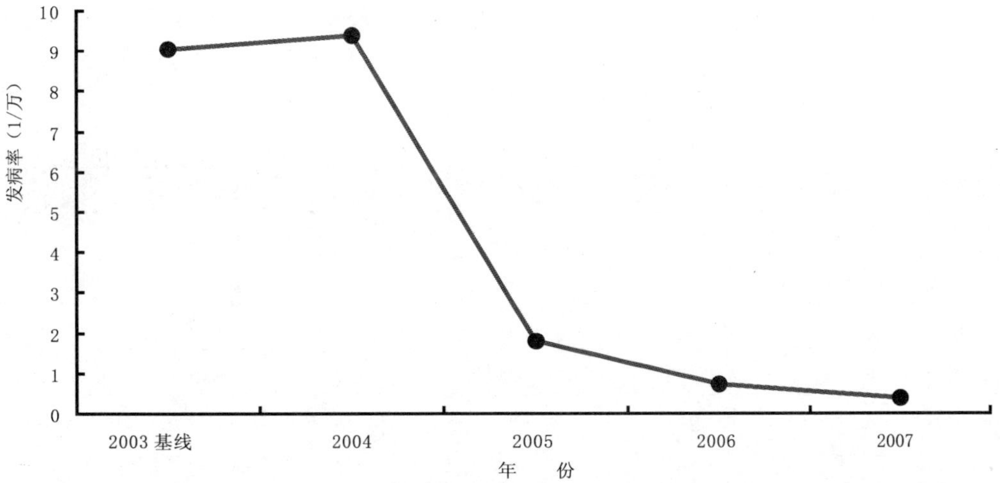

图 1–6　海南省 2003–2007 年恶性疟发病趋势图

5.3 中小学生能够正确回答至少 3 个与疟疾相关问题的比例：终期目标为 85%，终期调查结果为 89.39%，指标达标率 119.57%（详见表 1–28）。

表 1–28 海南省 10 个项目市县中小学生能够正确回答至少 3 个与疟疾相关问题的比例

县名 (1)	调查的中小学校数 (2)	调查的学生数 (3)	能正确回答三个疟疾相关问题的学生数 (4)	能正确回答三个疟疾相关问题的学生的比例(%) (5) = (4) / (3) ×100
万宁市	6	365	329	90.14
陵水县	6	939	843	89.78
保亭县	6	388	349	89.95
五指山	6	362	323	89.23
三亚市	6	360	327	90.83
乐东市	6	386	342	88.60
琼中县	6	394	348	88.32
白沙县	6	373	338	90.62
东方市	6	372	330	88.71
昌江县	6	376	328	87.23
合 计	60	4 315	3 857	89.39

5.4 发热病人在症状出现两天内求诊的比例：终期目标为 90%，终期调查结果为 85.27%，指标达标率 86.63%（详见表 1–29）。

表 1–29 海南省 10 个项目市县发热病人在症状出现两天内求诊的比例

县名 (1)	调查的行政村数 (2)	自述有发热史的村民数 (3)	自述有发热史的村民中发热两天内求诊的人数 (4)	发热病人在症状出现两天内求诊的比例(%) (5) = (4) / (3) ×100
万宁市	9	277	246	88.81
陵水县	9	480	424	88.33
保亭县	9	657	552	84.02
五指山	9	675	579	85.78
三亚市	9	596	507	85.07
乐东市	9	1 682	1 415	84.13
琼中县	9	632	542	85.76
白沙县	9	563	467	82.95
东方市	9	279	247	88.53
昌江县	9	166	143	86.14
合 计	90	6 007	5 122	85.27

5.5 拥有杀虫剂浸泡蚊帐（ITNs）的家庭比例：终期目标为30%，终期调查结果为52.38%，指标达标率151.18%（详见表1–30）。

表1–30 10个项目市县拥有杀虫剂浸泡蚊帐的家庭比例

县名 (1)	调查的行政村数 (2)	调查户数 (3)	拥有ITNs的户数 (4)	拥有ITNs户数的比例(%) (5)=(4)/(3)×100
万宁市	9	657	339	51.60
陵水县	9	273	140	51.28
保亭县	9	638	388	60.82
五指山	9	596	300	50.34
三亚市	9	611	334	54.66
乐东市	9	637	325	51.02
琼中县	9	635	311	48.98
白沙县	9	612	313	51.14
东方市	9	708	368	51.98
昌江县	9	587	301	51.28
合 计	90	5 954	3 119	52.38

5.6 网络直报疟疾病人的比例：终期目标为40%，终期调查结果为33.38%，指标达标率81.07%（详见表1–31）。

表1–31 海南省10个项目市县网络直报疟疾病人的比例

县名 (1)	调查的行政村数 (2)	走访调查的疟疾病例数 (3)	走访调查的疟疾病例中通过网络直报的病例数 (4)	疟疾病例通过网络直报系统报告的比例(%) (5)=(4)/(3)×100
万宁市	9	89	40	44.94
陵水县	9	155	39	25.16
保亭县	9	116	39	33.62
五指山	9	22	10	45.45
三亚市	9	52	23	44.23
乐东市	9	68	11	16.18
琼中县	9	90	22	24.44
白沙县	9	59	26	44.07
东方市	9	70	29	41.43
昌江县	9	13	6	46.15
合 计	90	734	245	33.38

6. 项目地区疟防投入

6.1 卫生行政部门组织和支持项目活动：海南省卫生厅和各项目市县卫生局非常重视本项目，将项目纳入全省和市县疟疾防治规划，制定年度疟疾防治计划时始终将项目工作作为疟疾防治规划的重要部分；卫生厅成立项目领导小组，厅长亲任组长，其成员均为各有关处室的主要领导；全程领导和关注项目的执行和进展。特别是厅疾控处的领导亲自参加项目的重要会议和重大督导，及时作出决策和指示，使项目始终在卫生行政部门的支持和领导下顺利开展，各项评估数字显示，项目进展顺利。

6.2 疟疾防治资金投入

项目执行 5 年内，项目地区疟防资金投入总额为 10 467 908.45 元，其中全球基金项目资金投入占 7.48 %，政府资金投入占 92.52 %。虽然全球基金项目资金投入仅占全省疟防资金的 7.48%，但项目管理规范，措施落实，效果显著，项目作为海南省疟疾防治活动的补充，显然起到了很好的作用，为海南省的疟防提供了宝贵的经验，给海南留下一批抗疟设备，同时也为海南培训了大量的疟防人员，增强了海南的疟防力量。项目执行 5 年来，疟疾总发病率从基线的 385/10 000 下降到 31.13/10 000，恶性疟发病率从基线的 9.06/10 000 下降到 0.40/10 000，达到了预期目标。

7．受益人群对项目的满意度

第一轮全球基金疟疾项目在海南省覆盖的疟疾病人及家属对项目提供的疟防服务的满意程度很高。

根据对白沙县、东方市、三亚市、保亭县和陵水县的调查，高疟区共访问 258 人，满意度在 60% 以下的 23 人占 8.91%，满意度在 60%-80% 的 59 人占 22.87%，满意度在 80% 以上的 176 人占 68.22%；中疟区共访问 255 人，满意度在 60% 以下的 16 人占 6.27%，满意度在 60%-80% 的 118 人占 46.27%，满意度在 80% 以上的 121 人占 47.45%；低疟区共访问 258 人，满意度在 60% 以下的 18 人占 6.98%，满意度在 60-80% 的 123 人占 47.67%，满意度在 80% 以上的 117 人占 45.35%。

合计共访问 771 人，满意度在 60% 以下的 57 人占 7.39%，满意度在 60-80% 的 300 人占 38.91%，满意度在 80% 以上的 414 人占 53.70%。

8．存在的问题

8.1 省项目办督促项目市县对在各级督导中发现的问题进行整改的力度尚嫌不足，部分县市发现的问题没有得到及时整改，同样的问题连续两个季度重复出现。

8.2 部分项目乡镇（场）少数数据的上报数与核实数不符。

8.3 部分项目乡镇（场）疟疾病人治疗处方没有分类保存。

8.4 由于乡村诊所个体医不具备镜检条件，大量的疟疾病人为临床诊断病例，镜检确诊的疟疾病人数和比例较低。

8.5 有些市县的季度活动资料保存混乱，不属于项目工作的常规抗疟资料也被放入项目资料档案里。

8.6 个别市县乡级资料没有完全按季度保存和装订成册，不便于数据查找。

8.7 由于项目药物采购滞后，致使基层药品供应不及时，影响病人治疗工作。

8.8 财务和物资管理方面，尚存在个别项目点固定资产辅助账中固定资产调拨未分项目点填写；项目物品辅助账中物品领用没有填写领用人；项目负责人审批用款申请书、结算单时未填写日期，部分经手人签字时也未填写日期；部分督导费用报销单上未填写督导地点，凭证后也未附相应的督导计划；市县级项目财务官员到下级督导没有督导记录等问题。

9．项目总体评价

第一轮海南省全球基金疟疾项目运转良好，措施落实，效果显著。项目考核的疟疾发病率、恶性疟发病率、目标地区中小学生能够回答至少 3 个与疟疾相关问题的比例、发热病人在症状出现 2 天内求诊的比例、拥有杀虫剂浸泡蚊帐（ITNs）的家庭比例、疟疾病例通过信息网络报告的比例六个指标中，发热病人在症状出现 2 天内求诊的比例稍低于 2007 年《监督评价（ME）计划与实施指南（第五年）》规定的指标，疟疾病例通过信息网络报告的比例这项指标由于部分市县乡镇级的疫情网络直报系统不够健全，致使病例漏报还比较严重，漏报率还比较高。其余指标均达到或超过规定的指标比例。

海南省全球基金疟疾项目办公室

2008 年 6 月

三、安徽省项目终期总结报告

在省卫生厅和省疾控中心的领导下，在全球基金一轮国家项目办的直接指导下，安徽省第一轮全球基金疟疾项目办按照全球基金疟疾项目管理的要求，按计划开展工作，自 2003 年 4 月起经过 5 年的运行，完成了项目各项工作内容和监督与评价计划。2008 年 4 月省项目办对 5 年来的工作进行了全面的总结和评估，现总结如下。

（一）项目概况

2003 年 4 月安徽省第一轮全球基金疟疾项目正式启动，安徽省前期两年度项目覆盖地区 2 个县，怀远县为控制疟疾暴发流行，执行各项目防治措施的落实及效果观察项目单位，五河县为疟疾监测单位，后三年仅怀远一个项目单位。安徽省按照国家项目办的要求，在省卫生厅的领导下，成立了由省疾病预防控制中心主任 / 副主任为项目主任、地寄科业务负责人为项目主管、财务科长为财务主管及相关业务人员组成的项目办公室。项目县也相应地成立了由卫生局领导、疾控中心领导及财务和相关业务人员组成的项目办公室。省项目办召开了项目启动会，并与项目县签订了项目责任书。

（二）项目剩余资金使用情况

费使用情况：5 年来共收到全球基金经费 978 243.13 元，其中目标二经费为 459 039.2 元，目标四经费为 519 130.86 元，下拨及使用经费 974 746.75 元，经费使用率为 99.65%。截至 2008 年 3 月 31 日，项目节余 3 396 元，按照项目结题计划于 6 月 1 日前支出网络信息费及审计费，项目经费全部支出，没有节余。

（三）项目设备物资盘点情况

5 年来，全球基金下拨和自购物资（详见表 1–32），2008 年 6 月前对所有资产进行处置。省项目办和怀远、五河县的物资移交省、县疾病预防控制中心使用。

表 1–32 固定资产和物资的盘点与处置计划

设备名称	数量	总金额	获得途径	目前运行情况	目前用途	目前使用部门	处置计划	处置时间	计划用途	计划使用部门
显微镜	12	47 681.61	拨入	良好	疟疾镜检	省、怀远、五河县项目办	移交其他部门	2008.6	疟疾镜检	省、怀远、五河县疾控
台式电脑	5	51 882.00	拨入	良好	项目专用	省、怀远、五河县项目办	移交其他部门	2008.6	疟疾防治	省、县疾控
笔记本电脑	3	43 500.00	拨入	良好	项目专用	省疾控 / 省项目办	移交其他部门	2008.6	疟疾防治	省疾控
复印机	1	14 800.00	自购	正常	项目专用	省疟疾项目办	移交其他部门	2008.6	疟疾防治	省疾控 / 第五轮
投影仪	1	19 800.00	自购	正常	项目专用	省疟疾项目办	移交其他部门	2008.6	疟疾防治	省疾控 / 第五轮
台式电脑	2	16 600.00	自购	正常	项目专用	怀远、五河县项目办	移交其他部门	2008.6	疟疾防治	县疾控 / 第五轮
笔记本电脑	1	10 700.00	自购	正常	项目专用	蚌埠市项目办	移交其他部门	2008.6	疟疾防治	市疾控 / 第五轮

（四）5 年工作总结

1. 项目管理。

省疾控中心设有项目办公室，共 4 人，均为兼职，怀远县设立项目办，共 5 人，有一名专职人员，兼职会计 1 名。

2. 监督与评价管理。

省及县项目办严格按照项目规划方案内容对县及各乡（镇）疟防工作进行督导，县项目办分别以每季度 9 个乡（镇）次的督导，督导内容包括乡村医生和镜检员培训、发热病人血检、病人治疗、媒介监测，并监督整改情况。省项目办依照督导程序对项目县，实施情况进行督导检查，依据项目评分标准，分项打分，对项目和财务执行情况进行评估，提出整改意见，写出督导报告。项目的专项督导保证了项目执行质量和资金的安全。2007 年 6 月第一轮全球基金国家项目办对安徽省项目执行情况进行的督导评估，认为安徽省项目整体执行情况良好，经费使用和资产管理符合全球基金的要求。

3. 财务管理。

财务管理严格按照《全球基金项目财务手册》以及相关规定执行，经费的支出根据项目计划开展，财务程序严格按照项目要求进行审核的同时，保障资金的快速、及时下拨，保障了工作的开展，并在每年省项目办都要对项目县开展项目财务专项督导。5 年来共收到全球基金经费 978 243.13 元，其中目标 2 经费 459 039.2 元，目标 4 经费 519 130.86 元，下拨及使用经费 974 746.75 元，经费使用率为 99.65 %，项目各项指标和预算执行率完成良好。

4. 物资采购管理。

固定资产 5 年来项目累计 185 265 元人民币，其中自购 2 台台式电脑，价值 16 600.00 元；笔记本电脑 1 台，10 700.00 元；投影仪 1 台，19 800.00 元；复印机 1 台，14 800.00 元。抗疟药品 49 750 人份（4.20 元 ×49 750），208 950 元，固定资产和物资累计收入 394 215 元人民币（表 1–33）。

表 1–33　安徽省累计固定资产和物资收支情况

设备名称	数量	金额（元）	支出数量	支出金额（元）
显微镜	12	47 681.61	12	47 681.61
台式电脑	7	64 482	7	64 482
笔记本电脑	4	54 200	4	54 200
复印机	1	14 800.00	1	14 800.00

续表

投影仪	1	19 800.00	1	19 800.00
抗疟药	49 750	208 850	49 750	208 850
合计	—	394 215	—	394 215

（五）项目执行进展

1. 疟疾调查推断发病率

采取分层随机整群抽样法。先将全县各乡镇按近 3 年（2005—2007 年）的疟疾发病率抽取了包集（高）、魏庄（中）、荆芡（低）3 个乡镇，再在这些乡镇中按近 3 年的疟疾发病率各抽取了 3 个行政村，分别为包集的包集（高）、滕元（中）、镇东（低）、魏庄的湖东（高）、年庙（中）、魏庄（低）和荆芡的沈郢（高）、牛王（中）、支湖（低），最后在上述行政村中共随机抽取了 10 个自然村，共走访居民 3 098 人，其中包集 1 031 人，荆芡 1040 人，魏庄 1027 人。疟疾病人 11 人，平均发病率为 35/ 万，网络报告 9 例，漏报率为 18.18%。怀远县 2007 年人口为 1 271 664，报告病例 626 例，根据捕获－再捕获法推算实际发病数为 765 例，发病率 6.02/ 万，与 2003 年报告病例 2 464 例，实际病例 9 258 相比分别下降了 222.09%和 1 110.19%。

2. 目标地区中小学生能够回答至少 3 个与疟疾相关问题的比例

采取分层随机整群抽样法，在全县抽取包集、魏庄、荆芡 3 个乡镇，每个乡镇（场）抽取中、小学校各 1 所，每所学校各 60 名学生（小学三年级到初中三年级）。对 360 名学生进行问卷调查能够正确回答三个疟疾相关问题的人数，结果为 100%，与 2003 年的 50%相比提高了 1 倍。

3. 发热病人在症状出现两天内求诊的比例

采取分层随机整群抽样法，在抽取的 10 个自然村中按照《第一轮中国全球基金疟疾项目居民家庭走访调查表》进行入户走访问卷调查村民中曾经发热病人数和 2 天内求诊的人数，平均求诊比例为 80.41%。

4. 网络直报疟疾病人比例

采取分层随机整群抽样法，在抽取的 10 个自然村中进行入户走访问卷调查，符合“血检阳性、典型临床症状、药物试治有效”其中之一即为疟疾病例。根据走访调查的疟疾病例名单，与县 CDC 网络直报疫情进行核对，网络直报疟疾病人比例为 54.55%。

5．主要项目指标执行情况

5.1 发热病人血检：怀远项目县建立了县中心镜检站和 29 个乡级镜检站。血检覆盖人口 127.166 万，共血检 135 627 人次，检出阳性 4 398 例，平均阳性率为 3.24%，血检率为2.14%。与项目启动前的2002年血检率0.39%相比提高了4.49倍(表1–34)。

表1–34　2003—2007年血检确诊病人比例（血检阳性率）

年份	血检人数	血检率(%)	检出阳性例数	血检阳性率(%)
2003	15 060	1.16	1 679	11.14
2004	31 721	2.52	867	2.73
2005	33 727	2.70	775	2.30
2006	27 097	2.13	741	2.73
2007	28 022	2.20	336	1.20

5.2 病人治疗：通过项目的实施，有效的推进了疟疾防治工作，疟疾病人得到了及时治疗，5年来治疗疟疾和疑似病人23 955例，疟疾病人的正规治疗率由项目启动前28.72%提高到2007年100.00%。

5.3 高危人群预防服药

5.3.1 疟疾的休止期治疗，2003—2007年分别对疟史、疑似病人、重点人群进行了休止期治疗共153 709人次，其中疟史病人10 136、疑似病人6 937人、重点人群104 180人、全民32 456人。

5.3.2 流行季节重点人群预防服药，2003—2007年，在流行季节对重点人群进行预防80 378人次。

5.4 人员培训:为提高疟疾诊断、治疗水平和项目的管理能力，2003—2007年省、县项目办分别举办了疟原虫镜检、疟疾防治技术、媒介、暴发流行控制及财务管理培训班。共举办培训班29个，培训各类人员1 032人次，接受疟疾防治知识培训率为96.17%。

5.5 项目督导：2005—2007年，按照全球基金项目活动的要求，每年省项目办对项目县及乡镇进行了一次以上的督导，项目县每年每月1次对3个乡镇进行1次疟原虫镜检、疟疾病人治疗、管理等各项防治措施落实情况进行督导，共督导37次81乡次，有效地保证了各项防治措施的落实和项目正常运转。

5.6 居民和中小学生疟防知识知晓情况：当地居民和中小学生的疟防知识知晓率分别从20.12%和40.45%，提高到89.18%和100.00%。

5.7 哨点主动监测

5.7.1 病例主动侦查，2005—2007年项目县每年一次8 000人以上的疟疾病人主动侦查，3年共调查了27 517人次，

5.7.2 间接荧光抗体试验（IFA）调查，2003—2007年，按照项目要求每年监测1 000人，项目县共监测5 619人次，检出阳性307人，平均阳性率为5.46%。

5.7.3 居民带虫率调查，共调查 4 122 人，阳性 32 人，平均阳性率为 0.78%。

5.7.4 媒介监测，为防制提供科学依据：从 2003 年起，6—10 月中旬开展每旬一次定点媒介监测，同时开展项目县 3 个定点以及专项疟疾媒介调查，对当地疟疾的种类、媒介按蚊的栖性、习性和季节分布等传疟因素有了系统的了解，5 年来监测结果显示没有发现嗜人按蚊，当地疟疾的传播媒介为中华按蚊。

种群比例调查 2003—2007 年每年 6 月中下旬，在怀远县选择了发病较高的万福、河溜的 6 个行政村，采取清晨全捕法，共捕获按蚊 6 373 只，经鉴定均为中华按蚊，中华按蚊的比例为 100%。

媒介密度监测 2003—2007 年，于 6 月下旬至 10 月上旬每旬一次 19:00-22:00，每旬一次进行了野外半通宵人诱饵捕，观察不同时间蚊虫密度。共观察 55 次，共捕获中华按蚊 1 314 只，平均密度为 12.41 只，平均人工小时密度为 5.72 只。

5.8 疟疾暴发的控制，2003—2007 年对疟疾疫情发生波动的 14 个乡镇 52 个村开展了人群服药和媒介防制的综合性防治措施，共对重点人群 13 301 人次，进行药物清理复治和预防服药，药物喷洒 79.2 万平方米，杀虫剂浸泡蚊帐 9 187 顶，有效地控制了疫情，经效果考核疟疾疫情得到了有效的控制。

获得的结果为项目 M&E 评价提供了依据。

5.9 设备与经费使用情况：5 年来共收到全球基金经费 978 243.13 元，其中目标二经费 459 039.2 元，目标四经费 519 130.86 元，下拨及使用经费 974 746.75 元，经费使用率为 99.65 %。电脑、显微镜等设备均为项目专用，项目各项指标和预算执行率完成良好。

（六）项目地区疟疾疫情现状

怀远县自项目运转以来，疟疾发病呈逐年下降的趋势，2003—2007 年怀远疫情报告分别为 2 464 例、1 321 例、1 218 例、1 170 例、620 例，2007 年疟疾病例约为 2003 年的 1/4；2003—2005 年曾不断出现以自然庄为单位的暴发点，通过项目的支持，2006—2007 年未出现暴发点，有效控制了疟疾的局部暴发流行。2003 年项目基线调查结果，用捕获－再捕获方法进行统计分析，全县估计发病人数为 9 258 例，估计漏报率为 88.20%。2007 年估计疟疾病人为 765 人，疟疾漏报率为 18.18%，估计发病人数下降为 2003 年的 1/2。

（七）第一轮疟疾项目对项目地区疟疾防治工作的影响

1. 降低了疟疾发病，控制了疟疾疫情：通过项目的开展，使项目县的疟疾发病比项目启动前的 2003 年有大幅降低，疟疾报告病例处于逐年下降的趋势 2004 年以来每年分别下降了 46.75%、7.16%、5.09%、46.49%，特别是 2005—2006 年安徽省与其毗邻的地区疟疾疫情呈高度大幅上升，而项目县的疫情处于稳中有降的势头。

2. 诊断能力及技术得以提高，借助全球基金的资助，提高了疟疾镜检人员、乡村防保医生、临床医生诊断能力与水平，培养了一批疟防专业技术人员，建立健全了疟防队伍。

3. 项目的管理模式提高了各级防病机构疾病的管理能力。

4. 通过健康宣传提高了群众的防病意识。

5. 全球基金疟疾项目在安徽省的实施，对当地疟疾经费是一个很大的补充，对疟疾防治工作的开展有很大的帮助，使疟疾防治效果更加显著。

（八）5 年项目执行评价

1. 评价

省项目办于 2008 年 4 月组成了终期专项评估组对怀远项目县的项目工作进行了评估，依据项目评分标准，分项打分，评估结果。(1) 县级评估：综合得分为 B 级 89 分；(2) 省级自评：安徽省全球基金第一轮疟疾项目自我评估综合评价为 A 级 92 分。结论是第一轮中国全球基金疟疾项目在本省实施 5 年中，在省卫生厅的领导下，在全球基金国家项目办的指导下，严格按照全球基金疟疾项目的计划、实施方案和制度要求开展工作，按照全球基金疟疾项目计划的要求使用经费，物资使用与管理符合项目用途。评估结果显示，较好地完成了全球基金第一轮疟疾项目规定的各项 M&E 计划指标。

2. M&E 指标完成情况

2.1 医生接受早期诊断和合理治疗（EDAT）培训的比例：项目实施前怀远项目乡、村级医生未接受过疟疾防治知识的培训，2004 年—2007 年乡村级医生接受疟疾防治知识培训为 1 032 人次，其中接受培训的村级医生 853 人次，受训率 100%。

2.2 对发热病人血检的能力：29 个项目乡镇，项目实施前仅有 14 个乡镇能正常开展镜疟原虫工作，血检率仅为 0.39% 2003 年项目启动后逐步在 29 个乡镇开展镜检工作，血检覆盖面逐年在扩大，5 年平均血检率为 2.14%，与项目启动前的 2002 年相比提高了 4.5 倍。

2.3 接受正规治疗的疟疾病人比例：2002 年漏报率为 88.20%，奎宁针剂使用普遍，疟疾病人的正规治疗率仅为 28.72%。通过项目的支持，开展培训、健康宣传和病人的管理，提高了乡村医生的诊断治疗水平与群众的防病意识，病人正规治疗率逐年提高，2007 年的规范治疗率达到 100%。

2.4 疟疾病例通过信息网络报告的比例：2003 年基线调查结果显示，2002 年全县疫情报告 1 906 例，落实病例 9 258 例，网络报告率为 20.58%，基线调查报告病例 114 例，落实病人数为 966 人，漏报率为 88.20%, 网络报告 11.80%，2003 年项目开展后自 2007 年全县疟疾疫情均通过网络报告，疟疾病例通过信息网络报告的比例逐年在提高，2007 年提高到 81.81%, 漏报率为 18.18%，与 2003 年相比疟疾病例通过信息网络报告的比例和漏报率，2004 年以后均高于 M&E 指标。

（九）成效与经验

5 年来安徽省第一轮全球基金疟疾项目在安徽省卫生厅和国家项目办的指导下，各项工作按计划如期开展、经费使用到位、基层疟防工作力度加大。通过五年的项目资助，使各项疟防工作上了一个台阶。

1. 发热病人血检数量有明显的增加，加强了对传疟媒介的监控力度，特别是项目地区疟原虫镜检能力得到了大幅度提高。

2. 项目工作也加强了疟防工作人员对防治工作的认识，现在许多常规工作也开始按项目化管理，有计划、有经费预算，工作过程按计划按预算落实，资料整理归档有序。

3. 项目工作不仅促进了安徽省疟疾防治工作，也使广大疟防工作人员学习到了项目规范化管理的经验。

4. 降低了疟疾发病，控制了疟疾疫情，第一轮全球基金疟疾项目仅在怀远县开展，通过 5 年项目的认真工作，怀远县网络直报病人数从 2003 年的 2464 例下降到 2007 年的 620 例，下降为 2003 年的 1/4，漏报率由 88.20% 降至 18.18%，网络直报的准确率在显著上升。

5. 通过健康教育，居民和中小学生疟防知识知晓情况：当地居民和中小学生的疟防知识知晓率分别从项目启动前的 20.12% 和 40.45%，提高到 89.18% 和 100.00%。

6. 正规治疗的疟疾病人比例：2002 年奎宁针剂使用普遍，疟疾病人的正规治疗率仅为 28.72%，通过项目的实施，开展培训、健康宣传和病人的管理，提高了乡村医生的诊断治疗水平与群众的防病意识，病人正规治疗率逐年提高，到 2007 年达到 100%。

（十）项目地区面临的挑战和应对思路

第一轮安徽省全球基金存在的不足之处为项目办缺乏项目管理经验，基本无专职项目管理人员，只是在疟疾防治工作中兼顾项目工作，没有完全按照项目要求进行项目管理，项目前 2 年计划性不够，物资药品不能按计划及时下拨，影响了第一轮安徽省全球基金项目的执行力度。项目县技术力量较薄弱，项目技术措施落实不到位；督导质量和效果不理想，尤其在及时发现问题、采取有效措施、跟踪整改进度，反馈利用效果等方面有一定差距。

通过一个阶段的工作积累，安徽省将更好地开展第五轮全球基金项目及其他项目化管理，克服已存在的缺陷。在卫生行政部门的领导和监管下，严格按项目协议、工作计划和指导手册认真落实项目任务，确保项目按计划、管理要求执行，确保项目措施得到有效落实；将进一步明确全球基金项目管理、财务、审计、采购管理和监督与评价等方面的要求和规范，使安徽省全球基金疟疾项目取得更好的成绩，为安徽省疟疾防治工作做出应有的贡献。

安徽省全球基金疟疾项目办公室

2008 年 5 月 27 日

四、河南省项目终期总结报告

（一）项目概况

第一轮全球基金河南省疟疾项目的实施，选择在信阳市的淮滨和商城县。淮滨作为疟疾控制县执行各项目防治措施的落实及效果观察；商城作为项目的监测县做项目计划的三个乡病原学监测及其中的一个乡蚊媒监测工作。

（二）项目剩余资金使用情况

经费使用情况：5 年来共收到全球基金经费 980 095.76 元，其中目标二经费 476 526.67 元，目标四经费 503 569.09 元，下拨至县级的经费 649 523.1 元，占总经费的 66.23%。项目各项指标和预算执行率完成良好。

截至 2008 年 3 月 31 日，项目节余 7 933.29 元，按照项目结题于 5 月 20 日支出 2007 年年会及结题会 7 500 元和网络信息费 433.29 元，项目经费全部支出，没有节余。

（三）项目设备物资盘点情况

5 年来，全球基金下拨和自购物资详见表 3–29，2008 年 6 月前对所有资产进行处置，省项目办和淮滨县的物资移交第五轮项目使用，商城县资产，1 台戴尔电脑移交给商城县第五轮全球基金疟疾项目办使用，其余移交县疾控中心（表 1–35）。

表 1–35 固定资产和物资的盘点与处置计划

设备名称	数量	总金额(美元)	获得途径	目前运行情况	目前用途	目前使用部门	处置计划	处置时间	计划用途	计划使用部门
显微镜	21	3 831.08	自购	15台良好,6台报废	疟疾镜检	项目乡镇卫生院	移交其他部门	2008.6	疟疾镜检	第五轮项目或原单位
显微镜	6	8 981.76	拨入	良好	疟疾镜检	省、县项目办	移交其他部门	2008.6	疟疾镜检	第五轮项目或原单位
显微镜	4	2 030.70	拨入	良好	疟疾镜检	县、乡项目办	移交其他部门	2008.6	疟疾镜检	第五轮项目或原单位
台式电脑	7	5 751.35	自购	良好	项目专用	省项目办	移交其他部门	2008.6	疟疾疫情报告	县 CDC
台式电脑	4	6 972.97	拨入	良好	项目专用	省项目办	移交其他部门	2008.6	第五轮项目	第五轮省项目办
笔记本电脑	1	1 878.38	拨入	良好	项目专用	省项目办	移交其他部门	2008.6	第五轮项目	第五轮省项目办
打印机	1	310.81	拨入	正常	项目专用	省疟疾项目办	移交其他部门	2008.6	第五轮项目	第五轮省项目办

（四）5 年工作总结

1. 项目管理

省疾控中心设有项目办公室，共 4 人，其中专职业务人员 2 名和专职或兼职会计各 1 名。

商城和淮滨县均设立项目办，有专职业务人员 1 名，兼职会计 2 名。

2. 监督与评价管理

两个县项目办严格按照项目规划方案内容对各乡（镇）疟防工作进行督导，全年两个县分别在每季度对 9 个乡（镇）进行督导，督导内容包括乡村医生和镜检员培训、发热病人血检、病人治疗、媒介监测、物资与财务管理等，对于不足之处，当场提出整改意见，并监督整改情况。每年 9 月中旬，县项目办进行了自查，同时将自查结果报省项目办和县卫生局，对发现的问题，诸如镜检员镜检技术较低、基层疟防意识淡薄和财务及物资管理提出了改进意见。9 月下旬，省项目办依照督导程序对两县项目实施情况进行督导检查，依据项目评分标准，分项打分，对项目和财务执行情况进行评估，提出整改意见，写出督导报告。项目的专项督导保证了项目执行质量和资金的安全。2007 年 6 月全球基金国家项目办对河南省项目执行情况进行的督导评估，认为河南省项目整体执行情况良好，经费使用和资产管理符合全球基金的要求。

3. 财务管理

5 年来共收到全球基金经费 980 095.02 元，其中目标 2 经费 476 526.67 元，目标 4 经费 503 569.09 元，下拨经费 649 523.1 元，占总经费的 66.23 %。项目各项指标和预算执行率完成良好。

财务管理严格按照《全球基金项目财务手册》以及相关规定执行，经费的支出根据项目计划执行，财务程序在严格按照项目要求进行审核的同时，保障资金的快速、及时下拨，保障了工作的开展，并且每年省项目办都要对项目县开展项目财务专项督导。

4. 物资采购管理

5 年来项目固定资产累计约合 220 127.00 元人民币，其中自购 21 台显微镜（价值 30 648.64 元）和 7 台台式电脑（价值 46 010.80 元）；抗疟药品 10 750 人份，价值 45 150 元（按 4.2 元 / 人份计算），固定资产和物资累计收入 265 277.00 元人民币。

固定资产累计支出 220 127.00 元，抗疟药品支出 6 950 人份，价值 29 190.00 元，剩余 3 800 人份，价值 15 960.00 元（还给省 CDC 疟疾防治库存），见表 1–36

表 1–36　河南省累计固定资产和物资收支情况

设备名称	数量	金额 (元)	支出数量	支出金额 (元)
显微镜	21	28 350.00	21	28 350.00
显微镜	6	66 465.00	6	66 465.00
显微镜	4	15 022.00	4	15 022.00
台式电脑	7	42 560.00	7	42 560.00
台式电脑	4	51 600.00	4	51 600.00
笔记本电脑	1	13 900.00	1	13 900.00
打印机	1	2 230.00	1	2 230.00
磷酸氯 / 伯喹片剂	10750	45 150.00	6 950	29 190.00
合计	–	265 277.00	–	249 317.00

5. 项目执行进展

5.1 建立项目组织、健全疟防专业队伍：省县两级成立了全球基金疟疾项目办公室，配备了专职或兼职的专业技术人员和财务人员。

5.2 培训人员、提高项目执行能力：5 年来共办镜检班 7 个，培训 192 人次；项目管理培训班 5 次，培训 159 人次；开办乡村医生疟疾防治知识、疫情报告和处理等培训班，项目县乡村医生共978名，受训1 332人次，平均受训1.36次，高于M&E指标的1.28平均受训人次。

5.3 宣传疟防知识，提高居民疟防意识：5年共张贴、悬挂宣传标语、宣传画2 059幅，下发宣传手册、传单5 000余份，电视宣传200余次，为疟疾防治工作创造了良好的舆论氛围。

5.4 2003年疟疾发病情况基线调查：2003年4月对淮滨县开展了疟疾发病等情况的基线调查工作，结果表明2002年全县疟疾理论估计发病人数为6 829人，估计漏报率为89.57%，经血检诊断病人36例，占理论估计病人的0.6%。疟防知识和诊疗能力调查70名乡村级医生3年内均未接受过疟防知识的专业培训，疟防意识淡薄，错诊、漏诊、用奎宁治疗以及其他不规范治疗等普遍存在；居民和中小学生对疟疾防治知识了解甚少，知晓率分别为14.36%和9.36%。

5.5 对项目县的高危人群进行预防性治疗：5年来于休止期治疗有疟史病人和疑似病人2 108人次。在疟疾流行季节，淮滨县重点放在沿洪河、淮河沿岸的疟史病人和患户家属及重点人群；商城县以外出海南、云南和安徽打工人员为主。两县采用氯、伯四日疗法进行预防性服药。5年共预防服药6 263人，正规率92.17%；休止期治疗5 847人次，正规率95.34%。休止期治疗和预防服药后县项目办都进行了考核，结果服药率和正规律均在90%以上。

5.6 开展血检疟原虫工作，提高诊断水平：5年共血检发热病人70 310人次，检出疟疾病人843人，血检确诊疟疾比例由2003年的33.16 %提高到2007年的60.31%。中心镜检站按照10%复查，共复查血片7 660张，2004年以后未发现漏检现象。

5.7 防蚊灭蚊，减少疟疾传播：2003年，对王岗乡发病率较高的村民组以及在洪河大坝上集中聚居的刘寨村、四河村的灾民帐篷、蚊帐，采用氟氯氰菊酯类杀虫剂进行药物喷洒帐篷、浸泡蚊帐，共喷洒帐篷232顶，面积为9 280m^2；浸泡蚊帐340顶，面积为6 120m^2；同时为居民发放免费蚊帐200顶，组织疫区群众广泛开展防蚊、灭蚊活动，降低了媒介按蚊密度。

5.8 做好媒介监测，为防制提供科学依据：从2003年起，6到10月中旬开展每旬一次定点媒介监测，同时开展项目县3个定点以及专项疟疾媒介调查，对当地按蚊的种类、媒介按蚊的栖性、习性和季节分布等传疟因素有了系统的了解，5年来监测结果显示没有发现嗜人按蚊，当地疟疾的传播媒介为中华按蚊，验证了20世纪80年代大面积使用有机磷滞留喷洒控制嗜人按蚊的效果，监测结果为疟疾媒介防治工作应以防制中华按蚊孳生，减少中华按蚊叮咬为主的针对性措施提供了依据。

5.9 开展主动病例侦查工作，提高控制暴发流行应急能力：从2005年起每年第

4 季度开展疟疾病例的主动侦查，深入了解了疟疾发病情况，及时发现和预防疟疾暴发点，例如 2006 年淮滨县王岗乡的主动监测中发现马寨村疟疾发病有上升的趋势后，及时结合常规疟疾防治，有效地控制了疟疾发病势头和范围，另一方面调查结果为 M&E 指标提供了依据。

5.10 疟疾暴发的控制：根据项目工作计划 2005—2007 年共开展了 4 次疟疾暴发的控制工作在 2 个项目县选发病高或有代表性的 3 个乡，每乡 1—3 个村作为观察控制点。进行疟疾疫情动态监测、疟疾媒介调查，对 4 000—8 000 人专项调查与居民 1 000 人的间接荧光抗体水平监测等。4 次共对 26 246 人次做了专项调查，2 828 人做了间接荧光抗体水平监测，同时做了 48 次疟疾媒介的密度和习性的观察。通过对观察结果的分析及时掌握了项目县的疟疾发病动态，对可能出现的疟疾暴发点及时采取预防措施，避免了疫情的扩大。

5.11 项目督导促进项目工作；为了进一步提高全球基金疟疾项目实施质量，两个县项目办严格按照项目规划方案内容对各乡（镇）疟防工作进行督导，全年两个县分别每季度开展 9 个乡（镇）次的督导，督导内容包括乡村医生和镜检员培训、发热病人血检、病人治疗、媒介监测、物资与财务管理等，对于不足之处，当场提出整改意见，并监督整改情况。每年 9 月中旬，县项目办进行了自查，同时将自查结果报省项目办和县卫生局，对发现的问题，诸如镜检员镜检技术较低、基层疟防意识淡薄和财务及物资管理提出了改进意见。9 月下旬，省项目办依照督导程序对两县项目实施情况进行督导检查，依据项目评分标准，分项打分，对项目和财务执行情况进行评估，提出整改意见，写出督导报告。项目的专项督导保证了项目执行质量和资金的安全。2007 年 6 月全球基金国家项目办对河南省项目执行情况进行的督导评估，认为河南省项目整体执行情况良好，经费使用和资产管理符合全球基金的要求。

（五）项目地区疟疾疫情现状

5 年来疟疾发病逐年降低，有效控制了疟疾的局部暴发流行。按淮滨县卫生防疫站 2002 年上报疫情统计，全县 2002 年疟疾病例为 57 例，均为间日疟，发病率 8.69/ 万。治疗病例 712 人。2003 年疟疾病人 1 105 人，根据项目基线调查结果，用捕获－再捕获方法（CRM）进行统计分析，全县估计发病人数为 6 829 例，发病率为 1.04%。CRM 估计漏报率为 89.57%。2007 年估计疟疾病人为 210 人，疟疾漏报率为 37.61%，估计发病人数比 2002 年下降了 96.92%。

商城县在开展监测的 3 个乡镇，仅在 2008 年发生了 1 例疟疾，但全县疟疾病人明显呈现上升，2004 年为 1 例、2005 年 7 例、2006 年 9 例、2007 年 20 例。

（六）第一轮疟疾项目对项目地区疟疾防治工作的影响

1. 使项目地区居民得到及时诊断与合理治疗，血检确诊疟疾比例由 2003 年的 33.16 % 提高到 2007 年的 60.31%。及时正规治疗比例提高到 73.28%。

2. 通过多次的主动侦察和暴发流行预防和控制工作，加强疟疾监测，对疟疾暴发点和流行趋势上升的疫点进行了有效的控制和预防，提高了应急反应能力。

3. 通过多种方式对居民和中小学生开展疟防知识宣传，提高社区居民有效预防和治疗疟疾的意识和需求，居民和中小学生的疟防知识知晓率分别达到了分别为 85.37 % 和 80.16 %。

4. 项目提高了管理能力，完善的管理理念和模式，很强的计划性，严格的财务管理和物资管理制度等对当前的疟疾防治工作提供了有益借鉴和帮助。

（七）5 年项目执行评价

省项目办于 2008 年 3 月 12 ~ 18 日组成了终期专项评估组对两个项目县的项目工作进行了评估，依据项目评分标准，分项打分，评估结果（1）县级评估：淮滨县综合得分为 B 级 86 分；商城县得分 B 级 81 分。（2）省级自评：河南省全球基金第一轮疟疾项目自河南评估综合评价为 A 级 92 分。

结论：第一轮中国全球基金疟疾项目在河南实施 5 年中，在省卫生厅的领导下，在全球基金国家项目办的指导下，严格按照全球基金疟疾项目的计划、实施方案和制度要求开展工作，按照全球基金疟疾项目计划的要求使用经费，物资使用与管理符合项目用途。

评估结果显示，河南省较好地完成了全球基金第一轮疟疾项目规定的各项 M&E 计划指标。

（八）成效与经验

1. 降低了疟疾发病，控制了疟疾疫情：通过项目的开展，使项目县的疟疾发病比项目启动前的 2002 年有大幅降低，2003 年的基线调查结果显示，2002 年估计的疟疾漏报率为 89.57%，2002 年估计疟疾病人为 6 829 人；2008 年 3 月终期评估调查，结果显示 2007 年估计疟疾病人为 210 人，疟疾漏报率为 37.61%，估计发病人数比 2002 年下降了 96.92%。

2. 培养了一批疟防专业技术人员，建立健全了疟防队伍：借助全球基金的资助，项目县、乡、村建立疟疾防治专业技术队伍，其中包括疟疾镜检人员、乡村防保医生、临床医生等，同时提供了镜检等诊断设备，为今后开展疟疾防治工作提供了人员、技术和物资保障。

3. 项目的管理模式为其他疾病的防治与管理提供了可借鉴的经验：全球基金项目的运作有一套较为完善的管理理念和制度，有很强的计划性，对今后开展工作减少主观性和盲目性有很好的借鉴作用。全球基金的财务管理和物资管理制度对提高管理水平亦有帮助。

4. 全球基金疟疾项目在河南省的实施，对当地疟疾经费是很大的补充，对疟疾防治工作的开展有很大的帮助，使疟疾防治效果更加显著。

（九）项目县简评

淮滨和商城县在实施第一轮中国全球基金疟疾项目5年工作中，按照项目计划开展工作，通过建立项目组织，健全疟防专业队伍，培养了一批疟防专业技术骨干，提高了县、乡、村各级疟疾防治的力度和水平；降低了疟疾发病率，控制了疟疾疫情，提高了居民疟防意识，完成了项目规定的各项M&E计划指标。

河南省全球基金疟疾项目办公室

2008年6月30日

五、湖北省项目终期总结报告

（一）项目概况

第一轮湖北省全球基金疟疾项目，执行时间为2003年4月1日至2008年3月31日，项目覆盖枣阳市（项目控制县）、曾都区（项目监测县）两市、区。项目旨在覆盖地区加强疟疾的及时诊断、规范治疗、疫情监测和有效防护，加强疟疾防治技术、项目管理培训和健康教育，遏制项目地区疟疾流行，降低疟疾发病，提高项目管理能力。项目自2003年4月启动以来，已执行了5年，按照项目计划开展了大量的疟疾病例诊断和治疗、暴发点的预防和控制、传疟媒介的监测和防制；对项目地区疟防专业人员、疟原虫镜检人员、财务管理人员进行了疟防知识、疟原虫镜检技术和财务管理的培训；省、县项目办分别对项目县、乡、村的执行力度和质量进行了督导；按照上级项目办的要求按时下发了抗疟药、灭蚊药、项目设备和疟防宣传画。通过项目的实施有效地遏制项目地区的疟疾流行，降低了疟疾发病，推动了湖北省疟疾防治以及其他疾病控制工作的开展，提高了项目管理及执行能力，取得了明显的成效。

（二）项目剩余资金使用情况

截止结题报告日，项目剩余资金零元。

（三）项目设备物资盘点情况

第一轮湖北省全球基金疟疾项目5年共收到国家项目办下发的Olympus显微镜13台（省项目办2台、下发项目县枣阳市疾控中心8台，曾都区2台）；笔记本电脑3台（省项目办2台、省厅1台）；台式电脑5台（省项目办2台、下发项目县枣阳市1台、曾都区1台，襄樊市疾控中心1台）；打印机1台（省项目办1台），以上设备均转为第五轮全球基金疟疾项目继续使用。收到国家项目办下发的抗疟药磷酸氯/伯喹片剂25 750人份，按时下发枣阳市（项目控制县）和曾都区（项目监测县）用于疟疾治疗；灭蚊药奋斗呐500公斤，下发枣阳市用于疟疾暴发点灭蚊。

（四）5年工作总结

1. 项目管理

1.1 成立项目领导小组、建立项目办。按照国家项目办的工作要求，2003年，省疾控中心和两个项目县于分别成立了以卫生行政部门、疾控中心主要领导和分管领导为负责人的全球基金疟疾项目工作领导小组和项目办，项目办具体负责项目工作的实施，办公室成员分工具体，责任明确，积极按计划组织督导检查和开展各项活动。

1.2 健全制度、明确职责，制订方案和计划。项目办制定了详细的项目管理制度和职责，制订了年度、季度工作计划和各项具体活动实施方案，在执行中工作有记录，年度和专项工作有总结，项目办网络运行畅通，能及时按计划上报项目季度工作报表和财务报表，报表填写规范，数据准确可靠，档案资料专人管理、专柜保存、分类存档。

2. 监督与评价管理

2.1 项目督导与检查。执行期间省项目办每年对两个县市不定期地进行项目执行情况的检查和一次综合督导评估，项目县对项目乡镇卫生院和村卫生室进行督导，实际完成督导率为97.80%（178/182次）。各级项目办督导检查后对存在的问题制定整改措施，下达整改意见书，督促各项目县、乡、村认真整改。

2.2 制定手册，规范管理。当第一轮和第五轮全球基金疟疾项目合并管理后，省项目办制定了“项目执行手册”，各地按照项目手册的要求，注重各项活动的痕迹资料管理，对各项数据认真核实，保证了上报数据的准确性和科学性。各级项目办对上报数据逐级汇总和上报，各项数据有来源，有据可查。

2.3 督促措施落实，评价项目实施效果。在项目实施期间，省项目办每年进行不定期的专项检查和督导，检查措施落实情况。项目控制县在项目执行的初期、中期和末期及项目监测县末期，均进行了项目效果评估调查，全面评价项目措施执行情况、疾病控制情况、物资管理情况、经费使用情况等。

3. 财务管理

项目办设立了全球基金疟疾项目专用账户，建立了财务管理制度，按项目活动专款专用，及时支付各项活动经费，报销凭据规范、合格。项目人员和财务人员积极联系，相互沟通，严格按照全球基金项目财务管理制度要求进行会计核算，内部控制制度健全；设立了分目标明细账，能够做到账账相符、账实相符、账表相符；根据工作计划开展项目财务管理培训，使县级财务人员了解全球基金项目财务核算、经费使用等问题的要求；根据工作计划开展财务督导活动，对督导发现的问题提出改进建议。

湖北省 5 年来共收到国家项目办下拨项目经费 1 029 864.33 元人民币，其中目标二收入 458 903.05 元人民币，目标四收入 570 961.28 元人民币。项目实际支出经费为 1 017 199.20 元人民币，其中目标二支出 450 042.00 元人民币，目标四支出 567 157.20 元人民币。

4. 物资采购管理

省项目办建立了项目物资专用账，对国家项目办下拨的物资进行验收、入库。物资的领用、下发实行项目负责人签字制度，手续完备，身份翔实。按照项目计划，省项目办购置灭蚊药溴氰菊酯 300 公斤，现症病人治疗药磷酸氯 / 伯喹片剂 4 900 人份，磷酸氯喹片剂 60 000 片，下发曾都区、枣阳市用于疟疾防治及暴发点处理。省项目办印制疟疾防治宣传画 10 000 张，按计划下发项目控制县和监测县。

5. 项目执行进展

项目自 2003 年 3 月至 2008 年 3 月共执行 5 年，按照计划在项目地区开展了居民的早期诊断和个人防护，优化疟疾控制项目的管理，具体完成情况如下：

5.1 项目地区居民发热病人血检：项目控制县和监测县共开展发热病人血检 69 907 人次，完成项目计划的 132.56%。实际经费支出 89 712.4 元人民币，经费预算执行率为 111.62%。

5.2 项目地区疟疾传染源和易感人群管理：项目控制县和监测县共治疗疟疾病

人 6 237 例（枣阳市治疗 5 500 例，曾都区治疗 737 例），报告治疗率 100%；开展高危人群预防服药 15 616 人次，实际开展预防服药 22 407 人次，完成计划的 143.49%。实际经费支出 41 203.4 元人民币，经费预算执行率为 107.92%。

5.3 疟疾暴发流行控制：项目控制县计划控制疟疾暴发点 147 村，实际完成控制 148 个村，完成率为 100.68%。实际经费支出 313 583.20 元，经费预算执行率为 92.13%。

5.4 项目地区哨点病例主动监测：项目控制县和和监测县计划哨点病例主动监测 25 900 人次，实际完成监测 25 972 人次，完成率为 100.28%。实际经费支出 72 534.06 元人民币，经费预算执行率为 109.92%。

5.5 项目地区媒介监测：项目控制县和和监测县设立的两个媒介监测点计划开展媒介监测 78 次，实际完成监测 83 次，完成率为 106.41%。实际经费支出 87 556.84 元人民币，经费预算执行率为 97.57%。

5.6 项目督导:项目控制县和和监测县计划开展镇卫生院、村卫生室督导 182 次，实际完成督导 178 次，完成率为 97.80%。省项目办对项目控制县和和监测县每年进行一次督导评估和不定期的专项活动检查,实际经费支出 304 623.80 元人民币，经费预算执行率为 93.52%。

（五）项目地区疟疾疫情现状

2003 年至 2007 年，项目控制县枣阳市共报告疟疾病例 5 500 例，年均报告发病率为 10.25/ 万(5 500/5/1 073 027)。其中各年分别报告疟疾病例为 3 052 例、1 036 例、401 例、570 例、441 例，项目结束时 2007 年度报告疟疾 441 例较 2003 年 3 052 例下降了 85.55%，但项目结束时局部地区仍有疟疾暴发点。项目监测县曾都区 2003 年至 2007 年疟疾疫情呈逐年下降趋势，疫情报告病例分别为 349 例、125 例、106 例、80 例、77 例。目前无暴发点出现。

（六）第一轮全球基金疟疾项目对覆盖地区疟疾防治工作的影响

1. 项目资金投入，提高了抗疟措施的执行力度。第一轮全球基金疟疾项目的实施，极大地提高了项目地区的疟疾防治工作能力，项目资金、药品和相关器材的投入极大地缓解了项目地区疟防资金、药品和相关器材的不足，提高了抗疟措施的执行力度，有效遏制局部地区疟疾暴发，降低了疟疾发病。

2. 项目培训提高了管理能力和防治水平。对项目管理人员的培训，大大提高了项目执行人员管理能力；疟防知识和镜检技术的培训，全面提高了项目县、乡疟防专业人员的防治水平和镜检员的镜检能力；对乡村医生的培训，提高了乡村医生村对疟疾的诊断水平和现症病人的正规治疗率。

3. 项目疟防知识宣传，提高了居民自我保护意识。项目覆盖地区广泛开展疟防知识的宣传，全面提高了广大居民和学生的疟防知识知晓率，增强了居民和学生的自我保护意识，夜晚睡眠挂蚊帐，居民住宅增添了防蚊设施，室内使用卫生杀虫剂，以及烟熏灭蚊等。

（七）5 年项目执行评价

项目执行 5 年来，培养了一大批疟防专业技术人才，提高了乡村医生的疟防专业知识和诊断治疗技能，更新了固有的疟疾防治理念，极大地促进了项目地区实施以消灭传染源为主的综合防治能力和疫情报告、监测能力，有效控制了河南省项目地区的疟疾流行，项目资金、药品、器材得到了合理、有效使用，为河南省实现消除疟疾的目标积累了丰富的经验。

（八）成效与经验

1. 项目执行 5 年来的成果与经验

1.1 树立了项目管理理念，提高了管理水平

实施全球基金项目，为我们引进了国际先进的管理经验和理念。项目刚开始启动时，由于对项目实施和管理了解很少，不知道如何按照项目管理的理念实施项目，仍然按原来的常规的思维方式和工作模式，走了一些弯路，产生了一些问题。随着项目工作的实施，参加项目管理培训，以及开展各级项目工作督导，逐步对项目实施和管理有了进一步的认识，对项目办的职责和运作模式有了明确的定位，全球基金项目就是以工作计划为支柱，实行严谨的财务制度来对整个项目的实施进行管理，从组织、协调、督导、培训、管理几方面来抓。通过这些先进的管理经验的应用，促进和更新了我们的观念，提高了我们的管理水平。

1.2 项目工作改善了项目县的工作条件，提高了疟疾防治工作的能力

全球基金疟疾项目的开展，不仅引进了国际资金，配备了一些仪器、设备、交通工具等，还利用各级的师资力量及项目经费，开展由国家培训省级，省级培训县级，县级培训乡镇级，乡镇培训村级的各类培训班。如项目管理、项目财务管理、疟疾疫情爆发流行的应急处理、疟原虫镜检、疟疾病例的发现、规范治疗、报告等培训班。项目实施一年以来，为省、项目县、项目实施乡镇和村培训了一批疟疾防治技术骨干，为省及项目县培训了一批项目管理及财务管理人才，规范了项目工作程序，提高了项目执行能力，提高了项目县的疟疾防治工作水平，同时也推动了全省疟疾防治工作。

1.3 有效遏制了项目地区疟疾暴发流行的趋势，降低了疟疾发病率。

项目执行 5 年来，枣阳市疟疾暴发点由项目执行前的 111 个降至项目结束后的 24 个，暴发点发生率下降了 78.38%。疟疾网络报告病例由项目执行前的 3052 例降至项目结束后的 441 例，报告发病率由执行前的 23.15/ 万降至 4.11/ 万，下降了 85.55%。曾都区 2003 年至 2007 年疫情报告疟疾病人分别为 349 人、125 人、106 人、80 人、77 人，发病率呈逐年下降的趋势。

1.4 培养了一大批疟防专业技术人才

项目实施 5 年来在国家项目办的高度重视和具体指导下，项目地区的发热病人血检、高危人群预防服药、现症病人正规治疗、疟防督导工作都得到了较好的落实，疫情报告网络健全畅通，疟疾疫情漏报率大幅度下降。培养和造就了一大批疟防专业技术人才，乡村医生的疟防诊治技能得到较大的提高。

1.5 提高了项目财务的执行能力

项目财务执行 5 年来，按照项目财务管理要求进行会计电算化核算，明确财务主管参与项目计划编制、报账审核，以及不同类别的财务审核程序，落实财务的审核责任。注重项目人员和基层财务人员的沟通，重视督导，及时纠偏，保障了财务管理的顺利运行，有效地提高了项目经费预算执行率。

2. 项目地区面临的挑战和应对策略

项目实施 5 年来，虽然项目地区疟疾暴发流行的态势得到遏制，各项抗疟措施得到了落实，居民和中小学生的疟防知识知晓率得到了提高。但是，由于受农村居住环境和生活习惯的限制，加上农村公共卫生防控体系的薄弱，抗疟药品抗药性、副作用以及疗程长等因素的影响，项目地区的疟防工作仍然任重道远。

在今后的疟防工作中，要改变上述状况，首先要进一步加大农村居民的健康教育，提高疟防知识知晓率，改善居民的生活条件和居住环境，消灭蚊虫孳生地，切断传播途径。其次，要改善乡（镇）、村疟防工作人员的工作报酬，提高疟防人员工作积极性。第三要加大乡村医生、镜检人员的培训力度，进一步提高疟疾诊断、治疗水平。

（九）项目县简评

枣阳市、曾都区项目实施 5 年来，疟疾疫情大幅度下降，现症病人正规治疗率、疟史病人正规休治率、居民和中小学生的疟防知识知晓率得到提高，疫情漏报率大幅度下降、各项抗疟措施得到有效落实。督导工作扎实进行，项目运行正常，疫情网络运行畅通，财务、物品、药品管理规范。总之，通过第一轮全球基金疟疾项目在枣阳市、曾都区的实施，有力推动并促进了项目地区疟疾防治工作的开展，为最终实现消除疟疾的目标奠定了坚实的基础。

湖北省全球基金疟疾项目办公室

2008 年 5 月 16 日

六、江苏省项目终期总结报告

第一轮江苏省全球基金疟疾项目在中国疾病预防控制中心中央执行机构（PR）、国家项目办和江苏省卫生厅的领导和支持下，省、县项目办已按计划组织实施并完成了第一轮全球基金疟疾项目工作任务。现将 5 年来的工作情况汇报如下：

（一）项目概况

2003 年 4 月 11 日江苏省与全球基金国家疟疾项目办公室签订“全球艾滋病、结核病和疟疾基金中国高传播区疟疾控制项目”协议后，江苏省启动了第一轮全球基金疟疾项目，项目地区为盱眙和泗洪两个县。

泗洪县 2000 年出现疟疾暴发流行，2001 年上报疟疾病人 788 例，实际发病人数超过 2 000 例，到 2003 年发病人数居全省首位。盱眙县曾在 1997 年出现疟疾暴发流行，走访调查发现疟疾病人超过 1 000 例。为此，江苏省第一轮全球基金疟疾项目办确定盱眙和泗洪 2 县为项目县，其中泗洪县确定天岗湖、上塘、位营、峰山、双沟、四河、瑶沟、归仁、梅花、石集、陈圩、曹庙、界集、青阳镇 14 个乡镇为项目乡镇；盱眙县确定仇集、桂五、王店、河桥、古桑、兴隆、穆店七个乡镇为项目乡镇。

项目总目标为初步控制项目县的疟疾暴发流行，其中，泗洪县的主要项目任务是控制疟疾暴发流行，盱眙县的主要项目任务是疟疾监测。项目的主要内容是加强高传播区疟疾控制与监测；加强流动人口疟疾管理与监测；加强健康教育与健康促进；加强疫情信息网络建设等。

主要项目活动包括发热病人查血片、项目县高危人群进行预防性治疗、开展“捕获－再捕获”法调查、疫情处理、疟疾暴发流行监测、进行哨点主动调查和媒介监测等。

（二）项目经费和使用情况

江苏省项目办收到第一轮全球基金疟疾项目经费总计 977 796.95 元。按预算省项目办经费 578 283.45 元，下拨各项目县经费 380 513.5 元，委托任务下拨经费 19 000 元，总计下拨经费 399 513.5 元（其中：盱眙 232 359.5 元，泗洪 167 154 元）。截至 2008 年 3 月末，除盱眙县结余经费 25 671.1 元外，其余经费已按计划使用完。

（三）项目设备物资和使用情况

按照项目要求，江苏省项目办有专人负责国家项目办采购部下拨各种物资的发放和管理，并按要求做好下拨物资的验收、入库、调拨工作。

1. 电脑

国家项目办共下拨台式电脑 4 台、笔记本电脑两台。其中 1 台台式电脑由省项目办主任使用，3 台台式电脑由省项目办官员使用；两台笔记本电脑原由省项目办官员使用。第五轮江苏省全球基金疟疾项目实施后，因其他项目县要求提供笔记本电脑，故经省项目办同意将其两台笔记本电脑与其他项目县（洪泽、六合两五轮项目县）调换使用。

2. 显微镜

国家项目办共下拨生物显微镜 9 台，体视显微镜 1 台。其中 2 台生物显微镜下拨至泗洪县项目办，其余都留在省项目办使用（表 1–37）。

表 1–37 国家项目办下拨物资清单

序号	设备名称	品牌型号	数量	设备状况	保管科室或人员
1	电脑	DELL-GX270SMT16"	2	良好	第一轮项目办
2	电脑	笔记本东芝 A100	2	良好	洪泽、六合县项目办
3	生物显微镜	OLYMPLUS CX21	5	良好	顾亚萍
4	体视显微镜	OLYMPLUS SZX9	1	良好	顾亚萍
5	电脑	DELL-OPTIPLEX GX280SMT17"	2	良好	第一轮项目办
6	生物显微镜	OLYMPUS CX 21	4	良好	两台省所，两台下拨泗洪

3. 抗疟药品

2004 年国家项目办下拨磷酸氯 / 伯喹片剂 12 500 人份，已全部用于两个项目县现场防治。2007 年 1 月 16 日国家项目办下拨磷酸氯 / 伯喹片剂 2 000 人份，已转第五轮江苏省全球基金疟疾项目办使用，用于补充病人治疗和休止期根治工作（休根工作）实际完成数超过计划任务数所需的药物缺口；2007 年 7 月 5 日国家项目办下拨磷酸氯 / 伯喹片剂 4 000 人份，归还江苏省寄研所，为 2003 至 2006 年任务完成超出计划数所需借调的药品。

4. 杀虫剂

2004 年国家项目办下拨氟氯氰菊酯 12 升，已全部用于两个县现场防治。

（四）5 年项目工作总结

1. 项目管理

2003 年召开项目启动会后，江苏省在卫生厅的领导下，成立了全球基金疟疾项目办公室，设立了专门的银行账户。并于 2007 年将第一轮疟疾项目工作与第五轮项目工作分开，由专人负责对第一轮项目进行管理，并制定了一系列的管理制度。第一轮全球基金两个县项目办也参照省项目办的管理制度成立了相应的管理机构，专人专职进行管理。

省项目办每季度定期召开省项目办人员协调会，交流情况，解决工作中存在的问题。经费到账使用和下拨均按计划执行，各项支付和报销符合财经管理制度和全球基金的要求。

2. 监督与评价管理

江苏省第一轮项目办在项目初期因未设县级项目办，对项目实施尚缺乏经验，项目管理和督查力度不足。第五轮项目实施后，结合县项目办的成立，加强了对项目的管理和督查。在国家项目办对江苏省督导后，根据国家项目办意见，江苏省第一轮和第五轮项目办分开，2 县项目办项目也第一轮和第五轮办分开，确定专人负责第一轮项目。

省项目办、项目县、项目乡镇的资料（项目工作资料、固定资产、项目进度季报表等资料）按照季度执行情况进行整理归档，第一轮、第五轮项目和常规疟疾防治工作资料能够分开进行分类归档。

按项目计划 2005 年 7 月、8 月和 9 月，省项目办官员泗洪县和盱眙县两县的项目工作进行了督导检查；2006 年 4 月省项目办的相关人员分别对泗洪县和盱眙县的休根工作进行了检查督导；7 月省项目办到盱眙县举办盱眙县全球基金药物灭蚊启动会并开展媒介监测调查；9 月对盱眙县全球基金疟疾项目第一轮工作进行了督导检查，并选择了近两年发病较高的仇集、鲍集两乡镇进行现场调查，发现县项目办对乡级的督导结果未及时反馈至被督导单位。

2007 年 5 月国家疟疾项目办对江苏省项目办和盱眙县进行项目管理和财务管理情况督导并就存在的问题提出了建议，省项目办在 7、8、9 月份分 3 次分别对盱眙和泗洪进行了项目专项督导检查；2007 年 10 月国家疟疾项目对江苏省项目办和盱眙县、泗洪县两县再次进行督查，肯定了江苏省项目办按照建议进行的迅速、有效的整改，认为省项目办与项目县的工作有明显的改进。

3. 财务管理

3.1 收入情况：截至 2008 年 3 月底，江苏省项目办收到第一轮全球基金疟疾项目经费总计 977 796.95 元。按预算下拨各项目县经费 380 513.5 元，委托任务下拨经费 19 000 元，总计下拨经费 399 513.5 元(其中盱眙 232 359.5 元，泗洪 167 154 元)。省项目办自留经费 578 283.45 元。利息收入 2 217.04 元。

3.2 支出情况：截至 2008 年 3 月底，该项目实际累计支出 954 342.89 元，完成预算 97.6%。

目标二：使目标地区居民得到更好的早期诊断和个人防护。累计支出 571 395.29 元，完成预算 100%。

目标四：疟疾项目控制管理 累计支出 382 947.6 元。完成预算 96.26%。

省本级项目专款支出总计 580 379.91 元，完成预算 100%。各项目县项目专款支出总计 373 962.98 元，其中：泗洪 167 274.58 元，完成预算 100%; 盱眙 206 688.4 元，完成预算 89%（表 1–38）。

表 1–38 江苏省项目办财务收支情况统计表

年度	收到拨款	利息收入	使用金额	经费结余
2003	90 253.21		66 052.00	24 201.21
2004	252 177.00	94.87	176 153.22	100 319.86
2005	172 502.90	843.51	266 918.72	6 747.55
2006	278 045.77	399.27	237 164.11	48 028.48
2007	184 818.07	879.39	140 886.70	92 839.24
2008			67 186.14	25 671.10
合计：	977 796.95	2 217.04	954 342.89	25 671.10

3.3 财务管理现状及经验总结

开展财务管理培训，认识全球基金财务管理的重要性，严格按照《全球基金项目财务管理手册》的要求，开设独立的银行账户，对拨入的全球基金专款进行有效的管理和监督，分项目工作目标进行财务核算。

加强项目财务督导，促使项目财务工作更加规范，通过国家项目办对省级、省级对县级的督导审计，及时整改存在问题，使项目实施中经费的使用更加合理合规，财务基础工作更加规范。

建立健全管理制度，提高项目财务管理水平，省项目办制定了财务管理制度、项目物资管理规定、内部控制制度，规范项目活动财务报账手续，做好固定资产和物品材料的辅助账，使项目资产账实相符。

做好财务报表的审核汇总上报，及时报送项目财务报表，加强财务与项目工作的配合，按计划合理使用项目经费。

4. 物资采购管理

第一轮江苏省全球基金疟疾项目 5 年设备小计为 198 576.88 元，物资小计 105 725.00 元，设备物资合计 304 301.88 元。其中省、县项目办自行采购金额为 92 630.00 元。

第一轮江苏省全球基金除了国家项目办下拨的物资外，还自行采购了一些物资和抗疟药用于江苏省第一轮全球基金项目工作，省项目办采购了电脑 1 台，数码照相机 1 台，投影仪 1 台；盱眙县项目办采购了电脑 1 台；泗洪县采购了显微镜 1 台。

国家项目办除在 2004 年分两次下拨了 12 500 人份磷酸氯 / 伯喹片剂，2005—2006 年第一轮全球基金国家项目办未下拨抗疟药，影响了第一轮全球基金江苏省项目办防治工作正常开展，故 2006 年江苏省全球基金疟疾项目办自购 1 万人份磷酸氯 / 伯喹片剂，用于盱眙和泗洪两县的全球基金疟疾项目工作（其中 4 000 人份为归还 2005 年向江苏省寄研所借药品）。分配情况为：2005 年盱眙、泗洪两县各 2 000 人份，2006 年分别为 1 000 和 2 000 人份，2007 年也分别为 1 000 和 2 000 人份。2007 年国家项目办二次下拨磷酸氯 / 伯喹片剂分别归还江苏省寄研所和转用于五轮全球基金的药品不足部分（表 1–39）。

表 1–39　江苏省项目办自行采购的固定资产一览表

设备名称	数量	总金额(元)	获得途径	购买时间	备注
电脑	1	8 060.00	自购	2005-11-30	盱眙县项目办
电脑	1	8 980.00	自购	2005-5-24	省本级
投影仪	1	19 200.00	自购	2004-2-18	省本级
数码机	1	3 840.00	自购	2003-6-30	省本级
显微镜	1	4 550.00	自购	2005-7-15	泗洪县项目办
磷酸氯 / 伯喹片剂	10 000	48 000.00	自购	2006-9-30	用于盱眙、泗洪 2 县
物资小计	–	92 630.00	–	–	–

江苏省第一轮全球基金项目办在物资采购管理前两年还存在一些不足之处，如下拨物资未有进出台账、省和县项目办自行采购物资用于一轮项目工作等。但通过 2007 年 5 月国家项目办督导后，江苏省项目办进行了物资管理整改，补全了物资进出台账，严格把控物资采购，2007 年省和县项目办未再发生自购物资现象。通过第一轮的物资管理的经验，现江苏省第五轮全球基金项目严格按照项目化管理执行，明确专人专管，做到物、帐两全。

5. 项目执行进展

江苏省项目办根据第一轮疟疾项目年度工作目标，严格按照项目计划任务书实施，其中目标二使目标地区当地居民得到更好的早期诊断和个人防护包括：项目地区居民发热病人血检、高危人群预防服药、疟疾暴发流行控制；目标四优化项目省的疟疾控制项目管理包括：项目地区哨点病例主动监测、项目地区媒介监测、省项目办年会和项目督导。具体执行情况如下：

5.1 项目地区居民发热病人血检

江苏省两个县 5 年计划对发热病人血检 48 000 人，实际血检 52 959 人，实际完成率 110.33%，查出阳性病人 287 例 , 阳性率 0.54%。

盱眙县 5 年计划发热病人血检 10 400 人次，实际完成数 11 211 人次，完成率 108%，发现阳性病人 16 例，阳性率 0.14%。其中：2003 年计划目标数 1 000 人次，实际完成数 763 人次，完成率 76.3%，发现阳性病人 11 例，阳性率 1.44% ；2004 年计划目标数 1 000 人次，实际完成数 852 人次，完成率 85.2%，发现阳性病人 5 例，阳性率 0.58% ；2005 年计划目标数 2 800 人次，实际完成数 2 702 人次，完成率 96.5%，未发现阳性病人；2006 年计划目标数 2 800 人次，实际完成数 4 240 人次，完成率 151%，未发现阳性病人；2007 年计划目标数 2 800 人次，实际完成数 2 654 人次，完成率 94.8%，未发现阳性病人。

泗洪县 5 年计划对发热病人血检 37 600 人，实际血检 41 748 人，实际完成率 111.03%，查出阳性病人 271 例 , 阳性率 0.65%。其中：2003 年计划血检 4 000 人，实际血检 4 157 人，完成率 103.93%，血检阳性 67 例，阳性率 1.61% ；2004 年计划血检 6 000 人，实际血检 6 302 人，完成率 105.03%，血检阳性 55 例，阳性率 0.87% ；2005 年计划血检 9 200 人，实际血检 9 525 人，完成率 103.53%，血检阳性 70 例，阳性率 0.73% ；2006 年计划血检 9 200 人，实际血检 9 251 人，完成率 100.55%，血检阳性 30 例，阳性率 0.32% ；2007 年计划血检 9 200 人，实际血检 12 513 人，完成率 136.01%，血检阳性 49 例，阳性率 0.39%（表 1–40）。

表 1–40 江苏省项目县发热病人血检情况表

年份	盱眙县				泗洪县			
	计划数	实际数	实际完成率	阳性数	计划数	实际数	实际完成率	阳性数
2003	1 000	763	76.3	11	4 000	4 157	103.93	67
2004	1 000	852	85.2	5	6 000	6 302	105.03	55
2005	2 800	2 702	96.5	0	9 200	9 525	103.52	70
2006	2 800	4 240	151	0	9 200	9 782	106.33	30
2007	2 800	2 654	94.8	0	9 200	12 513	136.01	49
合计	10 400	11 211	108	16	37 600	41 748	111.03	271

5.2 高危人群预防服药

根据项目计划任务书，高危人群预防服药仅在泗洪县开展，泗洪县五年计划对高危人群预防服药共 8 600 人，实际服药共 13 180 人。其中：2003 年计划预防服药 1 000 人，实际服药 4 217 人；2004 年计划预防服药 1 600 人，实际服药 2 985 人；2005 年计划预防服药 2 000 人，实际服药 2 214 人；2006 年计划预防服药 2 000 人，实际服药 2 430 人；2007 年计划预防服药 2 000 人，实际服药 1 334 人，主要原因为由于发病率下降，病人数减少后，相应所需要的服药人数减少。2003—2006 年超出计划数所需的药品由县项目办向江苏省寄研所从常规疟疾防治库存药品中借调。

5.3 疟疾暴发流行控制

5.3.1 人员技术培训

2005 年省项目办开展疟疾暴发流行监测与处理培训班，江苏省全球基金疟疾项目办公室于 2005 年 6 月 17–21 日在江苏省寄生虫病防治研究所举行省项目年会暨疟原虫镜检技术培训班，通过示教和带教，学员们基本掌握了疫点处理所必需的血片制作和染色、疟原虫镜检等技术。

5.3.2 盱眙县疟疾暴发流行监测和疫点处理

2003 年 7 个乡疫点处理病人(确诊病人和疑似病人)396 例、家属及四邻 3 684 人，全部服用了抗疟药。

2004 年 7 个乡疫点处理病人(确诊病人和疑似病人)248 例、家属及四邻 2 130 人，全部服用了抗疟药。

2005 年盱眙县开展“捕获 - 再捕获”调查，2005 年计划目标数调查 6 个乡 18 个村 3 600 人，实际完成数 6 个乡 18 个村 3 688 人，受调查人群中通过网络直报的疟疾病例数 8 例，走访调查出的疟疾病例数 41 例，走访调查出的疟疾病例中作为疫情网络直报的病例数 4 例，通过“捕获 - 再捕获”校正推算被调查人群实际疟疾病例数 75 例 , 推算病例数是网报病例数的 9 倍。疫点处理 7 个乡病人（确诊病人和疑似病人）167 例、家属及四邻 1 785 人。疟疾暴发流行后监测对小学生开展了 IFA 调查，共调查 2 乡 618 人，发现阳性 17 例。

2006 年盱眙县开展“捕获 - 再捕获”调查，2006 年计划目标数调查 3 个乡 9 个村 1 800 人，实际完成数 3 个乡 9 个村 1 848 人，受调查人群中通过网络直报的疟疾病例数 12 例，走访调查出的疟疾病例数 27 例，走访调查出的疟疾病例中作为疫情网络直报的病例数 5 例，通过“捕获 - 再捕获”校正推算被调查人群实际疟疾病例数 60 例。推算病例数是网报病例数的 5 倍。疫点处理 7 个乡病人（确诊病人和疑似病人）125 例、家属及四邻 849 人；疟疾暴发流行后监测对小学生开展间接荧光抗体试验（IFA）调查，共调查两乡 541 人，发现阳性有 12 人。

2007 年盱眙县开展疫点处理 2007 年 7 个乡病人（确诊病人和疑似病人）101 例、家属及四邻 942 人；疟疾暴发流行后监测对小学生开展 IFA 调查，共调查 1 乡 295 人，发现阳性 9 例。

5.3.3 泗洪县疟疾暴发流行监测和疫点处理

2003 年开展捕获－再捕获法，实际完成数 9 个乡 625 户 2 856 人，受调查人群中通过网络直报的疟疾病例数 32 例，走访调查出的疟疾病例数 45 例，走访调查出的疟疾病例中作为疫情网络直报的病例数 4 例，通过“捕获 - 再捕获”校正推算被调查人群实际疟疾病例数 302 例，推算病例数是网报病例数的 9.43 倍。疫情处理 13 个乡 129 例病人。疟疾暴发流行后监测对小学生开展 IFA 调查，共调查 1 乡 311 人，发现阳性 22 人。

2004 年开展捕获－再捕获法，实际完成数 9 个乡 685 户 3 282 人，受调查人群中通过网络直报的疟疾病例数 17 例，走访调查出的疟疾病例数 39 例，走访调查出的疟疾病例中作为疫情网络直报的病例数 4 例，通过“捕获 - 再捕获”校正推算被调查人群实际疟疾病例数 143 例，推算病例数是网报病例数的 8.41 倍。疫情处理 12 个乡 96 例病人。疟疾暴发流行后监测对小学生开展 IFA 调查，共调查 1 乡 281 人，发现阳性 21 人。

2005 年开展“捕获 - 再捕获”调查，2005 年计划目标数调查 9 个乡镇 18 个村，实际完成数 18 个村 1 412 户 6 742 人，受调查人群中通过网络直报的疟疾病例数 22 例，走访调查出的疟疾病例数 40 例，走访调查出的疟疾病例中作为疫情网络直报的病例数 4 例，通过“捕获 - 再捕获”校正推算被调查人群实际疟疾病例数 187 例，推算病例数是网报病例数的 8.5 倍。疫情处理 9 个乡 81 例病人；疟疾暴发流行后监测对小学生开展 IFA 调查，共调查两个乡 631 人，发现阳性 26 人。

2006 年开展“捕获 - 再捕获”调查，计划目标数调查 3 个乡 9 村，实际完成数 9 个村 642 户 2 945 人，受调查人群中通过网络直报的疟疾病例数 10 例，走访调查出的疟疾病例数 17 例，走访调查出的疟疾病例中作为疫情网络直报的病例数两例，通过“捕获 - 再捕获”校正推算被调查人群实际疟疾病例数 65 例，推算病例数是网报病例数的 6.5 倍；疫情处理 9 个乡 42 例病人；疟疾暴发流行后监测对小学生开展 IFA 调查，共调查 1 乡 208 人，发现阳性 11 人（表 1–41）。

2007 年泗洪县开展疫情处理 9 个乡 63 例病人；疟疾暴发流行后监测对小学生开展 IFA 调查，共调查 1 乡 315 人，发现阳性 7 人（表 1–42）。

表 1–41　江苏省项目县开展“捕获 – 再捕获”调查情况表

县名	年份	受调查人群中通过网络直报的疟疾病例数	走访调查出的疟疾病例数	走访调查出的疟疾病例中作为疫情网络直报的病例数	推算被调查人群实际疟疾病例数
盱眙	2005	8	41	4	75
	2006	12	27	5	60
泗洪	2003	32	45	4	302
	2004	17	39	4	143
	2005	22	40	4	187
	2006	10	17	2	65

表 1–42　江苏省项目县疟疾暴发流行后小学生 IFA 调查情况

年份	盱眙县			泗洪县		
	调查人数	阳性数	阳性率	调查人数	阳性数	阳性率
2003	-	-	-	311	22	7.07
2004	-	-	-	281	21	7.47
2005	618	17	2.75	631	26	4.12
2006	541	12	2.22	208	11	5.29
2007	295	9	3.05	315	7	2.22
合计	1 454	38	2.61	1 746	87	4.98

5.4 项目地区哨点病例主动监测

哨点病例主动监测工作仅在盱眙县开展，2005 年盱眙县开展带虫调查 8 000 人，发现病人 1 例；2006 年带虫调查 8 000 人，发现病人 2 例；2007 年带虫调查 8 000 人，发现病人 2 例。

5.5 项目地区媒介监测

媒介监测工作仅在盱眙县开展，2003 年计划任务 5 次，实际共开展 10 次，捕获到中华按蚊 152 只；2004 年计划任务 5 次，实际共开展 10 次，捕获到中华按蚊 80 只；2005 年计划任务 5 次，实际共开展 8 次，捕获到中华按蚊 55 只；2006 年计划任务 5 次，实际共开展 10 次，捕获到中华按蚊 66 只；2007 年计划任务 5 次，实际共开展 8 次，捕获到中华按蚊 56 只（表 1–43）。

表 1–43　江苏省盱眙县媒介监测情况表

年份	调查次数		捕获按蚊数		
	计划次数	实际次数	总按蚊数	中华按蚊数	嗜人按蚊数
2003	5	10	152	152	0
2004	5	10	80	80	0
2005	5	8	55	55	0

续表

2006	5	10	66	66	0
2007	5	8	56	56	0
合计	25	46	409	409	0

5.6 省项目办年会

省项目办每年定期召开项目年会，除常规总结和布置年度项目工作，还根据不同时期项目执行情况，组织项目工作人员进行专题研讨和交流。

2004年省项目年会于2005年6月17～21日在江苏省寄生虫病防治研究所召开，会议对2004年的工作进行了总结，指出了存在的问题，并明确落实了2005年的工作目标和任务。

2005年省项目年会于2006年4月17～20日在江苏省寄生虫病防治研究所召开，会议进行了2005年江苏省疟疾项目工作汇报和第一轮江苏省2006年工作计划，明确了省、县项目办内部要理顺内部工作机制，强调必须按照工作计划执行任务，严格按项目目标使用项目资金。

2006年省项目年会于2007年6月18～20日在江苏省寄生虫病防治研究所召开，参会人员有江苏省第一轮全球基金项目办公室和财务科人员，第一轮疟疾项目盱眙、泗洪县项目办主任、项目主管、项目官员和财务官员各1人。会上进行了2006年江苏省疟疾项目工作汇报，两个项目县也分别作了2006年工作总结汇报。会上还布置了“全球基金疟疾控制项目第一轮江苏省2007年工作计划和2008年评估总结计划”，省项目办还作了“项目县资料归档”及“财务整改情况”报告。省、县项目办应加强财务人员和项目人员的沟通和协调，尽快设立各自的固定资产和物资辅助账，并建立定期对账制度。

2007年省项目年会于2008年5月22～25日在江苏省寄生虫病防治研究所召开，会议主要内容为：第一轮江苏省全球基金疟疾项目2007年度进展情况；第一轮江苏省全球基金疟疾项目终期评估报告；交流第一轮江苏省全球基金疟疾项目终期专项调查情况；汇报第一轮江苏省全球基金疟疾项目财务管理和使用情况；汇报第一轮江苏省全球基金疟疾项目物资使用情况。

5.7 项目终期评估工作

终期评估动员与培训：2008年元月23日江苏省终期评估动员与培训会在盱眙县召开，会议由卫生厅疾控处蔡刚主持，高琪所长在会上对第一轮中国全球基金疟疾项目终期评估方案作了说明，省项目办对第一轮江苏省全球基金疟疾项目终期评估具体实施计划、要求和时间安排，以及终期评估财务项目评估提出了具体要求。

项目终期专项调查：按照国家项目办终期专项调查方案的要求，江苏省在盱眙县和泗洪县开展了终期评估专项调查，并及时将调查总结报告上报国家项目办。

（五）项目地区疟疾疫情现状

江苏省 2002—2007 年网络直报数疟疾病人发病数分别为 684、638、675、651、767 和 940 例。盱眙县 2002—2007 年网络直报数疟疾病人发病数分别为 84、81、58、25、54 和 42 例。泗洪县 2002—2007 年网络直报数疟疾病人发病数分别为 275、188、150、120、97 和 106 例。江苏省全省网络直报疟疾病人 2002—2006 年保持一个相对平衡的状态，从 2006 年起全省疟疾病人出现上升，2007 年全省疟疾病人将近千人，而同期两个全球基金项目县的网报病人数却呈下降态势。同时，根据专项调查结果，盱眙县 2005 年实际疟疾病例（确诊病例 + 疑似病例）是网报数的 9 倍，2007 年实际疟疾病例（确诊病例 + 疑似病例）是网报数的 7 倍。

2007 年江苏省共血检发热病人 438 704 人，检出阳性数为 686 人，阳性率为 0.156%；2007 年盱眙县共血检发热病人 12 607 人，检出阳性数为两人，阳性率为 0.016%；2007 年泗洪县共血检发热病人 21 273 人，检出阳性数为 66 人，阳性率为 0.310%。

（六）第一轮疟疾项目对项目地区疟疾防治工作的影响

5 年来江苏省第一轮全球基金疟疾项目在江苏省卫生厅和国家项目办的指导下，各项工作按计划实施，基层疟防工作力度加大。通过 5 年的项目资助，使各项疟防工作上了一个台阶。

通过全球基金疟疾项目实施，广大疟防工作人员学习到了项目规范化管理的经验，提高疟疾防治工作的水平。现在，常规疟疾防治工作也开始学习全球基金疟疾项目的项目化管理经验，有计划、有经费预算，工作过程按计划按预算落实，资料整理归档有序，促进了江苏省疟疾防治工作。

通过全球基金疟疾项目实施，项目县疟原虫镜检能力得到了大幅度提高，发热病人血检数量有明显的增加，对传疟媒介的监控力度显著增强，疟疾发病明显下降，暴发流行得到初步控制。

泗洪县网络直报病人数从 2003 年的 188 例疟疾病人下降到 2007 年的 106 例病人，疟疾病人数下降了 43.62%，盱眙县网络直报病人数从 2003 年的 81 例下降到 2007 年的 42 例，疟疾病人数下降了 48.15%。2005 年盱眙县采用捕获 - 再捕获方法推算出实际病例数（确诊病例 + 疑似病例）是网报数的 9 倍，2007 年终期评估采取同样方法推算出的病例数（确诊病例 + 疑似病例）是网络直报的 7 倍；泗洪县 2003 年采用捕获 - 再捕获方法推算出当年病例数是网报数的 9.4 倍，2007 年终期评估推算病例数（确诊病例 + 疑似病例）也有明显下降。与此同时，该两个县周边县近几年疟疾病人数不降反升，特别是与泗洪县相邻的睢宁县疟疾病人数从 2003 年的 13 例上升到 2007 年的 80 例，上升了 515.38%。通过 5 年来第一轮全球基金的各项活动，有效地降低了当地疟疾发病率，大大提高了当地中、小学生疟疾防治知晓率，明显增加了群众患病后求诊意识。泗洪县 2003 年中学生疟防知识平均合格率为 26.8%，小学生为 21.4%，现在疟防知识合格率为 84.38%，有明显的提高；2003 年正规治疗率为 20.0%，而 2007 年的正规治疗率达 100%。

（七）5 年项目执行评价

江苏省自项目实施 5 年来，得到了省卫生厅和省寄防所领导的高度重视，将项目工作目标纳入年度卫生工作考核目标，把项目目标任务按年度、按季度分配到各项目县，较好地完成了国家项目办下达的项目目标任务。在 5 年的项目实施过程中培养和锻炼了一批疟防专业队伍和实施人员，掌握了对项目工作的督导与评估的方法，项目资料的收集与整理规范要求，逐渐理解和领悟了全球基金项目的管理理念，把项目目标任务与项目资金紧密的联系起来，通过业务人员与财务人员的及时沟通与相互配合，确保项目资金的合理使用，项目目标工作任务顺利完成。

在项目执行的前期，由于对全球基金项目不是十分了解，在项目管理中存在一些问题，比如将项目工作和常规的疟疾病防治工作没有严格的分开，项目资金没有严格按照项目目标任务按季度下拨到项目县，导致项目资金的使用欠规范；在项目督导过程中，没有完全按照国家项目办下发的督导与评估指南开展督导与评估工作，对督导与评估中发现的问题，县项目没有及时反馈整改意见，省项目办也没有及时对整改情况进行跟踪督导。但这一些问题都在项目执行的过程终逐步得到了纠正和改进，为第五轮全球基金疟疾项目的执行和疟疾防治工作打下了坚实的基础。

（八）成效与经验

1. 江苏省第一轮全球基金所取得的成果及其经验

江苏省第一轮全球基金项目 5 年来，不仅遏制了项目县的疟疾流行程度，还更好地沟通了政府部门和卫生主管部门间的联系，全球基金项目归入当地疟疾防治规划的一部分。江苏省已把全球基金项目的目标和指标与江苏省疟防规划的目标和指标结合起来，卫生厅工作方案中也把全球基金疟疾项目作为一项考核内容。

项目使疟疾防治人员与财务人员学会了相互沟通，加强了项目与财务管理规范合理操作。项目实施还提高了基层的疾病预防控制的管理和规范化水平，为江苏省培训了一批基层防治疟疾的队伍。

2. 项目地区面临的挑战和应对思路

第一轮江苏省全球基金疟疾项目存在的不足之处为项目办工作人员缺乏项目管理经验，项目前两年计划性不够，物资药品不能按计划及时下拨，影响了第一轮江苏省全球基金疟疾项目的执行力度。同时，项目县技术力量较薄弱，项目技术措施落实不到位。另外，项目县的镜检能力和质量不高，督导质量和效果不理想，尤其在及时发现问题、采取有效措施、跟踪整改进度，反馈利用效果等方面能力较差。

通过一轮项目的工作积累，江苏省定能更好地开展第五轮全球基金项目及其他项目化管理工作，克服已存在的缺陷。江苏省第五轮全球基金疟疾项目将更好地与当地卫生行政部门加强沟通，及时汇报项目进展和存在的问题，在卫生行政部门的领导和监管下，严格按项目协议、工作计划和指导手册认真落实项目任务，确保项目按计划、管理要求执行，确保项目措施得到有效落实；将进一步明确全球基金项目管理、财务、审计、采购管理和监督与评价等方面的要求和规范，使江苏省全球基金疟疾项目取得更好的成绩，为江苏省疟疾防治工作作出应有的贡献。

（九）项目县简评

1. 泗洪县

泗洪县自项目实施 5 年来，得到了县政府和县卫生局的高度重视，将项目工作目标纳入年度卫生工作考核目标，把项目目标任务按年度、按季度分配到各项目乡镇，各项目乡镇按计划开展项目工作，较好地完成了项目目标任务，14 个项目乡镇的发热病人血检数从 2003 年的 4 157 例上升到 12 513 例，上升了 201.01%，网报发病数从 2003 年的 150 例下降到 2007 年的 81 例，下降了 46.36%，项目地区的疟疾病发病率有了较大幅度的下降。同时在 5 年的项目实施过程中培养和锻炼了一批县、乡两级项目管理和实施人员，掌握了对项目工作的督导与评估的方法和项目资料的收集与整理规范要求，逐渐理解和领悟了全球基金项目的管理理念，它是把项目目标任务与项目资金紧密的联系起来，通过业务人员与财务人员的及时沟通与相互配合，确保项目资金的合理使用，项目目标工作任务圆满完成。

但在项目执行的前期，县项目办由于对全球基金项目不是十分了解，在项目管理中存在一些问题，比如将项目工作和常规的疟疾病防治工作没有严格的分开，项目资金没有严格按照项目目标任务完成情况下拨到项目乡镇，导致项目资金的使用欠规范；在项目督导过程中，没有按照国家项目办下发的督导与评估指南开展督导与评估工作，对督导与评估中发现的问题，乡级没有及时反馈整改意见，县项目办也没有及时对整改情况跟踪督导。

泗洪县第一轮全球基金疟疾项目工作已经结束，虽然还存在一些不尽如人意的地方，但对基层的疟疾病防治工作的深入开展起到了很好的推进作用，同时积累了丰富的项目管理经验，为第五轮疟疾项目工作更好的实施打下了坚实的基础。

2. 盱眙县

盱眙县第一轮全球基金疟疾项目工作自2003年开展以来，经过县项目办和各乡镇项目办工作人员的共同努力，已完成了各项项目活动。7个项目乡镇的发热病人血检数从2003年的763例上升到2007年的2 654例，上升了247.83%，网报发病数从2003年的51例下降到2007年的26例，下降了49.02%，盱眙县经济条件相对较落后，人群文化水平低，外出务工人员较多，且受人员技术水平等条件的限制，对项目的部分活动完成质量和任务落实产生了一定的影响。5年来通过项目资助，使各项目乡镇的疟疾防治工作上了一个台阶，项目乡镇疟疾发病率也由2003年的2.56/万下降到2007年的1.28/万。项目工作也促使全县疟防工作人员对项目工作有了新的认识，许多常规工作也开始按项目化管理，做到有计划、有经费预算，工作按计划、预算落实，资料及时整理归档。第一轮全球基金项目使盱眙县疟疾防治工作有了较大进步。

江苏省全球基金疟疾项目办公室

2008年5月30日

七、广东省项目终期总结报告

第一轮全球艾滋病、结核病和疟疾基金广东疟疾项目自2003年2月全面实施以来，迄今已5年。在这5年的时间里，惠州和徐闻两个项目片在省项目办公室的领导和技术指导下，各项工作严格按协议和计划有关要求逐一开展。为了总结经验，更好地开展广东省疟防工作，现将广东疟疾项目五年来的工作情况总结如下：

（一）项目概况

第一轮全球基金广东省疟疾项目原计划是在广东省徐闻县和惠阳市进行，后因惠阳市行政区域的变更（已书面报告国家疟疾项目办），项目点增加了惠州市惠城区。这三个项目点一个位于广东省西南部与海南毗邻、另两个位于广东省珠三角，流动人口比较多。三个项目点历来均是广东省疟疾防治监测的重点县、区。第一轮全球基金广东疟疾项目的主要目标包括：（1）使项目地区居民得到更好的早期诊断和个人防护；（2）优化项目地区的疟疾控制项目管理等两个目标。

（二）项目工作及管理

1. 召开广东疟疾项目有关会议

为使项目工作能按协议和计划顺利开展，5 年来，省项目办共组织召开会议 5 次，每次与会人员均包括省卫生厅疾控处、省疾控中心有关领导及项目工作人员，管辖两个项目县的市卫生局、疾控中心有关领导，两个项目县卫生局、疾控中心有关领导等。每次年会，3 个项目点都对上一年的工作进行系统总结，对存在的问题及时进行解决，从而保证了整个项目计划的顺利完成。

2. 财务人员培训

5 年来惠州和徐闻两个项目片分别举办疟疾诊断和财务管理等培训班共 15 期，共培训医务人员 462 人次，财务人员 35 人次。通过培训和考核，有效提高了项目地区医务人员的疟疾诊断和治疗水平，提高了项目县财务人员的管理水平，加强了疟疾病例的网络直报工作，减少了疟疾病例的漏报。疟疾病人漏报率由实施前的 100% 到目前的 0；疟疾病人通过显微镜确诊的比例由实施前的 0 到目前的 100%。

3. 疟疾监测

惠阳和徐闻项目片严格按有关要求开展疟疾监测工作，特别是加强了流动人口发热病人疟原虫血检。3 个项目点 5 年共完成发热病人疟疾血检 117 945 人次，年血检率平均为当地总人口的 2.21%, 达到了预期的目标。通过监测，3 个项目点 5 年共发现疟疾病例 16 例并进行了正规治疗，真正做到了早发现、早治疗和早处理，有效地控制了项目地区的疟疾流行。正规治疗率由实施前的零提高到目前的 100%。

4. 卫生宣教

为使惠州、惠阳、徐闻的本地人群获得更好的早期诊断与个体保护，3 个项目点均以公共场所张贴宣传画、为中小学生上课通过广播、电视、报刊进行公益宣传等方式开展宣教工作。通过卫生宣教，使项目点的疟防工作上新台阶。中小学生疟防知识知晓率由实施前的 7.22% 提升到 90.33%；居民疟防知识知晓率由实施前的 5.13% 提升到 86.85%；居民发烧病人 2 天内求诊比例由 16% 提升到 95.09%。

5. 质量控制和督导

为保证项目的质量，根据各年度计划安排，省项目办对 3 个项目点共进行了 5 次工作质量和财务管理督导，每次督导完毕均有书面反馈督导报告，对存在不足，需要整改的问题都进行了跟踪。3 个项目点也按计划要求，每年各对 3 个镇督导 3 次，5 年共 135 次。通过这些督导，有效地保证了各项目点按计划开展工作，也及时解决了工作存在的问题。督导过程中，主要发现了以下问题：(1) 乡镇卫生院工作计划不够详细，各项指标没有细化。(2) 县对镇的血片复核缺少长期机制，今后应不定时抽查并将结果反馈被抽查单位。(3) 工作计划发生变更缺乏预先申请。(4) 财务报表和工作进度报表上报时间不够抓紧等。针对这些问题，省项目办已责成各项目办加以改进。

6. 项目管理

为保证项目的顺利实施，省项目办对项目管理制定了一系列措施。各项管理严格按照全球基金有关规定执行，一旦项目办人员发生调整，马上对新人进行培训。对县、镇一级项目办严格要求按项目计划开展工作。各项目办均实行网络直报和设备管理责任到人，从而保证了各项工作报表按时上报。3 个项目点的网络在五年时间里均运行良好，基本上能按时上报有关报表。

7. 指标完成情况（见表 1–44）

表 1–44 指标完成情况

关键指标		基线结果	第五年专项调查结果
项目主要目标二:使目标地区居民得到更好的早期诊断和个人防护			
1	发热病人血检计划完成的比例	人口总数的 0.16%	人口总数的 2.04%
2	通过显微镜确诊的疟疾病人比例	0	100.00%
3	接受正确治疗的疟疾病例比例	0	100.00%
4	发烧病人 2 天内就诊比例	16	95.09%
项目主要目标四:优化云南、海南及其他八个省的疟疾控制项目管理			
1	疟疾病例通过信息网络报告的比例	0	100.00%
2	疟疾病人漏报率	100.00%	0
3	居民疟防知识知晓率	5.13%	86.85%
4	中小学生疟防知识知晓率	7.22%	90.33%

（三）经费开支情况

1. 收入部分：2003 年收到拨款 90 253.21 元；2004 年收到拨款 151 526.00 元；2005 年收到拨款 117 881.16 元；2006 年收到拨款 299 781.89 元；2007 年收到拨款 139 103.47 元到目前为止，5 年共收到项目拨款 798 545.73 元。

2. 支出部分：2003 年总支出 90 253.21 元。2004 年总支出 151 526.00 元。2005 年总支出 114 319.13 元。2006 年总支出 282 151.80 元。2007 年总支出 128 396.50 元。2008 年总支出 32 647.67 元。以上各年总支出共 799 294.31 元（含 3 个项目办利息 748.58 元）。

（四）固定资产盘点与移交

经盘点，全球基金5年共下拨广东疟疾项目办固定资产约合人民币157 250.00元。项目于2008年3月31日结束后，广东省项目办于2008年5月对全球基金所有固定资产进行了清点。清点结束后，为了让项目县的疟防工作得以延续，我们把原先分配到各项目办使用的固定资产进行了财产移交并办妥了固定资产入账手续。各项目办资产情况见表1–45:

表1–45　全球基金广东疟疾项目固定资产辅助账（单位：元）

固定资产名称	固定资产型号	固定资产购置（PR赠送）			固定资产移交	
		时间	数量	总价	时间	单位
生物显微镜	Olympus Cx21	2004.12.1	8	40 000	2004.7.2（共6台）	广东省CDC（2台） 惠州CDC（2台） 惠阳CDC（2台） 徐闻CDC（2台）
便携式电脑	东芝 portege ra100	2004.12.1	2	33 800	2004.12..1（1台）	广东省CDC（1台） 广东省卫生厅疾控处(1台)
数码相机	Sony f717	2004.12.1	2	9 300	2004.12.1（1台）	广东省CDC（1部） 广东省卫生厅疾控处(1部)
激光打印机	Hp-1015	2004.12.1	2	4 900	2004.12.1（1台）	广东省CDC（1部） 广东省卫生厅疾控处(1部)
台式电脑		2004.12.1	5	47 250	2004.12.12（3台）	广东省CDC（2台） 惠州CDC（1台） 惠阳CDC（1台） 徐闻CDC（1台）
体视显微镜	Olympus Szx9	2004.12.1	1	6 000		广东省CDC
生物显微镜	Olympus Cx21	2007.1.23	4	16 000	2007.1.23（共3台）	广东省CDC（1台） 惠州CDC（1台） 惠阳CDC（1台） 徐闻CDC（1台）

（五）项目地区疟疾疫情现状

通过连续5年的项目实施，3个项目点的疟疾疫情得到了有效控制和巩固，连续5年均没有暴发流行点出现。监测结果显示，3个项目点疟疾年发病率目前均已控制在1/10万以下，其中徐闻2007年疟疾年发病率是0.16/10万（1例间日疟）；惠州惠城区2007年疟疾年发病率是0.25/10万（2例间日疟）；惠州惠阳区2007年疟疾年发病率是0.20/10万（1例间日疟）；流动人口疟疾病例得到及早地发现、治疗和处理。

（六）第一轮全球基金对项目地区疟疾防治工作的影响

5年项目的实施明显加强了项目地区政府和卫生行政部门对疟防工作的重视和投入；提高了各级卫生部门的疟疾诊断、治疗等技术平。通过项目的管理，提高了各级业务人员和财务人员的管理意识，从中吸取了先进的管理经验，为今后开展各项工作提供了宝贵经验。

（七）5年项目执行评价

结果显示，通过连续5年的项目实施，3个项目市、县基本达到预期的目标。项目市、县的疟疾发病率得到了有效控制，年发病率连续5年控制在1/10万以下；通过各种形式的卫生宣教，项目地区群众对疟疾防治知识由实施初期的几乎不懂到今日的基本掌握；项目地区的乡村医生和个体医生对疟疾的诊断水平也有了很大提高，对疟疾病例的管理和上报等意识得到了加强，疟疾病例漏报率由实施前的100%下降到目前的0；发热病人疟疾血检率由实施前的不足0.2%到现在的2%以上，大大地加强了项目市、县的疟疾监测工作；通过加强项目的管理和财务监督，使项目市、县相关人员的管理水平得到了显著提高。先进的国际管理经验，开拓了相关工作人员的视野，对工作的规范起到了积极的作用，如广东省的固定资产管理较为规范等。综合各种情况，我们认为省项目办和3个市、县项目办，以及参与项目地区的乡镇都是称职的，已完成了计划中的各项工作和管理，工作目标也达到了预期效果。

（八）成效与经验

5年项目的实施，其成效包括（1）项目地区疟疾疫情得到有效控制和巩固，年发病率连续5年控制在1/10万以下。(2)项目受益地区群众的防疟意识得到有效提高，发热人群2天内求诊的比例大幅提升。(3）项目地区医疗机构疟疾诊断和治疗水平得到了质的飞跃，监测质量和数量都大幅提高，基本实现了对疟疾病人实行早发现、早治疗、早处理的目标，减少了因误诊造成的浪费。(4）提高了项目地区的各种管理能力，对受益地区的疟疾防疫事业起到了示范作用。(5）减少了疟疾病人的漏报，从而对疟疾病例的动态情况掌握更为充分，为今后制定疟防措施提供更科学的依据。

广东省的3个项目点虽然按计划顺利完成各项工作，但今后面临的挑战仍然艰巨，具体表现在（1）卫生宣教工作力度和广度仍然有待进一步加强。（2）由于种种原因，3个项目点基层卫生院显微镜设备残旧或欠缺，镜检人员更换频繁，血检质量仍有待进一步提高，所以培训任务不能放松。（3）随着经济的发展，流动人口越来越多，流动性也越来越大，加强流动人口疟疾管理是今后疟防工作的重中之重。为了巩固抗疟成果，今后的思路应包括：（1）建议各级政府及卫生行政部门增加疟防经费投入；（2）加强技术人员培训和卫生宣教；（3）继续争取国际有关组织的援助，充分利用这些资金和技术推动广东省疟防事业的发展，只有这样才能巩固这3个项目点乃至全省的抗疟成果。

（九）项目县简评

通过5年项目工作的实施和终期评估，根据综合分数计算方法，惠州综合得分为90分；惠阳综合得分为89.1分；徐闻综合得分为90.2分。从综合得分可以可出，惠州市的项目工作完成相对较好，无论是卫生宣教还是疟疾病例的诊断、治疗和项目的管理、财务制度等都够为规范。徐闻在疟疾血检质量方面最为理想，卫生宣教和项目的管理、财务开支都能按计划执行。惠阳在卫生宣教方面较为理想，其形式的多样性开创了广东省疟疾卫生宣教工作新局面。惠阳的项目管理和财务开支也基本安计划执行，虽然期间项目人员有变动，但各项工作没有脱节，各种报表都能依时上报。

广东省疟疾项目办对参与第一轮全球基金广东疟疾项目的3个市、县的总评价是：其工作是认真的；管理是严格的；开支是规范的；成绩是肯定的。希望3个项目市、县今后能总结经验，发挥抗疟龙头作用，带动广东省疟防事业走向新高点。

广东省全球基金疟疾项目办公室

2008年5月

八、广西壮族自治区项目终期总结报告

（一）项目概况

广西百色市右江区位于北纬23° 32′—24° 17′，东经106° 07′—106° 56′，总面积3713km^{2}全区辖12个乡镇116个行政村844个自然村，总人口33.5万。主要传疟媒介有微小按蚊、中华按蚊和日月潭按蚊3种。2003年起第一轮中国全球基金疟疾项

目广西流动人口疟疾监测控制项目在右江区实施，项目执行5年来，开展了项目基线调查，县乡村防疫人员培训，发热病人血检侦查传染源，疟疾病人治疗，流动人口高危人群预防服药，项目督导和设备分发等工作，有效地防止了输入性疟疾病例的扩散，巩固了当地的疟疾防治效果，达到了项目计划的预期目标，现将项目实施以来的工作总结如下：

（二）项目剩余资金使用情况

截止2008年3月31日，本项目已无资金剩余，还超支了1 052.10元。

（三）项目设备物资情况

项目实施以来，共收到国家疟疾项目办公室调拨的物资有电脑4台（台式两台、笔记本电脑两台），生物显微镜11台，三目体视显微镜1台，抗疟药（磷酸氯/伯喹片剂）10 000人份，5%杀飞克12 000ml；疟疾宣传画4 000张，疟疾知识宣传小册子800本和印有全球基金疟疾项目的练习簿3 200本。省级采购数码相机两台，油镜头12个。目前生物显微镜3台，三目体视显微镜1台，数码相机1台在省级CDC，数码相机1台在卫生厅项目办。调拨给百色市疾病预防控制中心笔记本电脑1台，右江区乡卫生院显微镜8台，油镜头12个，5%杀飞克12 000ml及抗疟药约8 000人份。宣传画、小册子、练习簿全部分发到项目乡村学校。项目固定资产和药品的调拨和出入库手续均按照《中国全球基金项目物资采购与资产管理手册》和《全球基金财务管理手册》的要求进行固定资产和项目物资辅助账管理。

（四）5年工作总结

1. 项目管理

项目执行以来，卫生厅项目办指定了1名项目官员负责项目的日常管理和协调工作的开展，自治区CDC安排了1名专业技术人员专人负责项目年初计划制定、组织实施、督导，按季度收集、审核、汇总资料上报给国家项目办。做到季报表上报及时、填写规范、数据准确。

2. 项目监督与评价

2003—2007年，自治区CDC到百色市和右江区所有乡镇进行督导共18次40人次；市CDC到乡镇督导38次76人次。发现个别乡对“四热病人”存在血片制作染色质量差、疟防资料记录归档保存不规范等情况，对督导中发现的问题给予了及时纠正，保证了疟疾监测工作的效率和质量。2008年3月10—13日，厅卫生项目办组织有关人员对百色市右江区疟疾项目实施单位进行了项目评估，查看了市级

CDC项目执行5年来的有关文件、监测数据、总结以及督导报告，走访了汪甸、阳圩、永乐、龙川4个乡（镇）卫生院，实地察看了项目执行的有关情况，市级CDC以及右江区乡卫生院项目资料基本齐全，保管尚较完整，监测数据可信。该项目的实施对当地的疟疾防治起到了极大的促进作用，有效地巩固了疟疾防治成果，达到了预期的目标。

3．财务管理

厅卫生项目办指派两人分别兼任疟疾项目会计和出纳，负责项目财务收支及财务报表上报。财务人员与项目人员能经常进行有效沟通，及时交流项目经费使用和项目进展情况，同时制定了疟疾项目财务管理、物资管理相关制度，严格执行项目资金支出授权审批制度；项目资金使用合乎规范，无挤占挪用项目资金的情况；将全球基金的资金按照病种实行建账管理、按工作目标进行财务核算；按照《全球基金财务管理手册》规定的会计科目进行财务核算，科目使用合理。设置了独立银行账号，严格遵守中国人民银行颁布的《现金管理暂行条例》和《银行存款支付结算办法》；现金日记账和银行存款日记账做到账实相符。5年来收到国家项目办拨入经费共计人民币780 545.00元，其中目标区的疫情监测和报告356 745.70元、项目运行与管理423 799.30元。项目累计支出共计人民币781 597.10元，其中目标区的疫情监测和报告357 460.39元，目标四：项目运行与管理424 136.71元，包括：人员工资24 000.00元、病例报告管理费119 845.20元、信息监测费104 470.00元、印刷费8 830.90元、会议费35 250.50元、差旅费51 937.35元、设备购置费34 610.90元、物品材料费2 304.80元、培训费266 381.95元、交通费13 350.00元、项目监督检查评估费69 808.50元、财务培训监督检查费18 410.50元、其他支出32 396.50元。

4．项目执行进展

4.1 发热病人血检情况

2003—2007年右江区12个乡（镇）共血检当地居民发热病人71 891人次，检出间日疟原虫阳性2例，阳性率为0.00027%。流动人口监测12 034人次，检出疟原虫阳性20例，阳性率为0.166%，其中外来流动人口11 968人次，检出疟原虫阳性19例，间日疟18例，恶性疟1例；外出回归人员66人次，检出疟原虫阳性1例。从2005年到2007年，项目计划每年血检发热病人12 000人次，2003—2007年实际每年完成发热病人血检分别为11 653人次、13 510人次、12 344人次、17 147人次和17 237人次。

4.2 居民带虫调查

2005—2007年，项目计划每年完成居民带虫调查8 000人份，3年共24 000人，2004—2007年实际完成居民带虫调查22 922人次，完成任务数的95.51%，血检全部阴性。

4.3 高危人群预防服药

5 年来对查出的内源性病灶点和输入性病例的外源性病灶点病家及病家周围人群开展预防服药，在百罗高速公路工地民工和龙川镇竹凤村、阳圩镇的柳羊村、六茄甘蔗场、百色第二看守所等地的高危人群 2 208 人给予预防服药，其中 2004 年服药 578 人，2005 年服药 1 630 人，2006 年和 2007 年没有高危人群服药对象。

4.4 现症病人治疗

对 2003—2007 年血检阳性的 22 例疟疾现症病人，均给予磷酸氯喹 1.5g（基质）十磷酸伯氨喹 180mg 八天疗法正规治疗，治疗率和全程足量率均达到 100%。

4.5 人群疟防知识知晓情况调查

分别在那毕、汪甸、阳圩 3 个乡（镇）的福禄、连塘、百法、阳圩、平圩、六丰、汪甸、两琶、沙洪 9 个行政村和两所中小学进行疟防知识知晓情况调查，共调查村民 4 714 人，中学生 406 人，小学生 180 人，疟防知识知晓人数分别为 1 288 人，294 人、121 人，疟防知识知晓率分别为 27.32%、72.41% 和 67.22%，中小学学生疟防知识知晓率高于村民。

4.6 小学生和居民疟疾抗体调查

项目实施以来，对阳圩、那毕和汪甸 3 个乡 6 所小学 655 名小学生和居民 3 175 人采集滤纸血膜进行疟疾荧光抗体检测，结果全部阴性。

（五）项目地区疟疾疫情现状

在卫生厅项目办和百色市、区卫生局的领导下，右江区疟疾监测项目严格按照项目标书要求，采取目标管理，重点督导，发现问题，及时解决的有力措施，经过项目实施地区广大疟防工作者 5 年的共同努力，疟疾发病率继续控制在 1/ 万以下。2003 年以来每年血检未外出居民发热病人 1.1 ～ 1.7 万人次，仅检出当地感染疟疾病例 2 例，血检病灶点居民 22 980 人 次，未检出疟疾病人，血清学监测 3 175 份，也未检出疟疾抗体阳性，表明右江区采取的疟疾监测措施是可行的，疟疾防治成果继续得到巩固。

（六）疟疾项目成效与经验

1. 促进了人材培养

项目实施以来，对右江区乡级专业人员和村医生 248 人以及全自治区 84 个 CDC 的 154 名疟防人员分别进行了疟原虫镜检技术，疟疾信息管理和疟疾暴发流行应急处理技术等培训，有效地提高了基层防疫人员的专业技术水平。

2. 加强了疫情报告制度

通过疟疾信息管理人员培训、督查和改善公共卫生信息网络，市、县和乡级医疗卫生机构对网络直报疟疾疫情的重要性有了新的提高，全区每年监测发现的疟疾病人均通过网络上报，疟疾疫情信息报告达到了快捷畅通。

3. 提高了监测工作的质量

通过对项目地区发热病人采血、涂片、镜检，病人治疗，疫情报告等方面的督查和指导，基层防保人员的工作责任心得到进一步加强，提高了疟防监测工作的质量。

4. 有效地防止输入性疟疾扩散

2003—2007 年，项目地区共查出本地病例两例，输入性疟疾 20 例，由于及时发现和治疗病人及对病灶点进行了妥善处理。5 年来共血检病灶点本地居民 71 891 人次，流动人口 12 034 人次，居民带虫调查 22 922 人次，未发现输入性疟疾继发病例。

5. 促进了疟防工作的开展

右江区 12 个乡（镇）33.5 万人口的地区，5 年来当地感染疟疾发病率均控制在 1/10 万以下，百色水利枢纽工程和百罗高速公路施工工地疟疾疫情稳定，有效地保护了劳动力，保证了工程的顺利完成，促进了当地经济发展。

（七）项目地区简评

该项目实施 5 年来，百色市卫生局和右江区卫生局关心和支持全球基金右江区疟疾监测控制项目活动，将本项目作为当地疟疾防治规划的重要部分来抓，加强对该项目的领导和监管，派出官员与技术人员深入基层督导，及时解决疟疾监测工作中出现的问题，保证了该项目的顺利实施。同时右江区每年拿出 5.94 万元配套资金作为村医生从事疟防工作及其他防疫工作补助经费，有力地推动了当地的疟疾监测持续有效地进行，完成了项目的目标任务，巩固了当地疟疾防治成果，保护了人民身体健康，促进了当地社会经济发展，达到了预期的目标。

广西壮族自治区全球基金疟疾项目办公室

2008 年 6 月 30 日

九、四川省项目终期总结报告

四川省全球基金疟疾项目（2003 年 4 月 1 日～2008 年 3 月 31 日）在中国全球

基金疟疾项目办公室、四川省卫生厅的领导下严格按照项目工作计划组织实施，顺利完成了工作任务和目标，项目实施效果显著。现将四川省项目5年执行情况报告如下：

（一）项目概况

四川省全球基金疟疾项目2003年4月启动，项目覆盖宜宾市筠连县。筠连县地处四川盆地南缘，与云南省昭通地区接壤，全县面积1 256.13km^2，人口40.5万，辖20个乡。属国家级贫困县，是四川省的疟疾高发区之一。

项目为期5年，分二期执行。第一期项目为期2年(2003年4月—2005年3月)，第二期项目为期3年（2005年4月—2008年3月）。项目的总目标是及时发现和治疗输入性疟疾病例，减少由输入性病例导致的当地传播。两项具体目标包括使目标地区的居民得到更好的早期诊断和个人防护、优化疟疾控制项目管理。

四川省通过项目实施，重点加强项目县的疟疾控制与监测，预期目标是到2007年底项目县疟疾发病率（包括当地病例和输入病例）控制在1/万。

（二）项目执行情况

1. 项目管理

1.1 健全组织机构：2003年省、县分别成立了全球基金疟疾项目领导小组和办公室。项目执行期间根据工作需要不断充实调整了项目办人员。项目结题期间项目办运转正常，有专人负责项目工作。

1.2 落实责任：两期项目执行中省与项目县均签订了围绕项目目标制定的项目计划书；每年县项目办与项目乡镇签订“筠连县全球基金疟疾项目工作目标责任书”，明确目标、职责和任务。

1.3 信息管理：项目实施以来的各规定报表均在规定的时限内、完整准确上报；项目还以工作简讯、简报，通报项目工作进展情况等形式，加强工作信息交流与反馈。年度项目工作实施结束时及时进行总结。

1.4 督导检查：由省项目办和宜宾市疾控中心组成的省市联合督导组每年对项目县至少进行一次督导与年度考核。督导做到有计划、有记录，内容覆盖项目管理、防治工作、财务管理。形成的督导报告有分析、有反馈。项目县也按计划对项目乡镇进行季度督导。省、县项目办对项目实施中存在问题的整改情况也进行了追踪检查。

1.5 召开工作年会：2005—2007年每年4月召开四川省全球基金疟疾项目年会，总结经验，分析讨论工作中存在的问题和不足，布置下一年度的工作任务。项目2007年年会暨总结大会因受2008年5月四川汶川地震灾害影响延期至2008年6月召开。

2．项目活动

2.1 一期项目主要活动

2.1.1 基线调查：2003年7月按照基线调查技术方案，调查了筠连县的双腾镇、巡司镇、镇舟镇，共访问居民5 105人。调查1至3年级小学生453人。

2.1.2 强化疟疾疫情报告：自2004年开始，在全县范围内开展传染病防治法教育的基础上，全面推行疟疾疫情零报告、旬报告制度。

2.1.3 发热病人血检：2004年6月收到项目资助的显微镜，7月初镇舟、沐爱、乐义、落木柔、双腾、巡司等乡镇卫生院开展发热病人血检，2004年共血检2 090人。

2.1.4 业务培训：2003—2004年举办镇乡级培训班（会）4期，在11个镇乡开展村级医务人员培训13次，累计培训镇乡级医务人员122人次，村级医务人员239人次。

2.1.5 疟防知识宣传教育：在全县范围内开展了疟疾防治知识宣传教育，统一采用国家项目办公室下发的宣传资料，广泛进行宣讲。各乡、镇、村利用会议形式宣传。卫生院采用出壁报、墙报的方式宣传，广泛张贴疟防宣传画。2003—2004年220所中小学校进行了疟防知识宣传，进行宣传的学校数占全县中小学校的81%，受教育的学生约12 000人，占学生总数的76%。各镇、乡利用村组干部会议宣传76次，参会人员约1 800人次。张贴大小疟防知识画报3 800份。

2.1.6 疫点处理：2004年对2003年的20个疫点和2004年的98个疫点进行了灭蚊处理。在少数疫点对患者家属用氯喹、伯氨喹进行了预防服药。

2.2 二期项目主要活动

2005年7月二期项目启动，筠连县的乐义乡，镇舟镇，巡司镇，沐爱镇，双腾镇，落木柔镇，维新镇等7个乡镇被划为项目乡镇，人口187 283人。

2.2.1 发热病人血检：2005—2007共计开展发热病人血检31 087人次（详见表1–46）。

2.2.2 病人治疗及疫点处理：2005—2007年间共治疗病人67例，对所有疫点均进行了高危人群预防性服药及灭蚊处理。

2.2.3 高危人群预防性治疗：2005—2007年高危人群预防性治疗7 020人次，完成率117.00%（详见表1–46）。

2.2.4 技术培训：2005—2007年共举办疟疾防治、镜检培训班5期。培训县乡级疟防技术人员220人。

2.2.5 健康教育：2006年印制发放宣传画约30 000份、手册约30 000份，练习簿20 000册；2007年省项目办委托四川省疾控中心健康教育所制作了疟疾宣传科教片《关注健康、共抗疟疾》；2007年还制作了实用宣传品水杯、围裙、文件保护袋7 000余件，用于在居民、学生中开展疟防知识宣传教育。

2.2.6 监测调查：2005—2007年对7个项目乡镇24 976人进行了走访调查和血清抗体水平检测，其中走访调查23 571人。结果显示，居民的疟防知识知晓率逐年提高。蚊帐使用率下降与项目地区居民生活及居住条件改善有关。间接荧光抗体(IFA)试验检测1 405人次，抗体阳性率由2005年的3.53%降至2007年的0，表明防治措施有效，疟疾疫情得到控制（详见表1–48）。

表1–46 四川省全球基金疟疾项目2005年–2008年5月活动开展情况

	项目活动	计划任务	实际完成	完成率	备注
2005年	发热病人血检	12 000人次	6 681人次	55.68%	项目二期协议于2005年7月才签订，所以2005年上半年血检任务不明确，各乡镇卫生院仅按门诊常规医疗开展血检，故2005年血检人数远低于任务数。
	预防性治疗	2 000人次	2 845人次	142.25%	
	疫点人群带虫调查	8 000人	8 050人	100.63%	
	省级年会	1次	1次	100.00%	
	省级督导	1次	1次	100.00%	
	县级督导	21次	21次	100.00%	
2006年	发热病人血检	12 000人次	12 030人次	100.25%	
	预防性治疗	2 000人次	2 025人次	101.25%	
	疫点人群带虫调查	8 000人	8 181人	102.26%	
	省级年会	1次	1次	100.00%	
	省级督导	1次	2次	200.00%	
	县级督导	21次	21次	100.00%	
2007年	发热病人血检	12 000人次	12 376人次	103.13%	
	预防性治疗	2 000人次	2 150人次	107.50%	
	疫点人群带虫调查	8 000人	8 745人	109.31%	
	省级年会	1次	1次	100.00%	
	省级督导	1次	2次	200.00%	
	县级督导	21次	21次	100.00%	
2008年	终期专项调查	居民2 700人、学生360名	居民3 136人、学生387名	115.14%	
	省级自评估	1次	1次	100.00%	

2.2.7 项目终期专项调查　2008 年 3 月按照《四川省全球基金疟疾项目终期专项调查方案》，分层随机抽取了巡司镇的土房村、巡司村及黄荆村，双腾镇的鱼井村、两河村及沙坝村，沐爱镇的金坝村、尧坝村及楠坪村为调查点，共走访调查了 575 户，3 136 人。同期对 3 个乡镇的 387 名中小学生进行了疟防知识问卷调查(详见表 1–49)。

2.2.8 项目终期省级评估　2008 年 4 月由四川省卫生厅、四川省疾病预防控制中心和四川省疟疾防治技术指导组相关人员组成的四川省全球基金疟疾项目省级终期考评组，对项目 5 年的工作情况进行了综合评审。考评组对四川省全球基金疟疾项目的综合评价为 A。

（三）项目资金使用与管理

为了确保项目资金专款专用，我们严格按照《全球基金项目财务管理手册》的要求进行财务管理，实行独立建账，单独核算。项目活动做到有计划、有预算、有决算。在工作中，项目实施人员与财务管理人员能做到及时有效的沟通。在财务报销方面，严格实行财务审核制度，严格按照经费预算与工作计划执行情况使用经费，同时规范财务管理制度和使用制度。

1. 经费收入情况：

2003 年 ~ 2008 年 5 月共收到全球基金下拨经费 798 406.72 元，利息收入 1 747.82 元，其中目标 2 经费 288 862.73 元，目标 4 经费 511 291.81 元。

2. 经费支出情况：

2003 年 ~ 2008 年 5 月省项目办下拨筠连项目县工作经费 356 187.67 元。截至 5 月 23 日全省共计支出经费 758 051.66 元。

3. 经费结余情况：

截至 2008 年 6 月 30 日全省结余零元。

（四）物资管理

项目实施后，四川省收到国家项目办采购分发的电脑 8 台、Olympus 生物显微镜 12 台，体式显微镜 1 台，杀飞克 12 升和磷酸氯 / 伯喹片剂 12 000 人份。省、县项目办和项目乡镇按照全球基金物资管理要求对项目物资进行管理和使用；同时省、县项目办对物资管理反复督查。

四川省项目固定资产、物资盘点情况详见盘点表。

（五）项目地区疫情现状及项目成效

项目县筠连县是四川省的疟疾高发区之一，2002 年发病率为 1.66/ 万，2003 年基线调查结果表明，项目县疟疾疫情漏报严重，漏报率为 88.68%，居民的疟防知识知晓率仅 26.86%，学生的疟防知识知晓率为 36.87%。全县 20 个镇、乡卫生院仅 2 个卫生院开展了发热病人疟原虫镜检，卫生院基础设备差，人员素质低，疟疾防治技能不高。

项目的实施弥补了项目地区疟疾防治经费的缺口，补充了镜检器材，培养了一批疟疾防治及镜检专业人员，发热病人血检覆盖范围逐渐扩大，2007 年全县所有乡镇卫生院均能正常开展发热病人血检。

项目县 2007 年疟疾疫情：全县各级医疗机构报告疟疾病例 5 例，其中本地发病 4 例，输入性疟疾 1 例，发病率 0.12/ 万。2008 年的终期专项调查结果表明 2007 年疟疾疫情漏报率为 0。5 例疟疾病人均为血检确诊。对所有患者进行了及时、正规治疗。

四川省全球基金疟疾项目实施后极大地推动了筠连县的疟疾防治工作，提高了项目县疟疾防治水平，项目县的疟疾发病得到控制。2006 年疟疾发病率降至 0.49/ 万，2007 年疟疾发病率进一步降低至 0.12/ 万，分别较项目实施前 2002 年的 1.66/ 万下降了 70.48%、92.77%，提前实现了项目到 2007 年底疟疾发病率（包括当地病例和输入病例）控制在 1/ 万的目标。2007 年项目县通过显微镜确诊的疟疾病例为 100%，接受正规治疗的疟疾病例为 100%，两项指标均达到项目要求。项目终期专项调查结果显示，2007 年疟疾疫情漏报率由项目实施前的 88.68% 降至 0，学生的疟防知识知晓率由项目实施前的 36.87% 提高到 99.22%，居民的疟防知识知晓率由 26.86% 提高到 79.83%，分别提高了 169.11% 和 197.21%；97.74%的群众使用蚊香防蚊驱蚊。项目县居民疟疾防治知识知晓率显著提高，自我保护能力明显增强（见表 1–47、1–50，图 1–6、1–7）。

表 1–47 筠连县疟疾发病情况

发病情况	病例数	发病率（/ 万）	有发病的乡镇（个）	血检确诊病例数	通过显微镜确诊的疟疾病人比例（%）
2003 年	20	0.58	9	18	90
2004 年	98	2.47	13	61	62.24
2005 年	42	1.05	10	34	80.95
2006 年	20	0.49	3	15	75
2007 年	5	0.12	3（其中筠连镇病例为输入性，有本地发病的乡镇 2 个）	5	100

表 1-48 2005-2007 年居民监测调查结果

	调查户数	调查人数	疟防知识知晓率(%)			蚊帐使用率(%)	使用蚊香总户数	蚊香使用率(%)	IFA 检测		
			传播	治疗	预防				检测人数	阳性数	阳性率(%)
2005年	1 533	7 399	53.16（815/1 533）	67.25（1 031/1 533）	52.77（809/1 533）	82.89（6 133/7 399）	1 515	98.83	651	23	3.53
2006年	1 688	7 724	66.71（1 126/1 688）	75.89（1 281/1 688）	70.08（1 183/1 688）	80.15（6 189/7 724）	1 654	97.99	457	1	0.22
2007年	2 032	8 448	79.28（1 611/2 032）	78.15（1 588/2 032）	82.38（1 674/2 032）	42.92（3 626/8 448）	1 985	97.69	297	0	0

表 1-49 终期专项调查结果

乡镇名	调查村名	走访户数	调查村民数	疟史病例数	报告疫情例数	疟防知识知晓人数	疟防知识知晓率(%)	使用蚊帐人数	蚊帐使用率(%)	使用蚊香户数	蚊香使用率(%)
巡司	土房	58	320	0	0	46	79.31	238	74.38	56	96.55
	巡司	68	351	1	1	56	82.35	194	55.27	67	98.53
	黄荆	70	439	0	0	56	80.00	244	55.58	69	98.57
双腾	鱼井	64	307	0	0	49	76.56	190	61.89	61	95.31
	两河	56	327	0	0	43	76.79	174	53.21	53	94.64
	沙坝	81	388	0	0	58	71.60	240	61.86	80	98.77
沐爱	金坝	47	242	0	0	40	85.11	211	87.19	46	97.87
	尧坝	66	403	0	0	64	96.97	214	53.10	66	100
	楠坪	65	359	0	0	47	72.31	225	62.67	64	98.46
合计		575	3 136	1	1	459	79.83	1 930	61.54	562	97.74

表 1-50 基线调查与终期专项调查结果比较

	发病人数	发病率（1/万）	漏报率（%）	居民疟防知识知晓率（%）	学生疟防知识知晓率（%）	蚊帐使用率（%）	蚊香使用率（%）
项目实施前	64	1.66	88.68	26.86	36.87	69.19	未调查
项目实施后	5	0.12	0	79.83	99.22	61.54	97.74

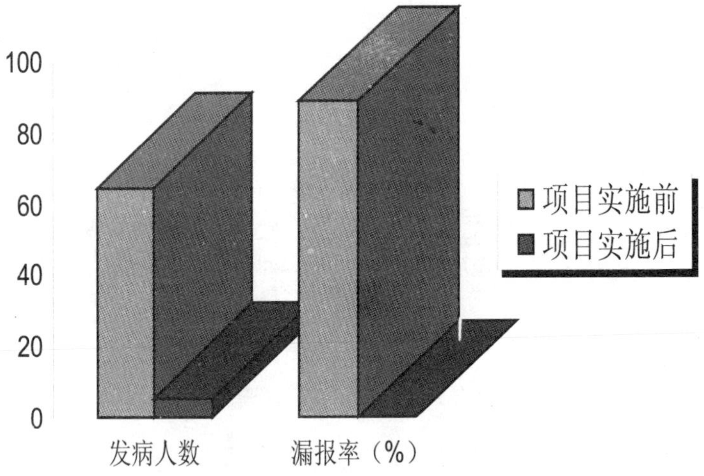

图 1-6 项目实施前后发病人数及漏报率比较

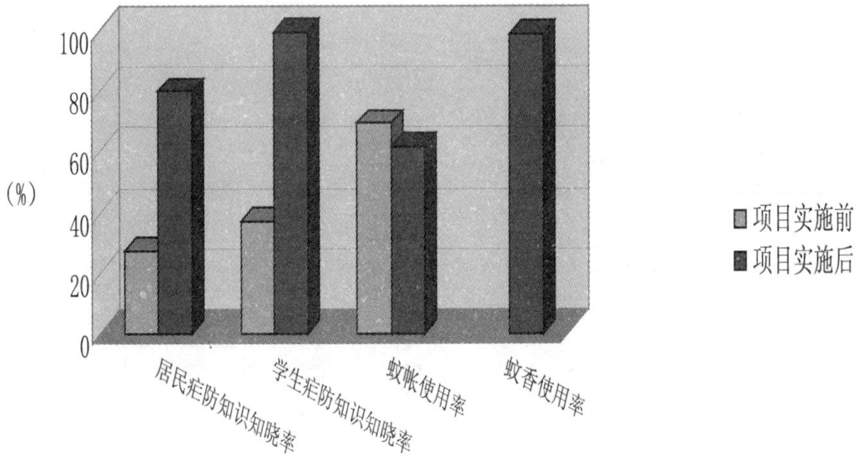

图 1-7 居民及学生疟防知识知晓率、蚊帐使用率、蚊香使用率比较

（六）项目执行评价

2008年4月，按照《第一轮中国全球基金疟疾项目终期评估方案》和《四川省全球基金疟疾项目终期评估方案》，由四川省卫生厅、四川省疾病预防控制中心和四川省疟疾防治技术指导组相关人员组成的四川省全球基金疟疾项目省级终期考评组对四川省全球基金疟疾项目5年的工作情况进行了综合评审。

考评组评估结果如下：四川省全球基金疟疾防治项目工作在实施过程中，得到了四川省卫生厅的大力支持和有效监管，筠连县卫生局对筠连县的项目工作也给予了积极支持。省级和县级项目机构健全，项目办公室管理有序，运转良好，项目信息系统运行正常，财务管理比较规范。所有的工作均按照项目计划执行，进展顺利。疟疾发病率、疟疾病人血检确诊率、流行季节重点人群预防性治疗人数等指标均达到或超过了项目要求。项目的实施也使基层疟疾防控机构和人员素质得到了整体提升，有力推动了项目县的疟疾防治，使该地区疟疾发病受到了有效控制，达到了预期的防治效果。由于全球基金项目的成功实施，也使得该县于2007年顺利通过了四川省基本消除疟疾达标考核，达到了卫生部颁布的《基本消除疟疾标准》，较《2006—2015年四川省疟疾防治规划》中2009年达标的要求整整提前了两年，取得了非常显著的社会经济效益。四川省全球基金疟疾项目综合评价为A。

项目县筠连县简评：筠连县的项目工作得到了县委、县政府和县卫生行政主管部门的大力支持；县级项目机构健全、项目办公室运转较好，项目信息网络运行正常，财务管理比较规范。按照项目计划开展发热病人血检、高危人群预防性服药等工作，项目进展顺利，实现了项目预期目标。

（七）项目经验

1. 全球基金项目的实施弥补了项目地区疟疾防治经费的缺口，同时国际项目的影响促使各级政府和卫生主管部门更加重视疟疾防治并从多方面积极支持，从而极大地推动了项目地区的疟疾防治工作。

2. 项目的实施培养了一批疟疾防治骨干和具有国际理念的项目管理人员，使疟疾防治工作制度化、科学化。

3. 针对项目地区疟疾流行特点采取了以控制传染源为主的综合性防治措施，全面加强防治。疟疾患者是主要传染源之一，通过对广大群众进行疟防知识宣传教育，并对临床医生进行疟疾诊治技能培训，使疟疾患者能及时主动就医，接受规范治疗，从而使患者及时治愈，不至于成为传染源。这对控制流行起了重要作用；通过建立发热病人镜检站、反复开展镜检人员培训，扩大血检覆盖范围使疟疾病人能早发现、早诊断，漏诊、误诊大大减少，亦对控制传染源、阻断传播起到了重要作用。

4. 疟疾防治离不开患者的密切配合与支持，离不开疫区群众的参与。项目实施中采用授课、会议宣讲、张贴宣传画、分发宣传册等多种形式开展全民疟防知识宣传教育，提高了广大群众的疟疾防治知识水平，增强了自我防病能力。群众对疟疾防治活动的依从性增强，患病后及时主动就医，积极主动配合预防工作。

5. 疫情漏报是疟防工作的老大难。项目实施中在对全县医务人员开展传染病防治法教育的基础上，全面推行疟疾疫情零报告、旬报告制度，强化疫情报告，使得项目县疫情漏报率逐渐降低。

6. 项目实施中充分的信息交流是发现问题、调控项目进度与质量的基础。通过与省、市、县政府和卫生行政部门加强沟通，获得了大力支持和密切合作，确保了项目工作顺利开展。省、市、县的逐级督导确保了项目实施质量的不断提高。

7. 项目实施中项目人员与财务人员及时、有效的沟通非常必要，既保证了资金的合理使用，又提高了资金的使用效率。

（八）今后工作建议

1. 由于全球基金项目的实施，筠连县的疟疾防治取得了显著成绩。但是疟疾具有传播快，易反复的特点，且疟疾流行的因素在当地尚未根本改变，仍然存在一些尚需解决的问题，主要表现为：乡村两级疟防人员不稳定，业务水平需进一步提高；部分乡、村专业人员对疟防工作产生了麻痹松劲思想；健康教育活动还需广泛深入地开展。因此，疟防工作不能松懈麻痹，需继续加强疟疾监测。密切关注当前疟疾传播与发病特点，及时调整防治策略，彻底消除残存病灶点，并加强基层卫生防疫人员的技术培训和流动人口的管理，防治疟情反弹。

2. 将全球基金的管理模式广泛地运用到全省的疾病防治工作中，进一步提高疾病防治的质量和管理的水平。

四川省全球基金疟疾项目办公室

2008 年 5 月 23 日

十、贵州省项目终期总结报告

贵州省全球基金疟疾项目办 5 年来在全球基金国家疟疾项目办的统一安排、统一管理下，在省卫生厅、省疾控中心各级领导的大力支持下，经过各级项目实施人员共同努力，基本圆满完成了项目的各项工作任务。通过项目的实施，贵州省项目县及项目乡镇疟防人员在技能上得到很大的提高，设备仪器也得到了一定的改善。积极推动和改善了项目地区的疟防工作。现将贵州省项目结题报告汇报如下：

（一）项目概况

贵州省第一轮全球基金疟疾项从2003年4月1日起开始实施，到2008年3月31日结束，共计5年时间，分为两个阶段实施。第一阶段为前两年，主要任务有：(1)项目工作人员培训；(2)项目疟疾基线调查；(3)项目地区居民疟疾的早期诊治及个人防护；(4)疟防知识的健康教育。第二阶段为后三年，主要任务有：(1)项目地区居民疟疾的早期诊治及个人防护；(2)流行季节主动监测；(3)疟疾暴发流行的控制；(4)疟疾控制项目的管理。总体来说，贵州省实施全球基金疟疾项目的目的是及时发现和治疗输入性疟疾病例，减少由输入性疟疾病例导致的当地传播。有效的遏制当地疟疾发病。

（二）项目剩余资金使用情况

项目资金截至结题之日，剩余金额零元。

（三）项目设备物资盘点情况

5年来，由国家项目办下拨到贵州省的物资主要有：三目多功能显微镜1台，双目生物显微镜9台，DELL台式电脑5台，东芝笔记本电脑2台，喷墨彩色打印机1台，SONY数码相机1台，传真机1台。由省项目办利用项目经费购买的物资主要有：联想电脑10台（下拨7台），联想激光打印机5台，东芝多媒体投影仪1台，松下传真机3台。目前所有设备都处于正常使用中。

（四）5年工作总结

1．项目管理

省项目办对项目的管理严格按照国家项目办编写的项目管理执行指导手册进行指导管理。贵州省项目管理主要采取：(1)项目常规管理：项目采取主任负责制；原始数据资料的归档管理等。(2)项目季度报表管理：季度数据核查；报表专人管理制；报表按时、如实上报。(3)项目重点业务活动执行管理：发热病人血检阳性片和阴性片的定时抽查；镜检培训；病人规范治疗及用药记录等。(4)经费使用管理：严格遵守《全球基金财务管理手册》，按计划、预算使用经费，专款专用等。(5)

物资管理：严格按照《全球基金物资管理和使用规定》执行；物资发放要有计划和方案等。

2. 监督与评价管理

省项目办严格按照国家项目办制定的督导评价计划执行方案进行监督和评价。如对目标二和目标四各项任务、指标的督导、考核、评价等。

3. 财务管理

5 年来，贵州省累计资金收入共 780 870.94，其中目标二累计收入 558 786.08 元，目标四累计收入 222 084.86 元。累计支出共 667 174.18 元，其中目标二累计收入 522 472.29 元，目标四累计收入 144 701.89 元。

在财务管理上，省项目办严格按照《全球基金项目财务管理手册》进行管理。严格按照工作任务、目标、计划专款专用，不搁置、截留和挪用，规范使用经费，账物对应，账目清楚。按时、如实上报财务季度报表，正常有序开展项目财务工作。

4. 物资采购管理

5 年来，省项目办累计收到的固定资产和物资主要有：三目多功能显微镜 1 台，双目生物显微镜 9 台，DELL 台式电脑 5 台，东芝笔记本电脑两台，喷墨彩色打印机 1 台，SONY 数码相机 1 台，传真机 1 台。折合人民币共计 173 934.4 元；累计下拨的固定资产和物资主要有：电脑 13 台，激光打印机 1 台，传真机 1 台。折合人民币共计 84 017.35 元。

贵州省项目对项目物资的采购严格按照国家统一招标正常渠道进行采购。遵照物资采购制度，使账物相互对应，保证项目资金的正确使用，以防项目经费挪用、他用、流失等不良现象发生。

5. 项目执行进展

项目执行 5 年来，各项项目活动、任务、指标都基本圆满完成。具体执行情况如下：

5.1 省项目办成立及项目启动：2003 年 5 月按国家项目办要求成立了由省卫生厅、省疾控中心共同组成的“全球基金贵州省疟疾项目办公室”。同时召开了第一阶段项目启动会。在 2005 年 7 月召开第二阶段项目启动会。

5.2 项目基线调查：2003 年 6 月在项目点榕江县，由省、州、县共 13 名调查人员经过 11 天奋战，共调查了 4 个乡镇 12 个行政村、1 030 户、4 738 人。按项目计划要求圆满完成基线调查工作。

5.3 基层医生培训：项目计划举办一次培训班、培训人数 29 人，实际举办培训班 5 次，共计培训 135 人。超计划完成了项目培训任务。大大提高了基层医生的疟防能力。

5.4 健康教育：省项目办严格按照项目计划要求在项目县完成各项健康教育工

作。在项目地区开展中小学生疟防知识健康教育，参加学生共计 2 366 人。组织群众健康教育座谈 1 次。与县电视台合作制作疟防知识专题宣教节目 1 期。在公共场所张贴疟疾宣传海报 1 360 张，发放宣传单 5 840 份，疟防知识手册 780 本，疟防知识练习本 2 366 本。进一步提高了当地群众的防疟能力。

5.5 按项目计划要求免费向居民发放杀虫剂浸泡蚊帐 126 顶，改善了部分居民防蚊设施条件，大大降低了这些居民的人蚊接触机会。

5.6 暴发点处理：省 5 年来由于在项目县未出现疟疾暴发点。因此在暴发点处理上未完成项目计划的暴发流行 20 次的任务。

5.7 发病情况：5 年共计发病 218 例，均为间日疟，其中血检阳性病例 87 例，临床诊断 131 例，治疗疟疾病人 218 人，治疗率 100%。在治疗病人上严格按照项目要求足量全程进行治疗。效果显著，基本无复发病例。

5.8 流动人口疟疾监测：计划外出回归人群血检 4 500 人实际完成 3 615 人，完成率 80.33%，计划外来人口血检 1 500 人实际完成 1 417 人，完成率 94.47%。血检发现阳性病例 12 例，临床诊断病例 8 例。实际血检数低于项目计划数，原因是在流动人口监测期间，由于外来人数和回归人数较少，低于计划监测人数，因此未完成项目计划监测任务。

5.9 居民发热病人血检：项目计划完成居民发热病人血检 50 868 人，实际完成 63 773 人，完成率 125.37%，血检发现阳性病例 49 例，临床诊断病例 99 例。超计划完成项目居民发热病人血检任务要求。

5.10 哨点主动监测：计划完成居民普查 18 000 人，实际完成 18 903 人，完成率 105.02%血检，发现阳性病例 16 例，临床诊断病例 24 例。哨点主动监测达到了项目计划任务要求。

5.11 保护高危人群：项目计划高危人群预防服药 6 000 人，实际完成高危人群预防服药 5 424 人，完成率 90.4%，未达到项目任务要求。主要原因是由于在 2005 年和 2006 年国家抗疟药供应相对缺乏。

5.12 项目计划召开年会 3 次，省项目办实际召开年会 3 次。召开项目年会达到项目计划要求。会议上省项目办按国家项目办及项目计划书的要求对项目工作进行了总结和评价。并对发现的问题进行整改。

5.13 项目督导：根据项目计划要求，县项目办 5 年来计划对乡镇进行督导 130 次，实际对乡镇进行督导了 139 次，完成率 106.92%，省项目计划对县项目办及其相关乡镇进行督导 9 次，实际督导 20 次。完成率 222.22%，省、县超计划完成项目计划督导任务。

5.14 存在的问题和建议：(1) 乡镇镜检员镜检水平较低，较难发现阳性疟疾病例，有待进一步加强专业培训；(2) 省、县项目办疟防资料存放不规整，有关疟疾项目资料收集不齐，有待改进；(3) 贵州省近年来疟疾暴发时有发生，疟防工作仍然艰巨，希望国家加大对贵州省疟防工作的支持。

（五）项目地区疟疾疫情现状

项目实施以来，项目地区疟疾发病数逐年呈上升状态。发病率由实施时 2003 年 0.52 ／万上升到 2007 年 4.21 ／万。这种现象是由于项目实施以后，疟疾防治工作逐步得到了地方政府卫生行政部门的重视，各项疟防措施逐步得到了具体落实，特别是疟疾的监测工作。使得该地区的疟疾疫情真正的显现出来。这打破了过去有病不报、怕报、瞒报，担心影响抗疟成绩，影响政绩的思想观念。从而出现了项目实施以后，发病率上升的现象。

（六）疟疾项目对项目地区疟疾防治工作的影响

项目的实施对项目地区疟疾防治工作的影响主要有 4 个方面：(1) 使疟疾防治工作进一步得到了地方各级政府卫生行政部门以及有关卫生部门的重视，确保了疟防工作的正常开展。为进一步具体落实各项疟防措施奠定了牢固的基础。(2) 项目的实施，为项目地区提供了部分的疟防经费以及必要的仪器设备（显微镜、电脑、玻片等）。为正常、有序、有效开展疟防工作提供了有力的保证。(3) 通过项目的实施不仅丰富了项目地区各级疟防人员的业务知识，同时也大大提高了项目地区各级疟防人员的业务技术能力。为项目地区疟防工作提供了技术保障。(4) 通过项目实施，项目地区积极开展了疟疾防治知识的健康宣传教育工作，大大提高了该地区居民的疟防知识知晓率。同时进一步提高了人民群众得病就诊的主动性。为疟防工作的顺利开展奠定了牢固的群众基础。

（七）5 年项目执行评价

项目实施 5 年来，通过各级项目工作人员的共同积极努力，项目各项任务、指标基本圆满完成。发热病人血检：任务完成率 125.37%，经费执行率 133.22%，评估得分 35 分；预防服药：完成率 90.40%，经费执行率 86.93%，评估得分 15 分；疟疾暴发流行控制：完成率 0，经费执行率 0，评估得分 0 分；疫情报告网络运行维护：经费执行率 124.75% ；省项目办日常管理：经费执行率 103.84% ；项目办年会：任务完成率 100%，经费执行率 124.88%，评估得分 10 分；项目督导：完成率为 106.67%，执行率 101.30%，评估得分 30 分。项目任务执行评估最终得分 90 分，因无暴发流行的发生，从而未完成5年项目计划控制疟疾暴发流行20次的任务被扣10分；其余的项目指标；项目的管理能力、项目的督导、评价管理能力、项目财务管理及物资管理评估得分都在90分以上。

省级项目总体评价得分92.2分，县级项目总体评价得分90.6分。项目综合评价得分91.24分，等级为A级。

（八）成效与经验

项目执行5年来，贵州省疟疾防治工作取得的成效和经验主要有4个方面：(1) 疟疾防治工作得到了政府卫生行政部门以及各卫生部门的重视；(2) 基层疟疾防治工作人员的业务知识和业务技能得到了大大的提高；(3) 通过健康宣传教育提高了群众的疟防知识知晓率，加深了群众对疟疾以及疟防工作的认识。为疟防工作的开展奠定了牢固的群众基础；(4) 项目的执行使各项疟防措施得到了具体落实，提高了病人的早期诊断、规范治疗以及个人防护能力，同时大大减少了疟疾的漏报。

项目执行后，项目地区得到了必要的经费、设备的支持，使该地区疟防工作得到了正常有效地开展。真实的疫情逐步得到了真实的体现。现在项目结束，而该地区虽然降低了一定的漏报，但漏报仍然存在，疟疾发病仍然严重。疟防工作仍需继续加强。从而项目地区面临的挑战是项目结束后，缺少项目经费等方面的支持，将如何继续做好项目地区的疟疾防治工作，降低漏报，遏制疟疾。

应对思路是：争取政府加大疟防经费的支持，业务上级部门继续加强对项目地区业务技术的指导，加强基层业务疟防队伍的建设和培训。使该地区疟防工作继续正常、有效、稳定的开展。降低漏报，遏制疟疾，降低疟疾发病，减少或控制疟疾暴发流行的发生。也希望国家今后加大对贵州省疟防工作的支持。

（九）项目县简评

贵州省项目县榕江县实施项目5年来，严格按照项目要求认真执行。根据项目要求基本圆满完成了项目的各项任务、指标。

发热病人血检：任务完成率125.37%，经费执行率133.22%，评估得分35分；预防服药：完成率90.40%，经费执行率86.93%，评估得分15分；疟疾暴发流行控制：完成率0，经费执行率0，评估得分0分；疫情报告网络运行维护：经费执行率124.75%；省项目办日常管理：经费执行率103.84%；项目办年会：任务完成率100%，经费执行率124.88%，评估得分10分；项目督导：完成率为106.92%，执行率101.30%，评估得分30分。项目任务执行评估最终得分90分，因无暴发流行的发生，从而未完成5年项目计划控制疟疾暴发流行20次的任务被扣10分；

其余的项目指标达标评估得分96分；项目的管理能力评估得分92分；项目的督导、评价管理能力评估得分93分；项目财务管理及物资管理评估得分90.05分。县级项目总体评价得分90.6分。

总体来说，榕江县执行项目5年来，工作上实事求是，踏实肯干。严格按照项目的任务、指标要求认真执行，遵守项目的各项规章制度。通过项目工作人员的共同积极努力，达到了项目实施的目的和要求。

贵州省全球基金疟疾项目办公室

2008年6月23日

第二章

终期评估报告

一、背景

2003年，第一轮中国全球基金疟疾项目—《中国高传播区疟疾控制项目》获得全球抗击艾滋病、结核病和疟疾基金（GF）资助，用于有效遏制项目省疟疾流行，阻断多重抗性恶性疟的传播与扩散。

项目预期执行5年（2003年4月1日至2008年3月31日），总预算6 406 659.00美元。覆盖云南省25个边境县，海南省有恶性疟传播的10个山区县，以及河南、湖北、安徽、江苏、广东、广西、四川、贵州8个省（区）各1—2个试点县，直接目标人群930万。项目旨在通过加强对项目地区疟疾的及时诊断、规范治疗和有效防护、加强云南边境地区流动人口疟疾管理、开展健康教育和健康促进、加强疟疾监测和项目管理能力等措施，遏制项目省疟疾流行，并有效控制多重抗性恶性疟的传播与扩散。

按照资助方GF的提议，委托中国国家协调委员会（CCM）组织评估组开展对第一轮中国全球基金疟疾项目的终期评估。在各项目省开展自评估的基础上，依据各项目省上报的自评估报告，评估组进行了认真的讨论与分析，选择项目主要覆盖省份—云南省和海南省，于2008年5月13日—5月31日，抽取这两个项目省的5个项目县11个项目乡镇进行了现场终期评估。其中在云南省分别抽查了省项目办、景洪市、陇川县、腾冲县，并抽查了3个项目县的6个项目乡（镇）及5个村卫生室；在海南省分别抽查了省项目办、白沙县、琼中县，并抽查了2个项目县5个项目乡（镇）及3个村卫生室。本次终期评估主要评估了项目计划和指标完成情况及工作质量，各级项目办的执行能力，以及项目对各级常规疟防的促进作用。

二、项目终期评估组成员

（一）云南组

组长：CCM疟疾专项工作组成员单位
　　阳光医生项目组　　徐东方
成员：中国CDC寄生虫病所　　潘嘉云
　　浙江省CDC寄生虫病防制所　　姚立农

中国 CDC 规财处　　　　　　　　　　赵桂英
中国 PR 采购部　　　　　　　　　　王　宇
陪同人员：国家项目办公室
项目主管：夏志贵
项目官员：贺杰、黄颖、金璟

（二）海南组

组长：CCM 疟疾专项工作组成员单位
中华预防医学会　　　　　　　　　　辛美哲
副组长：中国疾病预防控制中心（CCDC）审计处　袁灵华
成员：CCM 疟疾专项工作组成员单位
中国少数民族经济研究会　　　　　　刘世贵
全球基金中国地方代理机构　　　　　徐岭峰
中国 PR 采购部　　　　　　　　　　王　宇
陪同人员：国家项目办公室
项目主管：夏志贵
项目官员：贺杰、黄颖、金璟

三、项目终期评估目的

（一）评估项目计划和指标完成情况及工作质量。

（二）评估项目投入产出效果及对各级常规疟防的促进作用。

（三）为各级更好地落实国家疟疾防治规划和实施全球基金资助项目提供参考建议。

四、项目终期评估原则

（一）坚持独立、科学、客观、公正的评估原则。

（二）终期评估由各级卫生行政部门领导，各级疾病控制中心、寄生虫病预防控制所负责具体的组织实施，各级项目办配合评估实施并提供相关支持。

（三）为保证所抽查县（市）的代表性，使本次评估期间抽查的县（市）能代表项目两个主要项目省份（云南省和海南省）的整体情况，在云南省随机抽查 3 个项目县，即两个自评估县和 1 个非自评估县，每县抽查两个项目乡镇，即 1 个县项目办核实过资料的乡镇和 1 个县项目办未核实过资料的乡镇；在海南省随机抽查两个项目县，即 1 个自评估县和 1 个非自评估县，每县抽查两个项目乡镇，即 1 个县项目办核实过资料的乡镇和 1 个县项目办未核实过资料的乡镇；通过在各级抽查核实自评估的部分内容检验各级自评估的真实性和可靠性。

（四）根据抽查结果评价各级自评估的真实性和可靠性，在此基础上依据各级的自评结果做出整体评价。

五、项目终期评估的内容

（一）项目工作计划完成情况

按各级的项目工作计划内容进行计划完成率和预算执行率评估。

（二）项目考核指标达标情况

按终期专项调查结果评估以下 6 项指标。

1. 疟疾调查推断发病率；
2. 海南省项目县恶性疟调查推断发病率；
3. 中小学生能够正确回答至少 3 个与疟疾相关问题的比例；
4. 发热病人在症状出现两天内求诊的比例；
5. 拥有杀虫剂浸泡蚊帐的家庭比例；
6. 网络直报疟疾病人比例。

（三）项目管理及监督与评估管理

1. 项目管理能力

1.1 项目办公室建设和运转情况

1.1.1 项目办机构健全、规章制度完善；

1.1.2 各项目省、县按计划召开或参加项目年会、例会。

1.2 项目工作计划和总结

1.2.1 制定项目年度和季度工作计划；

1.2.2 制定各项具体活动的实施方案；

1.2.3 项目工作记录规范；

1.2.4 项目活动有总结；

1.2.5 按规定及时上报项目报表和报告。

1.3 项目培训

1.3.1 按计划开展项目培训活动；

1.3.2 项目管理和执行人员按要求参加有关的项目培训。

2．M&E 管理能力

2.1 有专人负责项目数据报表的收集、审核、汇总和上报工作；

2.2 项目季度报表上报及时、填写规范、数据准确；

2.3 项目办有 M&E 工作指南和模板；

2.4 组织开展或参加相关培训；

2.5 项目督导规范、有成效。

（四）项目财务管理及物资管理

1．项目财务管理能力

1.1 财务人员队伍建设

1.1.1 各级项目办财务人员配置是否齐全；

1.1.2 各级项目办财务不相容职务是否分人担任；

1.1.3 财务人员与项目人员是否经常沟通。

1.2 预算制订与预算执行

1.2.1 财务人员是否参与、了解项目预算；

1.2.2 项目支出标准是否符合预算；

1.2.3 项目资金的使用是否与工作计划相对应；

1.2.4 预算调整是否有批准。

1.3 项目资金管理

1.3.1 银行账号是否独立设置；

1.3.2 是否严格遵守中国人民银行颁布的《现金管理暂行条例》和《银行存款支付结算办法》；

1.3.3 现金日记账和银行存款日记账是否账实相符；

1.3.4 是否使用“全球基金项目空白票据购置、领用登记簿”，及时登记空白票据的购入、使用和结存。

1.4 项目财务管理

1.4.1 是否有项目财务管理、物资管理相关制度及实施情况；

1.4.2 项目资金支出是否严格执行授权批准制度，是否使用全球基金专用凭证；

1.4.3 项目资金使用是否合规；

1.4.4 是否将全球基金资金按照病种建账管理、是否分工作目标进行财务核算；

1.4.5 是否使用《全球基金财务管理手册》规定的会计科目进行财务核算，科目使用是否合理。

1.5 财务报表及会计档案管理

1.5.1 调阅财务季报、半年报和年报，是否账表相符；

1.5.2 省、市、县级项目每年是否进行了审计，是否有审计报告；

1.5.3 调阅项目开始至今的会计资料，检查财务票据、账簿、报表的装订和保管情况。

2．物资采购供应管理能力

2.1 项目固定资产和药品的采购是否按工作计划完成，是否及时下拨给省、县级项目点；

2.2 项目固定资产和药品的调拨、领用手续是否健全；

2.3 是否按照《全球基金财务管理手册》的要求，建立相应的固定资产和项目物品辅助账；

2.4 清点全球基金项目固定资产和药品，检查账实是否相符。

3．财务管理及物资管理评估的主要指标

3.1 资金管理情况分析：项目资金到位率、项目资金使用率；

3.2 预算执行情况分析：总预算执行率、未执行预算支出率、预算调整率；

3.3 会计核算情况分析：出纳核算差错率、会计记账差错率、库存现金准确率、银行存款准确率；

3.4 报表管理情况分析：财务报表上报及时率、财务报表上报准确率；

3.5 物资管理情况分析：项目物资采购完成率、固定资产完好率、项目药品使用率、存货完好率。

（五）项目地区疟防投入

1．卫生行政部门组织和支持项目活动

1.1 卫生行政部门将本项目作为疟疾防治规划的重要部分；

1.2 卫生行政部门对项目的支持与参与程度。

2．疟疾防治资金投入

（六）受益人群对项目的满意度。

六、项目终期评估的实施方法

采用逐级抽样的方法确定进行项目评估的项目点，按以下工作程序在省项目办和抽查的项目县进行现场评估：

1．听取该项目办自我评估报告，就关心的问题与座谈人员交流。

2．座谈后，以逐层抽查核实的方式，通过查阅项目活动、项目管理、财务与物资管理的工作记录、文件、资料等资料，或者咨询项目办工作人员抽查核实自评表的可靠性，并对评估表中各项内容评分。

3．在项目县，抽查两个项目乡镇（1 个县项目办核实过资料的乡镇和 1 个县项目办未核实过资料的乡镇）进行实地调查核实，通过考察乡卫生院血检登记、所保存血片的合格度、镜检员镜检能力、乡防保室、村诊所能否规范治疗疟疾病人等方式核实各项原始资料的汇总数据是否真实、准确。

4．根据核查结果完成现场评估表。

5．根据现场评估结果，与当地项目管理和实施机构进行反馈交流，并据此调整评分。

七、项目终期评估结果

（一）工作计划完成情况

1．本次评估对于工作计划完成情况的考核采用逐层抽查核实

1.1 在国家项目办审核各省自评报告，并与项目报表核对。

1.2 在云南省项目办和海南省项目办抽查核实自评估表中工作计划完成情况的部分数据。

1.3 在云南省第一轮项目的 25 个项目县内抽查景洪市、陇川县、腾冲县 3 个项目县，其中陇川县、腾冲县为云南省自评估县，景洪市为非自评估县；在海南省一轮项目的 10 个项目县内抽查白沙县、琼中县两个项目县，其中白沙县为海南省自评估县，琼中县为非自评估县。

1.4 云南省：在景洪市抽查了勐养镇卫生院、勐龙镇卫生院和勐龙镇曼伞村卫生室；在陇川县抽查了陇把乡卫生院、景罕镇卫生院、陇把乡弄安村卫生室和景罕镇曼面村卫生室；在腾冲县抽查了蒲川乡卫生院、固东镇卫生院、蒲川乡下甲村卫生室和固东镇河头村卫生室。

1.5 海南省：在白沙县抽查了白沙镇卫生院、元门乡卫生院和元门乡翁村；在琼中县抽查了长征镇卫生院、和平镇卫生院、乘坡农场卫生院、和平镇贝湾村以及乘坡农场 7 队卫生室。

2．抽查核实的内容

2.1 在国家项目办核对了各省自评报告与项目报表上报数值。

2.2 在云南省抽查核实了2006—2007年部分月份各级发热病人血检人数和疟疾病人得到规范治疗的人数。

2.3 在海南省抽查核实了2007年7至12月各级杀虫剂免费浸泡蚊帐数和本地居民疟疾病人得到规范治疗的人数。

3．核查结果

3.1 上报国家项目办的各省自评报告上报数与项目报表上报数基本一致。

3.2 云南省：省项目办、陇川县、腾冲县的各项目点自评汇总数据与核查数值基本一致。景洪市虽然市项目办自评汇总数据与核查数值基本相符，但是景洪市勐养镇卫生院由于被抽查月份血检登记和病人处方未标记区分流动人口和本地居民，不能很好的分别核查其血检与治疗人数，且其2006年11月血检总数与上报数值有偏差，被抽查月份血检上报数为450，核查数为263，疟疾病人治疗数上报数为155，核查值为110；勐龙镇曼伞村卫生室原始资料缺失，无法核查其疟疾病人治疗情况。（核查数值参见表2–1、表2–2）

根据抽查核实结果，虽然云南省各项目县自评汇总数据的准确性存在一定差异，但整体而言第一轮云南省全球基金疟疾项目省级自评和各项目县自评结果是准确可信的。

3.3 海南省：各级汇总上报数值和核查数值基本相符，根据抽查核实结果，第一轮海南省全球基金疟疾项目省级自评和各项目县自评结果是准确可信的。（核查数值参见表2–3、表2–4）

3.4 根据抽查核实结果，虽然被抽查的各项目县自评汇总数据的准确性存在一定差异，但就其整体而言仍然表明本次终期评估期间云南省和海南省省级自评和各项目县自评结果是准确可信的。因此，根据自评结果，第一轮中国全球基金疟疾项目基本上按照工作计划完成了有关项目工作，截至2008年3月31日，各项目省、县均按计划开展各项目活动，已累计培训乡村医生和镜检员12 305人次，累计血检发热病人2 530 245例，治疗疟疾病人493 403例，完成杀虫剂浸泡蚊帐365 039顶，公共场所张贴疟疾防治宣传画259 554份，开展中小学生疟疾知识培训12 644班次，经广播、电视进行疟防知识专题宣传516县次，各项项目工作有力地推动了中国的疟疾防治。（参见表2–5、表2–6）

（二）项目考核指标达标情况

2008年1月，按照项目工作计划，国家项目办安排云南省25个项目县和海南省10个项目县开展了终期专项调查，终期专项调查调查了“疟疾调查推断发病率”

等 6 项指标，终期专项调查结果显示第一轮云南省全球基金疟疾项目的总目标已基本完成，而第一轮海南省全球基金疟疾项目除发热病人在症状出现两天内求诊的比例稍低于项目终期目标，疟疾病例通过信息网络报告的比例这项指标由于部分市县乡镇级的疫情网络直报系统不够健全，致使病例漏报还比较严重，漏报率还比较高外，其余指标均达到或超过规定的指标比例，项目的总目标已基本完成。两省终期专项调查汇总结果显示：第一轮中国全球基金疟疾项目的总目标已经基本实现，云南省项目县疟疾调查推算发病率由 2002 年 195/ 万的基线下降到 65.88/ 万，下降了 66.22%；海南省项目县疟疾调查推算发病率和恶性疟调查推算发病率分别由 2002 年的 385/ 万和 9.06/ 万下降到 31.13/ 万和 0.40/ 万，分别下降了 91.91% 和 95.58%。

本次评估对于项目考核指标达标情况的考核采用逐层抽查核实，在核实云南省项目办和海南省项目办终期专项调查工作方案和汇总结果的基础上，抽查核实了云南省的景洪市项目办、陇川县项目办、腾冲县项目办的原始材料和海南省的白沙县项目办、琼中县项目办的原始材料，核查数值与上报数值基本无误差，根据核查结果，从对这 5 个项目县的抽查情况来看，第一轮中国全球基金疟疾项目的本次终期专项调查个项目县上报结果基本上是真实可信的，根据终期专项调查结果，第一轮中国全球基金疟疾项目已基本达到项目实施的总目标。（参见表 2–7、表 2–8）

（三）项目执行能力

本次评估通过对项目管理能力、监督与评估管理能力和财务及物资管理能力三个方面的考核评价云南省和海南省项目执行机构的项目执行能力，以此为基础对第一轮中国全球基金疟疾项目各级项目执行机构的项目执行能力做出综合评价。

在考核过程中，我们根据翻阅有关资料和与相关负责人员会谈、咨询所了解到的信息，对各级项目办就“项目终期评估的内容”中的“项目管理及监督与评估管理”和“项目财务管理及物资管理”给予考核评价。

根据对各级项目办的考核，各级项目办项目执行能力基本达到项目终期评估要求（参见表 2–12、表 2–18）：

1. 项目管理和监督与评估管理。各级项目办组织机构健全，制度基本完善，管理比较规范，工作有计划，活动有方案、有记录、有总结，并能够较好的保存原始支撑材料，项目报表上报及时，填写规范，对下级项目执行机构能按照工作计划开展项目督导，督导有成效。乡、村级项目执行机构大多数工作人员工作认真，有责任感，血检、治疗有登记有记录，基本完成上级项目办交办的任务。绝大多数村医能制作、送检血片，部分村医能开展镜检工作。但是在部分较薄弱的项目县，仍然存在着部分血检、治疗等活动数据与原始记录不一致，部分镜检员能力未完全过关，血片制片过程中涂片、染色不够规范等问题。需要督促这些县项目办提高项目执行能力，注意做好报表的审核工作，确保上报数据的准确性，并进一步加强乡村级的血检、疟疾治疗能力及项目管理能力建设。

2．财务管理。截至 2008 年 3 月 31 日，第一轮中国全球基金疟疾项目累计经费预算数为 6 406 659 美元，累计实际收入人民币 52 867 661.09 元（含利息收入），累计实际支出人民币 49 708 293.70 元，累计预算完成率为 97.13%，项目经费结余人民币 3 087 367.39 元；尽管在财务管理上还有需要加强的地方，但整体而言，各级项目办基本能够按照《全球基金财务管理手册》要求进行项目财务管理和会计核算工作，设立了全球基金独立银行账号，财务人员配置齐全，项目资金的使用基本与工作计划相对应，没有发现挤占挪用项目资金的情况；使用了全球基金项目空白票据购置、领用登记簿，及时登记了空白票据的购入、使用和结存；制定了相关的项目财务管理、物资管理制度，项目资金支出严格执行了授权批准制度，使用了全球基金专用凭证；对项目资金按照分工作目标进行财务核算，科目使用基本合理，基本能够做到账表相符、账实相符；省、市、县级的年度财务报表都进行了外部审计，并有审计报告存档；内部控制制度基本健全，会计档案管理规范。（参见表 2–9、表 2–10）

3．物资采购供应管理。目前，按照结题计划第一轮中国全球基金疟疾项目办正会同中国中央执行机构（PR）采购部进行物资清查，拟定物资处置方案，待物资清查完毕、确定物资处置方案后，将按照物资处置方案移交项目剩余物资。尽管在物资采购供应管理上还有需要加强的地方，但整体而言，各级项目办对项目物资的管理、使用、存储、发放情况总体情况良好。项目物资有专人管理，能够及时下拨给下级项目点。项目物资入库、领用、验收、调拨手续齐全。按照全球基金管理要求，建立了固定资产和物品辅助账。物资库存情况良好，项目物资单独、分类存放，库房清洁、干燥、防盗措施齐全，库存物资结余数量与辅助账核对无误。经过项目 5 年的运行，物资管理水平得到了大幅度提高。（参见表 2–11）

（四）项目地区疟防投入

根据与各级卫生行政部门领导及有关人员的座谈，我们发现：全球基金项目资金投入占各项目地区疟防资金的 52.70%，其中全球基金项目资金投入占云南省全省疟防资金的 87.43%，全球基金项目资金投入占海南省全省疟防资金的 56.75%；第一轮中国全球基金疟疾项目作为中国常规疟疾防治的重要补充，各级卫生行政部门都将其列入疟疾长期规划的重要组成部分，将项目的执行和实施作为重要的疟疾工作内容，并在其中直接参与并给予积极的支持，为项目的实施提供了必要和充足的行政保证。全球基金疟疾项目的实施，对当地的疟疾防治工作起到了有利的推动和积极的促进作用。

（五）受益人群对项目的满意度

第一轮中国全球基金疟疾项目覆盖的疟疾病人及家属对项目提供的疟防服务的满意程度很高。根据对各项目县开展抽样调查所抽取的 5 223 例项目受益人的调查结果，对免费抗疟治疗服务的满意率为 73.99%，对免费杀虫剂浸泡蚊帐服务的满意率为 96.40%，对免费获得宣传材料服务的满意率为 91.48%；整体满意度在 60% 以下的 57 人占 7.39%，整体满意度在 60-80% 的 300 人占 38.91%，整体满意度在 80% 以上的 414 人占 53.70%。

八、项目终期评估结论与建议

（一）结论

根据本次终期评估各项考核指标的考核结果，第一轮中国全球基金疟疾项目较好地完成了项目工作计划各项工作任务，基本达到了项目预期目标；虽然在项目执行过程中还存在着某些问题，但各级项目办的项目执行能力都得到了较大的提高。通过第一轮中国全球基金疟疾项目的实施，项目地区居民防疟、抗疟知识以及个人自我防护、主动就诊意识显著提高，项目地区拥有杀虫剂浸泡蚊帐的家庭比例也都有了很大提高，疟疾漏报率也有所降低；项目地区疟疾疫情得到了有效的控制，多重抗性恶性疟的传播与扩散得到了有效的控制。项目的实施还为各级疾控部门培养了大量的疟防人员，为各级疾控部门培养了一批项目管理人员，丰富了各级项目依托单位的管理理念和经验，提高了乡、村一级卫生人员的抗疟水平，留下了宝贵的经验，增强了疟防力量，为国家疟疾防治规划的实现提供了重要的补充。

项目执行过程中依然存在着一些问题与挑战，需要在今后的项目执行中给予关注、改进：

1. 多数项目县能很好的按照全球基金的要求，认真开展、完成项目活动，但个别项目县项目执行能力有待加强，其项目执行过程中的部分血检、治疗等活动数据与原始记录不一致，需要进一步做好报表的审核工作，确保上报数据的准确性。

2. 部分项目执行机构目前没有保留阴性血片备查，部分乡镇只保留了部分阳性血片，而按照项目要求应保留近期的部分阴性血片和全部的阳性血片；部分县、乡、村级项目执行机构血片制片过程中涂片、染色不够规范，部分乡镇镜检员能力未完全过关，对于低密度的原虫血片容易漏检，部分乡镇的村医不送检血片、未完好的保存病人处方和病例登记表。乡村级的血检、疟疾治疗能力及项目管理能力建设仍需要加强。部分乡镇的村医不送检血片。

3. 个别项目点存在有记账不及时，报销会议和培训费用附件不齐全，财务对下级项目点的督导力度不够，财务人员与项目人员缺乏有效沟通的问题。

4. 部分乡级卫生院物资管理文件、表格不够规范，存在物资下发、领用、库存登记情况不清晰的问题；部分乡级库管人员对项目了解不足，资料分类不清；个别项目点物品辅助账与实际库存情况部分有出入，部分下拨物资未作登记。个别项目点项目办人员对物资到货数量、领用分发、库存结余等情况了解不足。

（二）建议

1. 云南省应进一步加强对薄弱项目县的督导指导工作，加强其项目管理能力，督促县项目办注意做好报表的审核工作，确保上报数据的准确性。同时应该注意进一步加强乡村级项目执行机构的项目执行能力，提高其镜检、治疗操作的规范性及其项目管理能力。

2. 各级镜检机构应在今后的工作中按照有关规定保留更多的血片，以利于血片的复查。继续加强各级特别是乡镇卫生院镜检员能力的培训，不仅提高其判断疟疾血片的能力，也要规范其涂片、染色、镜检、保存等操作的规范性。

3. 在全球基金疟疾项目的财务物资管理方面，建议加强以下各项措施：

3.1 规范报销程序。支付培训、会议费的凭证后面要附有相关的培训、会议通知及承办宾馆开具的盖有公章的决算明细单，支付 1 万元以上的印刷费的凭证后面要附有相关的合同或工作协议，支付大额汽油费的凭证后面必须附里程单。

3.2 加强项目人员和财务人员的有效沟通，财务人员应了解项目预算，定期向项目人员提供项目资金的使用情况分析。

3.3 县项目办要加强对拨付给乡镇卫生院经费的监督，规范乡镇卫生院经费的使用，确保补助的领取和发放落实到个人。

3.4 各省、县项目办要按照《全球基金审计操作指南》的要求开展每年的项目审计工作，提高外部审计报告的质量。

3.5 加强财务人员和物资管理人员的沟通，财务人员对拨入的项目固定资产和药品要及时入账，并与物资管理人员建立定期（每季度或者每半年）对账制度。

3.6 将全球基金项目物资与常规疟防物资分开登记，以便管理和核对。

3.7 各级项目办要按照项目结题计划和终期评估方案的要求使用项目剩余资金，合理处置项目固定资产和剩余药品。

3.8 充分总结全球基金一轮疟疾项目的经验和教训，进一步提高项目财务管理和物资管理水平，使五轮、六轮疟疾项目的财务物资管理工作更规范。

4. 建议全面总结第一轮中国全球基金疟疾项目执行取得的成绩和存在的不足，并合理规划后续项目的设计和实施，注意加强对疟防工作的总体指导及对项目合作伙伴活动的协调管理作用，优化项目资源的配置和管理，确保各项疟防措施取得最佳效果，如长效蚊帐在村级的有效发放。

表 2–1　云南省发热病人血检核查结果

项目点	流动人口发热病人血检人数			本地居民发热病人血检人数			备注
	抽查月份自评汇总上报数	抽查月份实际核查数	符合度(%)	抽查月份自评汇总上报数	抽查月份实际核查数	符合度(%)	
项目点 1:云南省项目办	12 848	12 848	100.00	49 247	49 247	100.00	
项目点 2:景洪市项目办	4 636	4 636	100.00	21 890	21 890	100.00	
项目点 2.1:勐养镇卫生院	190	/	/	260	263	98.85	由于被抽查月份病人处方未标记区分流动人口和本地居民,不能很好的分别核查其血检人数。且其 2006 年 11 月血检总数与上报数值有偏差。
项目点 2.2:勐龙镇卫生院	21	21	100.00	354	343	96.89	
项目点 3:陇川县项目办	463	463	100.00	2 189	2 189	100.00	

续表

项目点 3.1:陇把乡卫生院	/	/	/	/	/	/	因为其乡镇部分村医病人血片直接送县 CDC 检查,但血检人数仍计入该乡镇,血检记录无法核对。
项目点 3.2:景罕镇卫生院	118	82	69.49	303	411	64.36	
项目点 3:腾冲县项目办	787	787	100.00	2 584	2 584	100.00	
项目点 3.1:蒲川乡卫生院	82	82	100.00	202	202	100.00	
项目点 3.2:固东镇卫生院	41	43	95.12	141	141	100.00	

表 2-2 云南省疟疾病人治疗核查结果

项目点	流动人口疟疾病人治疗人数			本地居民疟疾病人治疗人数			备注
	抽查月份自评汇总上报数	抽查月份实际核查数	符合度(%)	抽查月份自评汇总上报数	抽查月份实际核查数	符合度(%)	
项目点 1:云南省项目办	5 207	5 207	100.00	9 983	9 983	100.00	
项目点 2:景洪市项目办	1 360	1 358	99.85	3 658	3 650	99.78	
项目点 2.1:勐养镇卫生院	30	/	/	125	110	/	由于被抽查月份病人处方未标记区分流动人口和本地居民,不能很好的分别核查其治疗人数。

续表

项目点2.2：勐龙镇卫生院	22	22	100.00	27	27	100.00	
项目点2.2.1：勐龙镇曼伞村卫生室	原始资料缺失无法核查			原始资料缺失无法核查			该村卫生室原始资料缺失，无法核查其疟疾病人治疗情况。
项目点3：陇川县项目办	244	244	100.00	628	628	100.00	
项目点3.1：陇把乡卫生院	16	16	100.00	41	41	100.00	
项目点3.1.1：陇把乡弄安村卫生室	1	1	100.00	3	3	100.00	
项目点3.2：景罕镇卫生院	112	109	97.32	173	190	90.17	
项目点3.2.1：景罕镇曼面村卫生室	0	0	/	5	5	100.00	
项目点3：腾冲县项目办	396	396	100.00	1 597	1 597	100.00	
项目点3.1：蒲川乡卫生院	28	28	100.00	133	133	100.00	
项目点3.1.1：蒲川乡下甲村卫生室	0	0	/	10	10	100.00	
项目点3.2：固东镇卫生院	3	3	100.00	127	127	100.00	
项目点3.2.1：固东镇河头村卫生室	0	0	/	8	8	100.00	

表 2-3 海南省杀虫剂浸泡蚊帐数量核查结果

2007 年 7–12 月

项目点	上报上级项目办数值	核查数值	上报数据符合率(%)
海南省项目办	10 386	10 386	100.00
白沙县项目办	1 455	1 455	100.00
白沙镇卫生院	1 765	1 765	100.00
元门乡卫生院	2 036	2 034	99.90
琼中县项目办	1 654	1 654	100.00
长征镇卫生院	991	989	99.80
和平镇卫生院	1 274	1 272	99.84
乘坡农场卫生院	1 099	1 099	100.00
乘坡农场第七村卫生室	52	52	100.00

表 2-4 海南省规范治疗病人数核查结果

2007 年 7–12 月

项目点	上报上级项目办数值	核查数值	上报数据符合率(%)
海南省项目办	4 591	4 591	100.00
白沙县项目办	620	620	100.00
白沙镇卫生院	162	162	100.00
元门乡卫生院	194	193	99.90
琼中县项目办	707	707	100.00
长征镇卫生院	170	172	99.80
和平镇卫生院	228	228	99.84
乘坡农场卫生院	189	190	100.00
乘坡农场第七村卫生室	11	11	100.00

表 2-5 云南省项目工作计划完成情况

项目活动	云南省			景洪市			陇川县			腾冲县		
	计划	实际完成	完成率(%)	计划	实际完成	完成率(%)	计划	实际完成	完成率(%)	计划	实际完成	完成率(%)
目标Ⅰ:使云南的流动人口获得更好的诊断和治疗												
流动人口发热病人血检(人次)	116 000	155 480	134.03	6 245	8 340	133.55	6 195	5 892	95.11	6 565	14 243	216.95
流动人口疟疾病人规范治疗(例)	57 000	56 318	98.80	3 289	2 502	76.07	3 039	2 777	91.38	3 360	3 604	101.17
目标Ⅱ:使项目地区当地居民得到更好的早期诊断和个人防护												
项目地区居民发热病人血检(人次)	422 000	949 105	224.91	39 490	65 465	165.78	33 390	40 027	119.88	38 300	32 828	85.71
项目地区居民疟疾病人规范治疗(例)	224 880	198 912	88.45	12 845	11 663	90.80	16 460	8 436	51.25	17 560	11 137	63.42
乡、村医生/个体医生培训(人次)	5 525	11 614	210.21	440	440	100.00	200	363	226.88	200	350	140.00
疟原虫镜检员培训(人次)	280	251	89.64	2	2	100.00	14	14	100.00	15	13	86.67
杀虫剂浸泡(处理)蚊帐(顶)	225 000	228 443	101.53	5 900	13 686	231.97	10 700	12 281	114.78	11 450	11 594	101.26
目标Ⅲ:使云南省和海南省流行区居民更有效地采取疟疾预防措施												
健康教育材料印制(张、份)	135 500	135 500	100.00	/	/	/	/	/	/	/	/	/
项目市县用广播电视宣传疟疾知识(次)	225	320	142.22	40	85	212.50	5	30	600.00	5	7	140.00
给项目市县中小学生上疟防知识课(班次)	5 000	6 448	128.96	316	401	126.90	260	283	108.85	362	623	172.10
在公共场所张贴疟疾知识宣传画(张、份)	106 000	102 892	97.07	5 950	8 078	135.76	15 900	16 385	103.05	9 850	10 196	103.51
目标Ⅳ:优化云南、海南及其它八个项目省的疟疾控制项目管理												
项目地区哨点病例主动监测(人次)	120 000	126 310	105.26	6 360	6 378	100.42	6 360	7 417	116.62	7 200	7 200	100.00
项目地区药物抗性监测(点次)	4	4	100.00	/	/	/	/	/	/	/	/	/
项目地区专项调查(市县次)	31	31	100.00	1	1	100.00	2	2	100.00	4	4	100.00
召开项目会议(年会、例会)(次)	78	65	83.33	5	5	100.00	5	5	100.00	26	25	96.15
项目督导(市县次)	1 260	1 511	119.92	89	89	100.00	80	81	101.25	40	38	95.00

表 2-6 海南省项目工作计划完成情况

项目活动	海南省			白沙县			琼中县		
	计划	实际完成	完成率(%)	计划	实际完成	完成率(%)	计划	实际完成	完成率(%)
目标Ⅱ:使项目地区当地居民得到更好的早期诊断和个人防护									
项目地区居民发热病人血检(人次)	614 000	636 079	103.60	77 600	79 159	102.01	85 900	78 628	91.53
项目地区居民疟疾病人规范治疗(例)	59 980	56 447	94.11	14 460	14 919	103.17	15 480	12 881	83.21
乡、村医生 / 个体医生培训(人次)	2 400	3 049	127.04	320	333	104.6	160	160	100.00
疟原虫镜检员培训(人次)	330	427	129.39	/	/	/	/	/	/
杀虫剂浸泡(处理)蚊帐(顶)	90 000	112 235	124.71	13 000	20 964	161.26	12 800	18 210	124.71
高危人群预防服药(山寮巡诊 - 寮次)	900	714	79.33	90	70	77.78	90	70	77.78
目标Ⅲ:使云南省和海南省流行区居民更有效地采取疟疾预防措施									
健康教育材料印制(张、份)	125 000	125 000	100.00	/	/	/	/	/	/
健康教育人员培训(人次)	1 020	1 412	138.43	90	99	110	90	99	110.00
项目市县用广播电视进行疟疾知识宣传(次)	60	60	100.00	6	6	100.00	6	6	100.00
给项目市县中小学生上疟防知识课(班次)	2 550	3 673	104.82	300	327	109	305	311	101.97
在公共场所张贴疟疾知识宣传画(张、份)	50 000	52 936	105.87	5 800	5 781	99.67	6 000	6 500	108.33
目标Ⅳ:优化云南、海南及其它八个项目省的疟疾控制项目管理									
项目地区哨点病例主动监测(人次)	60 000	63 014	105.02	8 100	8 169	100.85	7 688	8 865	115.31
项目地区药物抗性监测(点次)	8	8	100.00	/	/	/	/	/	/
项目地区专项调查(市县次)	19	19	100.00	4	4	100.00	2	2	100.00
召开项目会议(年会、例会)(次)	4	4	100.00	10	10	100.00	11	11	100.00
项目督导(市县次)	110	131	119.09	237	237	100.00	255	269	101.57

表 2-7 第一轮云南省全球基金疟疾项目终期专项调查结果

项目点	疟疾调查推断发病率（1/万）		中小学生能正确回答至少3个与疟疾相关问题的比例（%）		发热病人在症状出现2天内求诊的比例（%）		拥有杀虫剂浸泡蚊帐的家庭比例（%）		网络直报疟疾病人比例（%）	
	基线调查值	终期调查值	基线调查值	终期调查值	基线调查值	终期调查值	基线调查值	终期调查值	基线调查值	终期调查值
云南省	196.63	65.88	58.2	94.83	37.95	92.36	4.30	32.36	8.80	45.30
富宁县	1.26	4.16	58.2	85.98	37.95	89.94	4.30	31.42	8.80	40.74
麻栗坡	5.18	17.00	58.2	87.36	37.95	90.63	4.30	31.80	8.80	46.67
澜沧县	84.59	30.33	58.2	99.48	37.95	93.60	4.30	33.38	8.80	40.98
泸水县	1.13	9.83	58.2	99.79	37.95	96.02	4.30	30.28	8.80	50.00
马关县	35.38	17.57	58.2	92.11	37.95	92.81	4.30	34.46	8.80	37.50
勐海县	296.30	36.18	58.2	96.20	37.95	97.20	4.30	35.45	8.80	46.67
福贡县	5.02	25.57	58.2	91.76	37.95	97.95	4.30	32.29	8.80	27.27
龙陵县	20.99	40.82	58.2	99.49	37.95	99.66	4.30	30.11	8.80	58.33
金平县	32.53	79.87	58.2	88.08	37.95	91.20	4.30	34.56	8.80	42.31
江城县	34.42	22.54	58.2	99.74	37.95	94.65	4.30	32.65	8.80	50.00
绿春县	8.54	17.18	58.2	88.78	37.95	92.90	4.30	30.12	8.80	42.86
镇康县	26.18	44.14	58.2	95.63	37.95	93.02	4.30	30.10	8.80	47.62
潞西县	12.94	153.77	58.2	95.82	37.95	97.47	4.30	32.76	8.80	46.88
沧源县	34.54	61.78	58.2	97.26	37.95	45.24	4.30	32.41	8.80	60.00
耿马县	22.51	45.39	58.2	97.29	37.95	93.95	4.30	36.98	8.80	33.33
河口县	28.85	87.73	58.2	96.10	37.95	93.62	4.30	32.27	8.80	46.67
腾冲县	187.19	36.43	58.2	100.00	37.95	90.82	4.30	31.42	8.80	56.76
盈江县	188.10	218.72	58.2	99.25	37.95	100.00	4.30	30.84	8.80	51.43
景洪县	399.90	4.45	58.2	85.46	37.95	93.37	4.30	38.34	8.80	47.62
孟连县	1 089.12	185.87	58.2	99.05	37.95	99.07	4.30	31.37	8.80	42.42
贡山县	27.58	142.1	58.2	99.44	37.95	93.41	4.30	31.31	8.80	35.00
勐腊县	445.36	131.58	58.2	93.11	37.95	52.48	4.30	24.12	8.80	40.54
陇川县	296.12	70.24	58.2	89.22	37.95	90.39	4.30	39.66	8.80	44.44
瑞丽市	273.67	380.43	58.2	96.98	37.95	95.92	4.30	31.60	8.80	48.39
西盟县	4 270.90	340.54	58.2	95.78	37.95	93.64	4.30	30.25	8.80	45.24

表 2-8 第一轮海南省全球基金疟疾项目终期专项调查结果

项目点	疟疾调查推断发病率(1/万)		项目县恶性疟调查推断发病率(1/万)		中小学生正确回答至少3个疟疾相关问题的比例(%)		发热病人在症状出现2天内求诊的比例(%)		拥有杀虫剂浸泡蚊帐的家庭比例(%)		网络直报疟疾病人比例(%)	
	基线调查值	终期调查值	基线调查值	终期调查值	基线调查值	终期调查值	基线调查值	终期调查值	基线调查值	终期调查值	基线调查值	终期调查值
海南省	385	31.33	9.06	0.4	62.57	89.39	54.61	85.27	38.91	52.38	5.02	33.38
万宁市	385	21.46	9.06	0.02	62.57	90.14	62.91	88.81	38.91	51.6	5.02	44.94
陵水县	385	42.4	9.06	0.12	62.57	89.78	56.76	88.33	38.91	51.28	5.02	25.16
保亭县	385	81.76	9.06	0.06	62.57	89.95	50.00	84.02	38.91	60.82	5.02	33.62
五指山	385	18.97	9.06	0.09	62.57	89.23	46.28	85.78	38.91	50.34	5.02	45.45
三亚市	385	5.21	9.06	0.79	62.57	90.83	62.32	85.07	38.91	54.66	5.02	44.23
乐东市	385	39.97	9.06	0.57	62.57	88.6	40.11	84.13	38.91	51.02	5.02	16.18
琼中县	385	61.89	9.06	0.1	62.57	88.32	62.81	85.76	38.91	48.98	5.02	24.44
白沙县	385	64.75	9.06	0.54	62.57	90.62	50.27	82.95	38.91	51.14	5.02	44.07
东方市	385	26.94	9.06	0.72	62.57	88.71	58.22	88.53	38.91	51.98	5.02	41.43
昌江县	385	14	9.06	0.3	62.57	87.23	53.68	86.14	38.91	51.28	5.02	46.15

表 2-9　云南省项目资金收支情况表

填表单位:第一轮云南省全球基金疟疾项目办公室　　　　填表日期:2008 年 3 月 31 日

周期序号	年度	科目	目标 1		目标 2		目标 3		目标 4		合计	
			人民币	百分比(%)	人民币	百分比(%)	人民币	百分比(%)	人民币	百分比(%)	人民币	百分比(%)
项目一期	2003-2004	预算	1 020 000.00	--	1 450 000.00	--	1 080 000.00	--	2 418 320.00	--	5 968 320.00	--
		到款	1 029 537.10	100.94	1 448 809.04	99.92	1 083 994.38	100.37	2 067 391.31	85.49	5 629 731.83	94.33
		支出	985 204.20	96.59	1 403 178.77	96.77	972 308.99	90.03	1 753 369.43	72.50	5 114 061.39	85.69
项目二期	2005	预算	122 560.00	--	1 058 720.00	--	320 800.00	--	902 000.00	--	2 404 080.00	--
		到款	72 346.20	59.03	450 643.30	42.56	174 763.45	54.48	979 200.12	108.56	1 676 953.07	69.75
		支出	137 868.24	112.49	510 141.60	48.18	211 342.33	65.88	1 165 273.46	129.19	2 024 625.63	84.22
	2006	预算	180 000.00	--	1 061 600.00	--	330 000.00	--	950 000.00	--	2 521 600.00	--
		到款	259 802.84	144.33	1 758 614.55	165.66	505 003.30	153.03	917 424.48	96.57	3 440 845.17	136.45
		支出	200 726.91	111.51	1 406 339.59	132.47	502 903.61	152.40	1 353 882.78	142.51	3 463 852.89	137.37
	2007	预算	111 200.00	--	748 000.00	--	104 000.00	--	902 000.00	--	1 865 200.00	--
		到款	117 903.51	106.03	728 965.87	97.46	107 114.13	102.99	1 860 011.02	206.21	2 813 994.53	150.87
		支出	108 492.06	97.56	714 944.42	95.58	109 530.95	105.32	766 356.86	84.96	1 699 324.29	91.11
	2008	预算	7 200.00	--	24 000.00	--	0.00	--	858 000.00	--	889 200.00	--
		到款	0.00	0.00	0.00	0.00	0.00	--	0.00	0.00	0.00	0.00
		支出	8 350.61	115.98	25 629.40	106.79	1 200.00	--	383 993.36	44.75	419 173.37	47.14
累计		预算	1 440 960.00	--	4 342 320.00	--	1 834 800.00	--	6 030 320.00	--	13 648 400.00	--
		到款	1 479 589.65	102.68	4 387 032.76	101.03	1 870 875.26	101.97	5 824 026.93	96.58	13 561 524.60	99.36
		利息	--	--	--	--	--	--	28 948.09	--	28 948.09	--
		支出	1 440 642.02	99.98	4 060 233.78	93.50	1 797 285.88	97.96	5 422 875.89	89.93	12 721 037.57	93.21
		结余	38 947.63	2.63	326 798.98	7.45	73 589.38	3.93	430 099.13	7.38	869 435.12	6.41

注：①预算数根据工作计划填写（折算汇率 1：8），到款数为实际收到 拨款数，支出数为实际支出数，结余数为截止 08 年 3 月 31 日项目资金结余数。

②预算拨付率＝到款数 / 预算数；预算执行率＝支出数 / 预算数；资金结余率＝结余数 / 到款数。

表 2-10 海南省项目资金收支情况表

填表单位:第一轮海南省全球基金疟疾项目办公室　　　　填表日期:2008 年 3 月 31 日

周期序号	年度	科目	目标 1 人民币	目标 1 百分比(%)	目标 2 人民币	目标 2 百分比(%)	目标 3 人民币	目标 3 百分比(%)	目标 4 人民币	目标 4 百分比(%)	合计 人民币	合计 百分比(%)
项目一期	2003—2004	预算	0.00	–	1 446 692.00	–	1 177 540.00	–	740 168.00	–	3 364 400.00	–
		到款	0.00	–	1 223 520.24	84.57	991 390.72	84.19	618 590.56	83.57	2 833 501.52	84.22
		支出	0.00	–	1 226 512.74	84.78	978 490.50	83.10	606 756.74	81.98	2 811 759.98	83.57
项目二期	2005	预算	0.00	–	424 320.00	–	113 600.00	–	363 600.00	–	901 520.00	–
		到款	0.00	–	414 901.84	97.78	287 374.13	252.97	538 142.16	148.00	1 240 418.13	137.59
		支出	0.00	–	405 661.51	95.60	273 708.50	240.94	474 447.07	130.49	1 153 817.08	127.99
	2006	预算	0.00	–	432 000.00	–	43 200.00	–	411 600.00	–	886 800.00	–
		到款	0.00	–	382 594.78	88.56	157 767.76	365.20	357 497.24	86.86	897 859.78	101.25
		支出	0.00	–	403 726.41	93.46	105 464.50	244.13	300 797.38	73.08	809 988.29	91.34
	2007	预算	0.00	–	361 600.00	–	41 600.00	–	363 600.00	–	766 800.00	–
		到款	0.00	–	320 506.04	88.64	18 127.00	43.57	572 084.87	157.34	910 717.91	118.77
		支出	0.00	–	383 397.40	106.03	42 626.00	102.47	344 529.36	94.76	770 552.76	100.49
	2008	预算	0.00	–	28 000.00	–	0.00	–	336 800.00	–	364 800.00	–
		到款	0.00	–	0.00	0.00	0.00	–	0.00	0.00	0.00	0.00
		支出	0.00	–	27 962.02	99.86	1 450.00	–	289 325.79	85.90	318 737.81	87.37
累计		预算	0.00	–	2 692 612.00	–	1 375 940.00	–	2 215 768.00	–	6 284 320.00	–
		到款	0.00	–	2 341 522.90	86.96	1 454 659.61	105.72	2 086 314.83	94.16	5 882 497.34	93.61
		利息	0.00	–	–	–	–	–	12 516.55	–	12 516.55	–
		支出	0.00	–	2 447 260.08	90.89	1 401 739.50	101.88	2 015 856.34	90.98	5 864 855.92	93.33
		结余	0.00	–	−105 737.18	0.00	52 920.11	3.64	82 975.04	3.98	30 157.97	0.48

注：①预算数根据工作计划填写（折算汇率 1∶8），到款数为实际收到拨款数，支出数为实际支出数，结余数为截止 08 年 3 月 31 日项目资金结余数。

②预算拨付率＝到款数 / 预算数；预算执行率＝支出数 / 预算数；资金结余率＝结余数 / 到款数。

表 2-11 海南省项目物资情况调查表

填表单位:第一轮海南省全球基金疟疾项目办公室			填表日期:2008 年 3 月 31 日	
物资名称	数量	总金额(元)	运行状况	备注
显微镜	173 台	712 488.09	良好	
计算机	16 台	169 400.00	良好	
打印机	12 台	27 600.00	良好	
4 轮驱动皮卡车	6 辆	520 800.00	良好	
125C 摩托车	152 辆	576 187.90	良好	
越野车 / 面包车	2 辆	440 649.53	良好	
多媒体投影仪	1 台	17 850.00	良好	
数码相机	1 架	7 840.00	良好	
固定资产小计	–	2 472 815.52	–	–
磷酸氯 / 伯喹片剂	68786 盒	189 485.20	–	
双氢青蒿素片剂	20000 盒	330 000.00	–	
蒿甲醚针剂	9200 盒	315 120.00	–	
复方磷酸哌喹片剂	50 罐	17 000.00	–	
一次性注射器	13500 支	5 900.00	–	
蚊帐	11980 顶	251 960.00	结余:400 顶	
杀飞克	104 瓶	15 912.00	–	
奋斗呐	2 吨	210 000.00	–	
ACT	5000 人份	75 000.00	结余:2000 人份	
药品及卫生产品小计	–	1 410 377.20	–	–
项目物资合计	–	3 883 192.72	–	–

表 2-12 第一轮中国全球基金疟疾项目终期评估现场评估表

被评估单位	第一轮云南省全球基金疟疾项目办公室			
项目点	省项目办	评估时间	2008 年 5 月 13-15 日	
评估项目	评估指标	评价	分值	得分
1. 项目工作计划完成情况(共 100 分)(A)	评估用表表 2 的真实准确性	由评估组指导国家项目办采取逐层抽查核实的方式完成；核查误差在 10% 以内，按照自评评分给分；	96	96
2. 项目考核指标达标情况(共 100 分)(B)	评估用表表 3 的真实准确性		100	100
3. 项目管理能力(共 100 分)(C)	项目办机构健全、规章制度完善(20 分)	项目办工作正常运行；项目办人员职责清晰，但评估期间项目信息管理员已更换，工作交结不到位；项目办工作规章制度齐全。	20	18
	按计划召开或参加项目年会、例会(10 分)	按照工作计划召开或参加会议；会议记录齐全。	10	10
	制定项目年度和季度工作计划(6 分)	制定了项目年度工作计划；制定了项目季度工作计划。	6	6
	制定各项具体活动的实施方案(4 分)	各项项目活动都有实施方案。	4	4
	项目工作记录规范(10 分)	项目工作有记录，但部分活动记录不齐全；项目工作记录细致清楚。	10	7
	项目活动有总结(4 分)	项目活动结束后都有总结。	4	4
	按规定及时上报项目报表和报告(6 分)	及时上报项目报表和报告；报表填写规范。	6	6
	按计划组织开展项目培训活动(15)	按工作计划开展或参加培训；培训内容针对当前项目需要；培训的记录、资料齐全。	15	15
	项目管理和执行人员按要求参加有关的项目培训(25)	根据项目执行人员培训覆盖率 ≥ 90%。	25	25
项目管理能力合计得分(C)			100	95

续表

4. M&E 管理能力(共 100 分)(D)	有专人负责项目数据、报表的收集、审核、汇总和上报工作(20 分)	收集、汇总、上报报表的人员不固定； 专人负责报表的审核。	20	12
	项目季度报表上报及时、填写规范、数据准确(20 分)	报表上报及时；报表填写规范；报表数据准确。	20	20
	项目办有制定或使用指导 M&E 工作的指南和模板(15 分)	有 M&E 工作的指南和模板；	15	15
	组织开展或参加相关培训(15 分)	组织开展或参加相关培训；培训记录、资料齐全，内容有针对性。	15	15
	项目督导规范、有成效(30 分)	按照工作计划开展督导；有督导通知、但部分督导无督导报告； 督导过程有记录；部分督导后未及时跟踪整改情况，督导发现问题仍存在。	30	25
M&E 管理能力合计得分(D)			100	87
5. 项目财务与物资管理能力(100 分)(E)	财务人员队伍建设情况	无失分	10	10
	预算制订与预算执行情况	财务人员对项目预算了解不多	10	10
	项目资金管理能力	无失分	10	10
	项目财务管理能力	无失分	10	10
	报表及审计情况	无失分	10	10
	会计档案管理能力	财务票据报表装订不完全符合要求	10	8
	项目物资管理能力	无失分	10	10
	培训及督导完成情况	未按照开展所有督导	10	7
	内部控制制度评估	无失分	10	10
	根据项目点具体情况，提出其他评估要求和内容	其他	10	9
项目财务物资管理能力合计得分(E)			100	94
评估合计得分(T)=(A)*0.4+(B)*0.2+(C)*0.1+(D)*0.1+(E)*0.2				95.4
评估等次	■A(>80)□B(70-80)□C(60-70)□D(50-60)□E(<50)			

表 2-13 第一轮中国全球基金疟疾项目终期评估现场评估表

被评估单位	第一轮景洪市全球基金疟疾项目办公室			
项目点	景洪市项目办	评估时间	2008 年 5 月 16 ~ 18 日	
评估项目	评估指标	评分标准	分值	得分
1. 项目工作计划完成情况(共 100 分)(A)	评估用表表 2 的真实准确性	由评估组指导国家项目办采取逐层抽查核实的方式完成;核查误差超过 20%,按照自评评分 *0.8 给分	66	52
2. 项目考核指标达标情况(共 100 分)(B)	评估用表表 3 的真实准确性		100	100
3. 项目管理能力(共 100 分)(C)	项目办机构健全、规章制度完善(20 分)	项目办工作正常运行;项目办人员职责清晰;项目办工作规章制度不齐全。	20	10
	按计划召开或参加项目年会、例会(10 分)	按照工作计划召开或参加会议; 会议记录齐全。	10	10
	制定项目年度和季度工作计划(6 分)	制定了项目年度工作计划; 制定了项目季度工作计划。	6	6
	制定各项具体活动的实施方案(4 分)	部分项目活动没有实施方案。	4	2
	项目工作记录规范(10 分)	项目工作有记录,但部分活动记录不齐全 ;部分项目工作记录与活动总结不符。	10	5
	项目活动有总结(4 分)	部分项目活动结束后没有总结。	4	2
	按规定及时上报项目报表和报告(6 分)	及时上报项目报表和报告; 报表填写规范。	6	6
	按计划组织开展项目培训活动(15)	按工作计划开展或参加培训;培训内容针对当前项目需要;培训的记录、资料齐全。	15	15
	项目管理和执行人员按要求参加有关的项目培训(25)	根据项目执行人员培训覆盖率≥ 90%,但是培训效果不让人满意,部分村医水平没有完全达到项目要求。	25	15
项目管理能力合计得分(C)			100	71

续表

4. M&E管理能力（共100分）（D）	有专人负责项目数据、报表的收集、审核、汇总和上报工作（20分）	专人负责收集、汇总、上报报表； 专人负责报表的审核，但有时报表没有审核。	20	15
	项目季度报表上报及时、填写规范、数据准确（20分）	报表上报及时；报表填写规范；报表数据不够准确。	20	15
	项目办有制定或使用指导M&E工作的指南和模板（15分）	有M&E工作的指南和模板；	15	15
	组织开展或参加相关培训（15分）	组织开展或参加相关培训；培训记录、资料不齐全。	15	10
	项目督导规范、有成效（30分）	按照工作计划开展督导；有督导通知、但部分督导无督导报告； 督导过程有记录；部分督导后未及时跟踪整改情况，督导发现问题仍存在。	30	20
M&E管理能力合计得分（D）			100	75
5. 项目财务与物资管理能力（100分）（E）	财务人员队伍建设情况	无失分	10	10
	预算制订与预算执行情况	财务人员对项目预算了解不多	10	9
	项目资金管理能力	无失分	10	10
	项目财务管理能力	无失分	10	10
	报表及审计情况	财务账表有部分出入	10	9
	会计档案管理能力	财务票据报表装订不完全符合要求	10	9
	项目物资管理能力	物资辅助账不完善，物资调拨手续不完全	10	8
	培训及督导完成情况	未按照开展所有督导	10	7
	内部控制制度评估	无失分	10	10
	根据项目点具体情况，提出其他评估要求和内容	其他	10	8
项目财务物资管理能力合计得分（E）			100	90
评估合计得分（T）=（A）*0.4+（B）*0.2+（C）*0.1+（D）*0.1+（E）*0.2				73.4
评估等次	□A（>80）■B（70-80）□C（60-70）□D（50-60）□E（<50）			

表 2-14 第一轮中国全球基金疟疾项目终期评估现场评估表

被评估单位	第一轮陇川县全球基金疟疾项目办公室			
项目点	陇川县项目办	评估时间	2008 年 5 月 18 ~ 20 日	
评估项目	评估指标	评分标准	分值	得分
1. 项目工作计划完成情况(共100分)(A)	评估用表表 2 的真实准确性	由评估组指导国家项目办采取逐层抽查核实的方式完成。 核查误差在 10% 以内,按照自评评分给分。	96	96
2. 项目考核指标达标情况(共100分)(B)	评估用表表 3 的真实准确性		100	80
3. 项目管理能力(共 100 分)(C)	项目办机构健全、规章制度完善(20 分)	项目办工作正常运行;项目办人员职责清晰;项目办工作规章制度齐全。	20	20
	按计划召开或参加项目年会、例会(10 分)	按照工作计划召开或参加会议; 会议记录齐全。	10	10
	制定项目年度和季度工作计划(6 分)	制定了项目年度工作计划; 制定了项目季度工作计划。	6	6
	制定各项具体活动的实施方案(4 分)	各项项目活动都有实施方案。	4	4
	项目工作记录规范(10 分)	项目工作有记录,但项目前期部分活动记录不齐全;项目工作记录细致清楚。	10	7
	项目活动有总结(4 分)	项目活动结束后都有总结。	4	4
	按规定及时上报项目报表和报告(6 分)	及时上报项目报表和报告; 报表填写规范,但血检数据有一定出入。	6	4
	按计划组织开展项目培训活动(15)	按工作计划开展或参加培训;培训内容针对当前项目需要;培训的记录、资料齐全。	15	15
	项目管理和执行人员按要求参加有关的项目培训(25)	根据项目执行人员培训覆盖率≥ 80%。	25	20
项目管理能力合计得分(C)			100	90

续表

4. M&E 管理能力(共 100 分)(D)	有专人负责项目数据、报表的收集、审核、汇总和上报工作(20 分)	专人收集、汇总、上报报表；专人负责报表的审核。	20	20
	项目季度报表上报及时、填写规范、数据准确(20 分)	报表上报及时；报表填写规范；部分季度报表有误。	20	15
	项目办有制定或使用指导 M&E 工作的指南和模板(15 分)	有 M&E 工作的指南和模板；	15	15
	组织开展或参加相关培训(15 分)	组织开展或参加相关培训；培训记录、资料齐全，内容有针对性。	15	15
	项目督导规范、有成效(30 分)	按照工作计划开展督导；有督导通知、督导报告；督导过程有记录；部分督导后未及时跟踪整改情况，督导发现问题仍存在。	30	25
M&E 管理能力合计得分(D)			100	90
5. 项目财务与物资管理能力(100 分)(E)	财务人员队伍建设情况	财务与项目人员有效沟通不够	10	9
	预算制订与预算执行情况	财务未参与项目预算的制定，部分项目支出与工作计划、预算不符	10	7
	项目资金管理能力	现金日记账与银行存款日记账有出入	10	9
	项目财务管理能力	无失分	10	10
	报表及审计情况	部分报表与账目有出入	10	9
	会计档案管理能力	无失分	10	10
	项目物资管理能力	物资辅助账不完善，物资调拨手续不完全	10	8
	培训及督导完成情况	未按照开展所有督导	10	8
	内部控制制度评估	财务电子信息系统建设有待加强	10	9
	根据项目点具体情况，提出其他评估要求和内容	无失分	10	10
项目财务物资管理能力合计得分(E)			100	89
评估合计得分(T) = (A) *0.4+ (B) *0.2+ (C) *0.1+ (D) *0.1+ (E) *0.2				90.2
评估等次	■ A (>80) □ B (70-80) □ C (60-70) □ D (50-60) □ E (<50)			

表 2–15 第一轮中国全球基金疟疾项目终期评估现场评估表

被评估单位	第一轮腾冲县全球基金疟疾项目办公室			
项目点	腾冲县项目办	评估时间	2008 年 5 月 21 ～ 23 日	
评估项目	评估指标	评分标准	分值	得分
1. 项目工作计划完成情况（共 100 分）（A）	评估用表表 2 的真实准确性	由评估组指导国家项目办采取逐层抽查核实的方式完成；核查误差在 10% 以内，按照自评评分给分。	92	92
2. 项目考核指标达标情况（共 100 分）（B）	评估用表表 3 的真实准确性		100	100
3. 项目管理能力（共 100 分）（C）	项目办机构健全、规章制度完善（20 分）	项目办工作正常运行；项目办人员职责清晰；项目办工作规章制度齐全。	20	20
	按计划召开或参加项目年会、例会（10 分）	按照工作计划召开或参加会议； 会议记录齐全。	10	10
	制定项目年度和季度工作计划（6 分）	制定了项目年度工作计划； 制定了项目季度工作计划。	6	6
	制定各项具体活动的实施方案（4 分）	各项项目活动都有实施方案。	4	4
	项目工作记录规范（10 分）	项目工作有记录，但部分活动记录不齐全 ；项目工作记录细致清楚。	10	8
	项目活动有总结（4 分）	项目活动结束后都有总结。	4	4
	按规定及时上报项目报表和报告（6 分）	及时上报项目报表和报告； 报表填写规范。	6	6
	按计划组织开展项目培训活动（15）	按工作计划开展或参加培训；培训内容针对当前项目需要；培训的记录、资料齐全。	15	13
	项目管理和执行人员按要求参加有关的项目培训（25）	根据项目执行人员培训覆盖率≥ 90%。	25	25
项目管理能力合计得分（C）			100	96

续表

4. M&E 管理能力(共 100 分)(D)	有专人负责项目数据、报表的收集、审核、汇总和上报工作(20 分)	专人收集、汇总、上报报表；专人负责报表的审核。	20	20
	项目季度报表上报及时、填写规范、数据准确(20 分)	报表上报及时；报表填写规范；报表数据准确。	20	20
	项目办有制定或使用指导 M&E 工作的指南和模板(15 分)	有 M&E 工作的指南和模板；	15	15
	组织开展或参加相关培训(15 分)	组织开展或参加相关培训；培训记录、资料齐全，内容有针对性。	15	15
	项目督导规范、有成效(30 分)	按照工作计划开展督导；有督导通知、督导报告； 督导过程有记录；部分督导效果不理想，应进一步加强乡镇对病例的管理。	30	25
M&E 管理能力合计得分(D)			100	95
5. 项目财务与物资管理能力(100 分)(E)	财务人员队伍建设情况	财务与项目人员有效沟通不够	10	9
	预算制订与预算执行情况	财务未参与项目预算的制定，部分项目支出与工作计划、预算不符	10	8
	项目资金管理能力	无失分	10	10
	项目财务管理能力	无失分	10	10
	报表及审计情况	部分报表与账目有出入	10	9
	会计档案管理能力	无失分	10	10
	项目物资管理能力	物资辅助账不完善，物资调拨手续不完全	10	10
	培训及督导完成情况	未按照开展所有督导	10	8
	内部控制制度评估	无失分	10	10
	根据项目点具体情况，提出其他评估要求和内容	其他	10	8
项目财务物资管理能力合计得分(E)			100	92
评估合计得分(T)=(A)*0.4+(B)*0.2+(C)*0.1+(D)*0.1+(E)*0.2				94.3
评估等次	■A(>80)□B(70-80)□C(60-70)□D(50-60)□E(<50)			

表 2-16 第一轮中国全球基金疟疾项目终期评估现场评估表

被评估单位	第一轮海南省全球基金疟疾项目办公室			
项目点	省项目办	评估时间	2008 年 5 月 26 ~ 28 日	
评估项目	评估指标	评价	分值	得分
1. 项目工作计划完成情况(共 100 分)(A)	评估用表表 2 的真实准确性	由评估组指导国家项目办采取逐层抽查核实的方式完成;核查误差在 10% 以内,按照自评评分给分;	98	98
2. 项目考核指标达标情况(共 100 分)(B)	评估用表表 3 的真实准确性		92	92
3. 项目管理能力(共 100 分)(C)	项目办机构健全、规章制度完善(20 分)	项目办工作正常运行;项目办人员职责清晰;项目办工作规章制度齐全。	20	20
	按计划召开或参加项目年会、例会(10 分)	按照工作计划召开或参加会议; 会议记录齐全。	10	10
	制定项目年度和季度工作计划(6 分)	制定了项目年度工作计划; 制定了项目季度工作计划。	6	6
	制定各项具体活动的实施方案(4 分)	各项项目活动都有实施方案。	4	4
	项目工作记录规范(10 分)	项目工作有记录;项目工作记录细致清楚。	10	10
	项目活动有总结(4 分)	项目活动结束后都有总结。	4	4
	按规定及时上报项目报表和报告(6 分)	及时上报项目报表和报告; 报表填写规范。	6	6
	按计划组织开展项目培训活动(15)	按工作计划开展或参加培训;培训内容针对当前项目需要;培训的记录、资料齐全。	15	15
	项目管理和执行人员按要求参加有关的项目培训(25)	根据项目执行人员培训覆盖率≥ 90%。	25	25
项目管理能力合计得分(C)			100	100

续表

4. M&E 管理能力（共 100 分）（D）	有专人负责项目数据、报表的收集、审核、汇总和上报工作（20 分）	专人收集、汇总、上报报表；专人负责报表的审核。	20	20
	项目季度报表上报及时、填写规范、数据准确（20 分）	报表上报及时；报表填写规范；部分季度报表有误。	20	20
	项目办有制定或使用指导 M&E 工作的指南和模板（15 分）	有 M&E 工作的指南和模板；	15	15
	组织开展或参加相关培训（15 分）	组织开展或参加相关培训；培训记录、资料齐全，内容有针对性。	15	15
	项目督导规范、有成效（30 分）	按照工作计划开展督导；有督导通知、督导报告；督导过程有记录；部分督导后未及时跟踪整改情况，督导发现问题仍存在。	30	27
M&E 管理能力合计得分（D）			100	97
5. 项目财务与物资管理能力（100 分）（E）	财务人员队伍建设情况	财务与项目人员有效沟通不够	10	9.5
	预算制订与预算执行情况	部分支出与预算不符	10	9.5
	项目资金管理能力	无失分	10	10
	项目财务管理能力	无失分	10	10
	报表及审计情况	部分审计报告内容不完全符合 PR 颁布的要求	10	9
	会计档案管理能力	无失分	10	10
	项目物资管理能力	物资辅助账不完善，物资调拨手续不全	10	9
	培训及督导完成情况	无失分	10	10
	内部控制制度评估	无失分	10	10
	根据项目点具体情况，提出其他评估要求和内容	其他	10	10
项目财务物资管理能力合计得分（E）			100	97
评估合计得分（T）=（A）*0.4+（B）*0.2+（C）*0.1+（D）*0.1+（E）*0.2				96.7
评估等次	■A（>80）□B（70-80）□C（60-70）□D（50-60）□E（<50）			

表 2–17 第一轮中国全球基金疟疾项目终期评估现场评估表

被评估单位	第一轮白沙县全球基金疟疾项目办公室			
项目点	白沙县项目办	评估时间	2008 年 5 月 28 ~ 29 日	
评估项目	评估指标	评分标准	分值	得分
1. 项目工作计划完成情况(共 100 分)(A)	评估用表表 2 的真实准确性	由评估组指导国家项目办采取逐层抽查核实的方式完成;核查误差在 10% 以内,按照自评评分给分。	98	98
2. 项目考核指标达标情况(共 100 分)(B)	评估用表表 3 的真实准确性		97	97
3. 项目管理能力(共 100 分)(C)	项目办机构健全、规章制度完善(20 分)	项目办工作正常运行;项目办人员职责清晰;项目办工作规章制度齐全。	20	20
	按计划召开或参加项目年会、例会(10 分)	按照工作计划召开或参加会议; 会议记录齐全。	10	10
	制定项目年度和季度工作计划(6 分)	制定了项目年度工作计划; 制定了项目季度工作计划。	6	6
	制定各项具体活动的实施方案(4 分)	各项项目活动都有实施方案。	4	4
	项目工作记录规范(10 分)	项目工作有记录,但部分记录缺失;项目工作记录细致清楚。	10	8
	项目活动有总结(4 分)	项目活动结束后都有总结。	4	4
	按规定及时上报项目报表和报告(6 分)	及时上报项目报表和报告; 报表填写规范。	6	6
	按计划组织开展项目培训活动(15)	按工作计划开展或参加培训;培训内容针对当前项目需要;培训的记录、资料齐全。	15	13
	项目管理和执行人员按要求参加有关的项目培训(25)	根据项目执行人员培训覆盖率≥ 90%。	25	25
项目管理能力合计得分(C)			100	96

续表

4. M&E 管理能力(共100分)(D)	有专人负责项目数据、报表的收集、审核、汇总和上报工作(20分)	专人收集、汇总、上报报表；专人负责报表的审核。	20	20
	项目季度报表上报及时、填写规范、数据准确(20分)	报表上报及时；报表填写规范；部分季度报表有误。	20	20
	项目办有制定或使用指导 M&E 工作的指南和模板(15分)	有 M&E 工作的指南和模板。	15	15
	组织开展或参加相关培训(15分)	组织开展或参加相关培训；培训记录、资料齐全，内容有针对性。	15	15
	项目督导规范、有成效(30分)	按照工作计划开展督导；有督导通知、督导报告；督导过程有记录；部分督导后未及时跟踪整改情况，督导发现问题仍存在。	30	24
M&E 管理能力合计得分(D)			100	96
5. 项目财务与物资管理能力(100分)(E)	财务人员队伍建设情况	财务与项目人员有效沟通不够	10	8
	预算制订与预算执行情况	财务未参与项目预算的制定	10	9
	项目资金管理能力	无失分	10	10
	项目财务管理能力	财务物资管理制度不够完善	10	9.5
	报表及审计情况	部分审计报告内容不完全符合 PR 颁布的要求	10	9
	会计档案管理能力	无失分	10	10
	项目物资管理能力	物资辅助账不完善，物资调拨手续不全	10	9
	培训及督导完成情况	无失分	10	10
	内部控制制度评估	项目内控制度不完善	10	9.5
	根据项目点具体情况，提出其他评估要求和内容	其他	10	10
项目财务物资管理能力合计得分(E)			100	94
评估合计得分(T)=(A)*0.4+(B)*0.2+(C)*0.1+(D)*0.1+(E)*0.2				96.6
评估等次	■A (>80) □B (70-80) □C (60-70) □D (50-60) □E (<50)			

表 2–18 第一轮中国全球基金疟疾项目终期评估现场评估表

被评估单位	第一轮琼中县全球基金疟疾项目办公室			
项目点	琼中县项目办	评估时间	2008 年 5 月 29 ~ 30 日	
评估项目	评估指标	评分标准	分值	得分
1. 项目工作计划完成情况(共 100 分)(A)	评估用表表 2 的真实准确性	由评估组指导国家项目办采取逐层抽查核实的方式完成;核查误差在 10% 以内,按照自评评分给分。	96	96
2. 项目考核指标达标情况(共 100 分)(B)	评估用表表 3 的真实准确性		82	82
3. 项目管理能力(共 100 分)(C)	项目办机构健全、规章制度完善(20 分)	项目办工作正常运行;项目办人员职责清晰;项目办工作规章制度齐全。	20	20
	按计划召开或参加项目年会、例会(10 分)	按照工作计划召开或参加会议; 会议记录齐全。	10	10
	制定项目年度和季度工作计划(6 分)	制定了项目年度工作计划; 制定了项目季度工作计划。	6	6
	制定各项具体活动的实施方案(4 分)	各项项目活动都有实施方案。	4	4
	项目工作记录规范(10 分)	项目工作有记录; 项目工作记录细致清楚。	10	10
	项目活动有总结(4 分)	项目活动结束后都有总结。	4	4
	按规定及时上报项目报表和报告(6 分)	及时上报项目报表和报告; 报表填写规范。	6	4
	按计划组织开展项目培训活动(15)	按工作计划开展或参加培训;培训内容针对当前项目需要;部分培训的记录、资料不齐全。	15	13
	项目管理和执行人员按要求参加有关的项目培训(25)	根据项目执行人员培训覆盖率≥ 90%。	25	25
项目管理能力合计得分(C)			100	98

续表

4. M&E管理能力(共100分)(D)	有专人负责项目数据、报表的收集、审核、汇总和上报工作(20分)	专人收集、汇总、上报报表；专人负责报表的审核。	20	20
	项目季度报表上报及时、填写规范、数据准确(20分)	报表上报及时；报表填写规范；部分季度报表有误。	20	20
	项目办有制定或使用指导M&E工作的指南和模板(15分)	有M&E工作的指南和模板；	15	15
	组织开展或参加相关培训(15分)	组织开展或参加相关培训；培训记录、资料齐全，内容有针对性。	15	15
	项目督导规范、有成效(30分)	按照工作计划开展督导；有督导通知、督导报告；督导过程有记录；部分督导后未及时跟踪整改情况，督导发现问题仍存在。	30	26
M&E管理能力合计得分(D)			100	96
5. 项目财务与物资管理能力(100分)(E)	财务人员队伍建设情况	财务与项目人员有效沟通不够	10	9
	预算制订与预算执行情况	财务未参与项目预算的制定，部分项目支出与工作计划、预算不符	10	8.5
	项目资金管理能力	现金管理不够完善，现金日记账与银行存款日记账有出入	10	7
	项目财务管理能力	无失分	10	10
	报表及审计情况	部分审计报告内容不完全符合PR颁布的要求	10	9.5
	会计档案管理能力	无失分	10	10
	项目物资管理能力	物资辅助账不完善	10	8
	培训及督导完成情况	部分财务督导活动未按照计划开展	10	9
	内部控制制度评估	无失分	10	10
	根据项目点具体情况，提出其他评估要求和内容	其他	10	10
项目财务物资管理能力合计得分(E)			100	91
评估合计得分(T) = (A) *0.4+ (B) *0.2+ (C) *0.1+ (D) *0.1+ (E) *0.2				92.4
评估等次	■A (>80) □B (70-80) □C (60-70) □D (50-60) □E (<50)			

第三章

专项调查报告

第一节 基线调查报告

2003年我国成功获得了全球基金的资助，在以云南、海南两省为重点，兼顾疟疾发病较多的中部安徽、湖北、河南和江苏四省以及南部广东、广西、四川和贵州4省，共计覆盖10个省实施全球基金疟疾控制项目。于2003年10月项目完成基线调查，现将基线调查的结果汇总如下。

一、调查内容与方法

（一）调查范围

在云南省25个项目县（市）和海南省10个项目县（市），经分层随机整群抽样，进行回顾性调查。

（二）调查时间

2003年5月21日至6月20日。

（三）调查指标与方法

1.疟疾调查推断发病率

1.1 分母：被调查县（市）当年人口总数。

1.2 分子：项目县（市）当年疟疾推算实际病例数。

1.3 调查方法：分层随机整群抽样，回顾性调查。

1.3.1 抽样方法：采取分层随机整群抽样法。第一层：按近3年（2005—2007年）的疟疾发病率，将全县（市）的各乡镇按发病率高、中、低分为3类。在每类乡镇中随机抽取1个乡镇为调查点。第二层：以抽取的乡镇为单位，按近3年的疟疾发病率，将全乡镇的各行政村按发病率高、中、低分为3类。在每类行政村中随机抽取1个行政村。第三层：在每个抽中的行政村中随机抽取1—3个自然村或村民组。即全县（市）共3个乡镇9个行政村9—27个自然村，每一行政村调查村民数不少于300人，总人数不少于2 700人。

1.3.2 调查对象：被调查县 CDC、乡镇卫生院、村诊所和被调查村民。

1.3.3 调查内容与实际疟疾发病率推算方法：(1) 采用捕获 - 再捕获方法（CMR）推算被调查乡镇实际疟疾发病例数。在被调查县（市）CDC 疫情网络直报系统上获得被调查村疟疾病例数（C 值）；符合“血检阳性、典型临床症状、药物试治有效”其中之一即为疟疾病例，挨户走访调查当年有疟史的居民数（R 值）；核对走访调查中发现的有疟史者名单和被调查村的上报疟疾病例名单，记录相符的疟疾病例数（M 值）；按公式 N=[（C+1）（R+1）/（M+1）]-1 推算各县（市）被调查村的疟疾实际发病数。(2) 推算项目县（市）实际疟疾病例数 = 项目县（市）报告疟疾病例总数 ÷（项目县（市）被调查村疟疾报告病例数 /N）。(3) 从统计局获得项目县（市）人口总数。(4) 推算项目县（市）实际疟疾发病率 = 推算项目县（市）实际疟疾病例数 / 项目县（市）当年人口总数 ×10000/ 万。

1.3.4 汇总表

被调查县人口数(1)	被调查县上报疟疾病例数(2)	受调查人群中通过网络直报的疟疾病例数(C值)(3)	走访调查出的疟疾病例数(R值)(4)	走访调查出的疟疾病例中作为疫情网络直报的病例数(M值)(5)	推算被调查人群实际疟疾病例数(N值)(6)	推算被调查县(市)实际发病数(7)=(2)/{(3)/(6)}	推算被调查县(市)实际发病率(1/万)(8)=(7)/(1)×10000

填表人：　　　　　　　　填表日期：

2. 海南省 10 个项目县（市）的恶性疟发病率

2.1 分母：被调查项目县（市）当年人口总数。

2.2 分子：项目县（市）当年恶性疟推算实际病例数。

2.3 调查方法：分层随机抽样，回顾性调查。

2.3.1 抽样方法：采取分层随机整群抽样法。按近三年的恶性疟发病率将全县(市)的各乡镇分为恶性疟流行重、中、轻三类，每类中随机抽取 1 个乡镇。即全县（市）抽取 3 个乡镇。

2.3.2 调查对象：被调查县（市）CDC 和乡镇卫生院。

2.3.3 调查内容与实际恶性疟发病率推算方法：(1)采用捕获 - 再捕获方法(CMR)

推算被调查乡镇实际恶性疟发病例数。在被调查县（市）CDC疫情网络直报系统上获得被调查乡镇恶性疟病例数（C值）；核查被调查乡镇卫生院恶性疟病例登记数（R值）；核对恶性疟病例登记名单和上报名单，记录相符的恶性疟病例数（M值）；按下列公式推算各县(市)被调查乡镇实际恶性疟病例数N=[(C+1)(R+1)/(M+1)]-1。(2)推算项目县（市）实际恶性疟病例数＝项目县（市）报告恶性疟病例总数 ÷（项目县（市）被调查乡镇恶性疟报告病例数/N)。(3) 从统计局获得项目县（市）人口总数。(4) 推算项目县（市）实际恶性疟发病率＝推算项目县（市）实际恶性疟病例数/项目县（市）当年人口总数 ×10000/万。

2.3.4 汇总表

被调查县人口数(1)	被调查县上报恶性疟病例数(2)	被调查乡镇卫生院恶性疟疫情报告数数(C 值)(3)	被调查乡镇恶性疟病例登记数(R 值)(4)	恶性疟名单相符的病例数(M 值)(5)	推算被调查乡镇实际恶性疟病例数(N 值)(6)	推算被调查县(市) 实际恶性疟病例数(7) = (2) / {(3) / (6)}	推算被调查县(市) 恶性疟实际发病率(1/万)(8)= (7)/ (1) ×10000

填表人：　　　　　　　　　　填表日期：

3. 目标地区中小学生能够回答至少3个与疟疾相关问题的比例

3.1 分母：抽查的中小学生数。

3.2 分子：调查出能正确回答3个疟疾相关问题的中小学生数。

3.3 调查方法：采取分层随机整群抽样法，全县（市）抽取3个项目乡镇（场），每个乡镇（场）抽取中、小学校各1所，每所学校各60名学生。即每县（市）3个乡镇（场）6所学校共360人（小学三年级到初中三年级）。通过问卷调查能够正确回答三个疟疾相关问题的人数。

3.4 汇总表

乡镇名（1）	调查的中小学校数（2）	调查的学生数（3）	能正确回答三个疟疾相关问题的学生数（4）	能正确回答三个疟疾相关问题的学生的比例（%）（5）=（4）/（3）×100
合计				

填表人：　　　　　　　　填表日期：

4. 发热病人在症状出现两天内求诊的比例

4.1 分母：调查的发热病人数。

4.2 分子：发热病人在症状出现两天内求诊的人数。

4.3 调查方法：采取分层随机整群抽样法，方法同 1，即每县（市）共 3 个乡镇（场）9 个行政村（作业区）9—27 个自然村（队）。入户走访调查村民中曾经发热病人数和 2 天内求诊的人数。

4.4 汇总表

乡镇名（1）	调查的行政村数（2）	自述有发热史的村民（3）	自述有发热史的村民中发热 2 天内求诊的人数（4）	发热病人在症状出现 2 天内求诊的比例（%）（5）=（4）/（3）×100
合计				

填表人：　　　　　　　　填表日期：

5. 拥有杀虫剂浸泡蚊帐（ITNs）的家庭比例

5.1 分母：走访调查的户数。

5.2 分子：走访调查出的拥有药浸蚊帐（ITNs）户数。

5.3 调查方法：分层随机整群抽样，方法同 1.，即每县（市）共 3 个乡镇（场）9 个行政村（作业区）9—27 个自然村（队），入户走访调查。

5.4 汇总表

乡镇名(1)	调查的行政村数(2)	调查户数(3)	拥有 ITNs 的户数(4)	拥有 ITNs 户数的比例(%)(5) = (4) / (3) ×100
合计				

填表人：　　　　　　　　　　填表日期：

6. 网络直报疟疾病人比例

6.1 分母：走访调查出的疟疾病例

6.2 分子：走访调查出的疟疾病例中通过网络直报的人数

6.3 调查方法：采取分层随机整群抽样法，方法同 1.，即全县（市）共 3 个乡镇（场）9 个行政村（作业区）9—27 个自然村（队）。入户走访调查，符合“血检阳性、典型临床症状、药物试治有效”其中之一即为疟疾病例（分母）。根据走访调查的疟疾病例名单，与县 CDC 网络直报疫情进行核对，相符者为分子。

6.4 汇总表

乡镇名(1)	调查的行政村数(2)	走访调查的疟疾病例数(3)	走访调查的疟疾病例中通过网络直报的病例数(4)	网络直报疟疾病人比例(%)(5) = (4) / (3) ×100

二、调查结果

云南省将所有 25 个项目县（市）全部作为调查县，问卷调查了 25 县 75 个乡镇 386 个行政村的 24 628 户居民 71 771 人和 144 所中小学校的 8 825 名学生，入户调查了 386 个行政村的居民疟史、蚊帐使用情况。

海南省将所有10个项目县（市）全部作为调查县，问卷调查了10县30个乡镇55个行政村的9 574户居民33 563人和60所中小学校的6 175名学生，入户调查了55个行政村的居民疟史、蚊帐使用情况。

（一）云南省25个项目县和海南省10个项目县疟疾调查推断发病率

基线调查方案设计了在调查县内各乡镇按疟疾流行的重、中、轻分成三类，按分层随机抽样法，直至选中的自然村为调查点（3乡9村）。运用捕获—再捕获方法（CMR），以走访调查有疟史者核算实际发病人数。

根据走访调查的结果，云南省疟疾调查推断发病率为196.62/万（113 066/5 750 344）。海南省疟疾调查推断发病率为385/万（119 267/3 100 000）。

（二）海南省10个项目县恶性疟发病率

海南省10个项目县（市）恶性疟流行区人口数为1 093 818人，恶性疟991例，恶性疟发病率为9.06/10 000。

（三）目标地区中小学生能够正确回答至少3个与疟疾相关问题的比例

学生调查对象采取本人填写问卷调查表方式进行问卷调查，被调查者在5个疟疾基本知识问题中能正确回答3个以上者视为知晓疟疾防治知识。

目标地区能正确回答至少3个与疟疾相关问题的学生比例为60.00%（9 000/15 000），其中云南省为58.20%（5 136/8 825），海南省为89.39%（3 857/4 315）。

（四）发热病人在症状出现两天内求诊的比例

目标地区发热病人在症状出现两天内求诊的比例为44.12%（24 721/56 031），其中云南省为37.95%（13 385/35 274），海南省为54.61%（11 336/20 757）。

（五）拥有杀虫剂浸泡蚊帐（ITNs）的家庭比例

项目地区拥有ITNs的居民家庭比例为13.98%（4 783/34 202）。其中云南省为4.30%（1 058/24 628），海南省为38.91%（3 725/9 574）。

（六）疟疾病人通过信息网络报告的比例

项目地区疟疾病人通过疟疾监测网络报告的比例为7.12%（496/6 963）。其中云南省为8.80%（341/3 877），海南省为5.02%（155/3 086）。

表 3–1 项目指标基线调查结果汇总表

	指标	云南			海南			合计		
		分子	分母	比例	分子	分母	比例	分子	分母	比例
1	云南省25个项目县和海南省10个项目县疟疾调查推断发病率	113 066	5 750 344	196.62/ 万	119 267	3 100 000	385/ 万	-	-	-
2	海南省恶性疟调查推断发病率	-	-	-	991	1 093 818	9.06/ 万	-	-	-
3	目标地区中小学生能够回答至少3个与疟疾相关问题的比例	5 136	8 825	58.20%	3 864	6 175	62.57%	9 000	15 000	60.00%
4	发热病人在症状出现2天内求诊的比例	13 385	35 274	37.95%	11 336	20 757	54.61%	24 721	56 031	44.12%
5	拥有杀虫剂浸泡蚊帐(ITNs)的家庭比例	1 058	24 628	4.30%	3 725	9 574	38.91%	4 783	34 202	13.98%
6	疟疾病人通过信息网络报告的比例	341	3 877	8.80%	155	3 086	5.02%	496	6 963	7.12%

第二节 全球基金疟疾项目2004年度调查报告

全球基金第一轮中国疟疾项目第2年度（2004年4月1日至2005年3月31日）工作已经结束，根据项目监督与评价（M&E）计划，国家项目办组织云南省项目办和海南省项目办制定了2006年度专项调查具体实施方案，并开展了相关指标的年度专项调查。

一、调查内容与方法

（一）调查时间：2005年3月。

（二）补充调查时间：2005年7月。

（三）调查范围：云南省25个项目县（市），海南省10个项目县（市）；时间范围2004年1—12月。

（四）抽样方法：采取分层随机抽样法。

第一层：以被调查县为单位，根据近三年的疫情报告，将全县各乡镇按发病率高低分类。在每类乡镇中随机抽取1个乡镇为调查点。

第二层：以抽取的乡镇为单位，根据近三年的疫情报告，将全乡镇各行政村按发病率高低分类。在每类行政村中随机抽取1个行政村为调查点。

第三层：以抽取的行政村为单位，随机抽取1—3个自然村或村民组为调查点。

（五）调查对象：以被调查县CDC、乡镇卫生院、村诊所以及被调查村民为对象。

（六）调查内容与方法：统一调查方案，统一培训调查员，使用统一的调查表格，进行回顾性调查。

1. 流动人口中发热病人正确诊断并规范治疗的比例：从被抽到的乡镇卫生院门诊登记中收集就诊的流动人口发热病人资料作为分母，然后核对发热病人血检登记和处方，统计分母中得到正确诊断和规范治疗的疟疾病人数作为分子。

2. 疑似病人通过医疗机构确诊为疟疾病人的比例：核查被抽到的乡镇卫生院和村诊所门诊记录与处方，收集疑似疟疾病人数（分母）。调查核对乡镇卫生院发热病人血检登记，统计分母中血检阳性人数（分子）。

3. 血检（镜检或快速诊断试条诊断）阳性的疟疾病人中给予规范治疗的比例：核查被抽到的乡镇卫生院血检登记，统计血检阳性数（分母）。核对乡镇卫生院处方，统计分母中得到规范治疗的疟疾病人数（分子）。

4. 贫困家庭拥有杀虫剂处理蚊帐（ITNs）的比例：在被抽到的村，从村民小组组长处得到该村贫困家庭数量（分母）和清单，然后逐户走访调查，同时获取该村贫困家庭中拥有杀虫剂处理蚊帐的家庭数（分子）。

5. 求医行为改变（发热病人在症状出现两天内求诊的比例）：在被抽查的村进行走访调查，同时获得曾经发热病人数和两天内就诊的人数（分母和分子）。

6. 自我防护行为的改变（拥有 ITNs 的居民正确使用 ITNs 的比例）：在被抽查的村进行走访调查，同时获得拥有 ITNs 的居民数和正确使用 ITNs 的居民数分别作为分母和分子。正确使用指：蚊帐每天使用，蚊帐无破损，蚊帐使用时无缝口。

7. 疟疾病人通过监测系统报告的比例：在被抽查的村进行走访调查，获得实际疟疾病例数（血检确诊、典型临床症状、药物试治有效者）作为分母，根据走访调查的疟疾病例名单，与县 CDC 上报疫情进行核对，名单中姓名、性别、年龄、地址相符者为分子。

8. 目标地区当地居民和中小学生能够回答至少 3 个与疟疾相关问题的比例：被抽查的村民和中小学生数为分母。采用问卷调查，其中能够正确回答出至少三个疟疾相关问题的村民和学生数为分子。

二、调查结果

云南省将所有 25 个项目县（市）全部作为调查县，问卷调查了 25 县 75 个乡镇 286 个行政村的 17 089 户居民 41 499 人，入户调查了 286 个行政村的居民疟史、蚊帐使用情况。

海南省将所有 10 个项目县（市）全部作为调查县，问卷调查了 10 县 30 个乡镇 54 个行政村的 2 876 户居民 33 626 人，入户调查了 54 个行政村的居民疟史、蚊帐使用情况。

（一）流动人口中发热病人正确诊断并规范治疗的比例

云南省共调查 7 872 例流动人口中的发热病人，其中正确诊断并规范治疗了 1 371 例，正确诊断并规范治疗的比例为 17.42%。

（二）疑似病人通过卫生机构确诊为疟疾病人的比例

项目地区疑似病人通过卫生机构确诊为疟疾病人的比例为 8.15 %（3 879/47 617）。其中云南省为 17.88%（2 501/13 991），海南省为 4.10%（1 378/33 626）。海南省疑似疟疾病人确诊为疟疾病人的比例较低，既反映了疟疾流行的地区差异性，也表明不同地区间乡村医生、乡镇卫生院防保组人员项目工作水平和工作质量存在一定差异。

（三）血检阳性的疟疾病人中给予规范治疗的比例

项目地区血检阳性的疟疾病人中给予规范治疗的比例为 74.32%（3 601/4 845）。其中云南省为 75.25%（1 931/2 566），海南省为 73.28%（1 670/2 279）。

（四）贫困家庭拥有药浸蚊帐的比例

项目地区贫困家庭拥有药浸蚊帐的比例为 24.86%（1 736/6 982）。其中云南省为 7.43%（305/4 106），海南省为 49.76%（1 431/2 876）。云南省贫困家庭拥有 ITN 的比例较低，主要是由于药物浸帐不是云南省的主导防治措施，而且为贫困家庭提供药物浸帐也不是项目工作重点，两年来项目提供的蚊帐数量（14 973 顶）和杀虫剂的数量均有限。

（五）求医行为变化（发热病人在症状出现 2 天内求诊的比例）

项目地区发热病人在症状出现 2 天内求诊的比例为 66.77%（8 801/13 182）。其中云南省为 70.98%（6 388/8 999），海南省为 58.88%（2 463/4 183）。

（六）自我防护行为的变化（拥有 ITNs 的居民正确使用 ITNs 的比例）

项目地区拥有 ITNs 的居民正确使用 ITNs 的比例为 69.93%（5 246/7 502）。其中云南省为 92.56%（1 941/2 097），海南省为 61.15%（3 305/5 405）。

（七）疟疾病人通过疟疾监测网络报告的比例

项目地区疟疾病人通过疟疾监测网络报告的比例为 18.45%（349/1 892）。其中云南省为 6.31%（83/1 316），海南省为 46.18%（266/576）。云南省该指标较低，主要原因是与乡村医生和个体私人诊所不报告病例有关，也与基层镜检水平低下、理解不到位和政府干预有关。由于交通不便，大量疟疾病人经乡村医生和个体私人医生治疗，乡医和个体私人诊所不报告疫情一直是疟疾疫情报告工作中的难点。

（八）目标地区当地居民和中小学生能够回答至少 3 个与疟疾有关问题的比例

目标地区当地居民和中小学生能够回答至少 3 个与疟疾有关问题的比例为 43.73%（22 596/51 668）。其中云南省为 41.09%（17 054/41 499），海南省为 54.50%（5 542/10 169）。

表 3-2 项目指标 2004 年度专项调查结果汇总表

指标		云南			海南			合计		
		分子	分母	比例(%)	分子	分母	比例(%)	分子	分母	比例(%)
1	流动人口中发热病人正确诊断并规范治疗的比例	1 371	7 872	17.42	-	-	-	1 371	7 872	17.42
1.1	流动人口发热病人正确诊断的比例	1 567	7 872	19.91	-	-	-	1 567	7 872	19.91
1.2	流动人口发热病人规范治疗的比例	1 375	7 872	17.47	-	-	-	1 375	7 872	17.47
2	疑似病人通过卫生机构确诊为疟疾病人的比例	2 501	13 991	17.88	1 378	33 626	4.10	3 879	47 617	8.15
3	血检阳性的疟疾病人中给予规范治疗的比例	1 931	2 566	75.25	1 670	2 279	73.28	3 601	4 845	74.32
4	贫困家庭拥有药浸蚊帐的比例	305	4 106	7.43	1 431	2 876	49.76	1 736	6 982	24.86
5	求医行为变化(发热病人在症状出现 2 天内求诊的比例)	6 338	8 999	70.98	2 463	4 183	58.88	8 801	13 182	66.77
6	自我防护行为的变化(拥有 ITNs 的居民正确使用 ITNs 的比例)	1 941	2 097	92.56	3 305	5 405	61.15	5 246	7 502	69.93
7	疟疾病人通过疟疾监测网络报告的比例	83	1 316	6.31	266	576	46.18	349	1 892	18.45
8	目标地区当地居民和中小学生能够回答至少 3 个与疟疾有关问题的比例	17 054	41 499	41.09	5 542	10 169	54.50	22 596	51 668	43.73

第三节　全球基金疟疾项目 2005 年度调查报告

为全面了解全球基金第一轮中国疟疾项目 2005 年度项目实施效果，根据项目监督与评价（M&E）计划要求，国家项目办组织云南和海南省项目办制定了 2005 年度专项调查具体实施方案，并开展了相关指标的年度专项调查。

一、调查内容与方法

（一）调查时间

海南省 2005 年 12 月 26—31 日，云南省 2006 年 1 月 7—20 日。

（二）调查方法

统一调查方案，统一培训调查员，使用统一的调查表格，通过分层随机抽样，进行回顾性调查。

（三）调查范围

经分层随机抽取的云南省和海南省各 3 个项目县(市)9 个项目乡镇 27 个行政村；时间范围：2005 年 1—12 月。

（四）抽样方法

根据 2003-2005 年疟疾发病率（其中海南为恶性疟发病率）高低，采取分层随机抽样法。第一层：将全省各项目县（市）按发病率分为重、中、轻 3 类，在每类县（市）中随机抽取 1 个县（市）为调查县。第二层：以被调查县为单位，将全县各乡镇按发病率分为重、中、轻 3 类。在每类乡镇中随机抽取 1 个乡镇为调查点。第三层：以抽取的乡镇为单位，将全乡镇各行政村按发病率分为重、中、轻 3 类。在每类行政村中随机抽取 1 个行政村为调查点。以抽取的行政村为单位，随机抽取 1—3 个自然村或村民组为调查点。即每县调查 3 个乡 9 个行政村 9—27 个自然村。

（五）调查对象

以被调查县 CDC、乡镇卫生院、村诊所以及被调查村民、中小学生为对象。每一行政村调查村民数不少于 300 人，每县不少于 2700 人；每个乡镇抽取中、小学校各 1 所，每所学校各 60 人，共 120 人，全县 3 个乡镇共 360 人（小学三年级到初中三年级）。

（六）调查内容

1. 通过显微镜确诊的疟疾病人比例：核查被抽到的乡镇卫生院门诊记录与处方，符合“血检阳性、典型临床症状、药物试治有效”其中之一即为疟疾病例（分母），调查核对乡镇卫生院发热病人血检登记，统计血检阳性人数（分子）。

2. 目标地区中小学生能够正确回答至少 3 个与疟疾相关问题的比例：问卷调查被抽查的中小学生中能够正确回答出至少 3 个疟疾相关问题的人数。

3. 目标地区居民能够正确回答至少 3 个与疟疾相关问题的比例：问卷调查被抽查的居民中能够正确回答出至少 3 个疟疾相关问题的人数。

4. 求医行为改变（发热病人在症状出现两天内求诊的比例）：在被抽查的村进行走访调查，同时获得曾经发热病人数和两天内就诊的人数（分母和分子）。

5. 自我防护行为的改变（拥有 ITNs 的居民正确使用 ITNs 的比例）：在被抽查的村进行走访调查，同时获得拥有 ITNs 的居民数和正确使用 ITNs 的居民数分别作为分母和分子。正确使用指：蚊帐每天使用，蚊帐无破损，蚊帐使用时无缝口。

6. 疟疾病人通过信息网络报告的比例：在被抽查的村进行走访调查，符合“血检阳性、典型临床症状、药物试治有效”其中之一即为疟疾病例（分母），根据走访调查的疟疾病例名单，与县 CDC 网络直报疫情进行核对，名单中姓名、性别、年龄、地址相符者为分子。

7. 云南省疟疾调查推断发病率：根据捕获－再捕获的方法，采用公式 N=[（C+1）（R+1）/（M+1）]-1（其中 C：受调查人群中上报的疟疾病例数；R：走访调查出的疟疾病例数；M：走访调查出的病例中作为疫情报告的病例数）分别推算各抽样县被调查人群实际疟疾病人数及其漏报率，以被调查人群的疟疾漏报率推算 3 个项目县的实际疟疾发病人数和发病率。

8. 海南省恶性疟调查推断发病率：根据捕获 - 再捕获方法（CMR）推算被调查乡镇实际恶性疟发病例数（N=[（C+1）（R+1）/（M+1）]–1）：(1) 在县（市）CDC 疫情网络直报系统上获得被调查乡镇恶性疟病例数（C 值）；(2) 核查被调查乡镇卫生院恶性疟病例登记数（R 值）；(3) 核对恶性疟病例登记名单和上报名单，

记录相符的恶性疟病例数（M 值）。依据公式：项目县实际恶性疟病例数 = 项目县报告恶性疟病例总数 ÷（被调查乡镇恶性疟报告病例数 /N），推算出项目县实际恶性疟病例数（分子），从统计局获得项目县人口总数（分母）。

二、调查结果

云南省从重、中、轻度流行区中分别抽取西盟县、腾冲县和绿春县作为调查县，问卷调查 3 县 9 个乡镇 27 个行政村的 9 192 名居民，12 所中小学校的 1 167 名学生，调查了 9 个乡镇卫生院和抽样村卫生室门诊处方、发热病人登记和门诊日志。

海南省从重、中、轻度流行区中分别抽取东方市、白沙县和万宁市作为调查县，问卷调查 3 县 9 个乡镇 27 个行政村的 1 667 名居民，18 所中小学校的 1 189 名学生，调查了 9 个乡镇卫生院和抽样村卫生室门诊处方、发热病人登记和门诊日志。

（一）通过显微镜确诊的疟疾病人比例

目标地区通过显微镜确诊的疟疾病人比例为 30.37%（539/1 775），其中云南省为 16.35%（162/991），海南省为 48.09%（377/784）。云南省通过显微镜确诊为疟疾病人的比例较低，该省基层疟防人员的镜检能力需要加强。

（二）目标地区中小学生能够正确回答至少 3 个与疟疾相关问题的比例

能正确回答至少 3 个与疟疾相关问题的学生比例为 74.32%（1 751/2 356），其中云南省为 75.58%（882/1 167），海南省为 73.09%（869/1 189）。

（三）目标地区居民能够正确回答至少 3 个与疟疾相关问题的比例

能正确回答至少 3 个与疟疾相关问题的居民比例为 40.89%（4 290/10 491），其中云南省为 37.14%（3 277/8 824），海南省为 60.77%（1 013/1 667）。云南省该指标较低，与调查对象对问题的理解差异及少数民族地区健康教育程度有关。

（四）求医行为变化（发热病人在症状出现 2 天内求诊的比例）

目标地区发热病人在症状出现 2 天内求诊的比例为 67.44%（2 924/4 336），其中云南省为 63.90%（1 864/2 917），海南省为 74.70%（1 060/1 419）。

（五）自我防护行为的变化（拥有 ITNs 的居民正确使用 ITNs 的比例）

项目地区拥有 ITNs 的居民正确使用 ITNs 的比例为 73.14%（2 546/3 481）。其中云南省为 64.10%（75/117），海南省为 73.45%（2 471/3 364）。

（六）疟疾病人通过信息网络报告的比例

项目地区疟疾病人通过疟疾监测网络报告的比例为 17.11%（143/836）。其中云南省为 6.35%（39/614），海南省为 46.85%（104/222）。云南省该指标较低，与基层镜检人员欠缺、镜检水平低下和政府干预有关，同时少数民族多名字以及当地居民自诊自疗特别是少数民族患病不就医等现象一定程度上也影响了该指标。

（七）云南省疟疾调查推断发病率

云南省疟疾调查推断发病率为 148.09/ 万（13 295/897 800），尚未达到 136/ 万的预定目标。由于云南情况比较特殊，腾冲的疟疾病例大多存在于外出缅甸的当地居民中，调查时，此部分居民大量外出，故通过走访调查能够找到疫情上报相符的病例很少。绿春和西盟的情况则不同，少数民族通常会有几个名字，再因为根据译音记录，随着调查或记录人员的不同，记录的汉字也有出入，因此很难对两种方法得来的资料进行准确匹配，找到相符的人数也很少。

（八）海南省恶性疟调查推断发病率

海南省恶性疟调查推断发病率为 1.79/ 万（201/1 125 144）。该省中、轻度恶性疟流行县已达到基本消除恶性疟标准，但各乡镇间恶性疟流行程度差异很大，如轻度恶性疟流行区万宁市，其南桥乡恶性疟实际发病率为 14.42/ 万，为此，2008 年全省项目地区恶性疟发病率达 1/ 万以下的总目标任务仍艰巨。

结论

全球基金第一轮疟疾项目实施以来，疟疾控制效果逐步显现。2005 年度海南省各指标均达到预期效果，但地区间发展不平衡，疟疾病例通过信息网络报告的比例难以进一步提高等问题需引起重视；云南省的居民求医行为、居民自我保护行为、学生疟防知识等指标都有明显提高，但疟疾病人通过显微镜确诊的比例、居民疟防知识、疟疾病人通过信息网络报告比例、疟疾调查推断发病率等指标完成不足，初步分析与少数民族地区健康教育程度不高以及基层疟防人员专业技术水平低相关，项目下阶段对此将认真研究，重点解决。

表 3-3 项目指标 2005 年度专项调查结果汇总表

	指标	云南			海南			合计		
		分子	分母	比例(%)	分子	分母	比例(%)	分子	分母	比例(%)
1	通过显微镜确诊的疟疾病人比例	162	991	16.35	377	784	48.09	539	1 775	30.37
2	目标地区中小学生能够回答至少3个与疟疾相关问题的比例	882	1 167	75.58	869	1 189	73.09	1 751	2 356	74.32
3	目标地区居民能够回答至少3个与疟疾相关问题的比例	3 277	8 824	37.14	1 013	1 667	60.77	4 290	10 491	40.89
4	求医行为改变(发热病人在症状出现2天内求诊的比例)	1 864	2 917	63.90	1 060	1 419	74.70	2 924	4 336	67.44
5	自我防护行为的变化(拥有ITNs的居民正确使用ITNs的比例)	75	117	64.10	2 471	3 364	73.45	2 546	3 481	73.14
6	疟疾病人通过疟疾监测网络报告的比例	39	614	6.35	104	222	46.85	143	836	17.11
7	云南省疟疾调查推断发病率	13 295	897 800	1.48	-	-	-	-	-	-
8	海南省恶性疟调查推断发病率	-	-	-	201	1 125 144	0.018	-	-	-

第四节　全球基金疟疾项目 2006 年度调查报告

为全面了解第一轮中国全球基金疟疾项目 2006 年度项目实施效果，根据项目监督与评价（M&E）计划要求，国家项目办组织云南省项目办和海南省项目办制定了 2006 年度专项调查具体实施方案，并开展了相关指标的年度专项调查。

一、调查内容与方法

（一）调查时间

海南省 2007 年 1 月 14—31 日，云南省 2007 年 1 月。

（二）调查方法

统一调查方案，统一培训调查员，使用统一的调查表格，通过分层随机抽样，进行回顾性调查。

（三）调查范围

经分层随机抽取的云南省和海南省各 3 个项目县(市)9 个项目乡镇 27 个行政村；时间范围：2006 年 1—12 月。

（四）抽样方法

根据 2004—2006 年疟疾发病率（其中海南为恶性疟发病率）高低，采取分层随机整群抽样法。第一层：将全省各项目县（市）按发病率分为重、中、轻 3 类，在每类县（市）中随机抽取 1 个县（市）为调查县。第二层：以被调查县为单位，将全县各乡镇按发病率分为重、中、轻 3 类。在每类乡镇中随机抽取 1 个乡镇为调查点。第三层：以抽取的乡镇为单位，将全乡镇各行政村按发病率分为重、中、轻 3 类。在每类行政村中随机抽取 1 个行政村为调查点。以抽取的行政村为单位，随机抽取 1—3 个自然村或村民组为调查点。即每县调查 3 个乡 9 个行政村 9—27 个自然村。

（五）调查对象

以被调查县 CDC、乡镇卫生院、村诊所以及被调查村民、中小学生为对象。每一行政村调查村民数不少于 300 人，每县（市）不少于 2 700 人；每个乡镇抽取中、小学校各 1 所，每所学校各 60 人，共 120 人，全县 3 个乡镇共 360 人（小学三年级到初中三年级）。

（六）调查内容

1. 云南省 25 个项目县和海南省 10 个项目县疟疾调查推断发病率

根据捕获 - 再捕获的方法，采用公式 N=[（C+1）（R+1）/（M+1）]–1（其中 C：受调查人群中上报的疟疾病例数；R：走访调查出的疟疾病例数；M：走访调查出的病例中作为疫情报告的病例数）分别推算各抽样县被调查人群实际疟疾病人数及其漏报率，以被调查人群的疟疾漏报率推算 3 个项目县的实际疟疾发病人数和发病率。

2. 海南省 10 个项目县恶性疟发病率

根据捕获 - 再捕获方法（CMR）推算被调查乡镇实际恶性疟发病例数（N=[（C+1）（R+1）/（M+1）]-1）：(1) 在县（市）CDC 疫情网络直报系统上获得被调查乡镇恶性疟病例数（C 值）；(2) 核查被调查乡镇卫生院恶性疟病例登记数（R 值）；(3) 核对恶性疟病例登记名单和上报名单，记录相符的恶性疟病例数（M 值）。依据公式：项目县实际恶性疟病例数 = 项目县报告恶性疟病例总数 ÷（被调查乡镇恶性疟报告病例数 /N），推算出项目县实际恶性疟病例数（分子），从统计局获得项目县人口总数（分母）。

3. 拥有杀虫剂浸泡蚊帐（ITNs）的家庭比例

在被抽查的村进行走访调查，同时获得居民家庭户数和拥有 ITNs 的居民家庭户数分别作为分母和分子。

4. 目标地区中小学生能够正确回答至少 3 个与疟疾相关问题的比例

问卷调查被抽查的中小学生中能够正确回答出至少 3 个疟疾相关问题的人数。

5. 发热病人在症状出现两天内求诊的比例

在被抽查的村进行走访调查，同时获得曾经发热病人数和两天内就诊的人数（分母和分子）。

6. 疟疾病人通过信息网络报告的比例

在被抽查的村进行走访调查，符合“血检阳性、典型临床症状、药物试治有效”其中之一即为疟疾病例（分母），根据走访调查的疟疾病例名单，与县 CDC 网络直报疫情进行核对，名单中姓名、性别、年龄、地址相符者为分子。

二、调查结果

云南省从重、中、轻度流行区中分别抽取盈江县、龙陵县和沧源县作为调查县，问卷调查了3县9个乡镇27个行政村的8 797名居民和18所中小学校的1 057名学生，入户调查了27个行政村的居民疟史、蚊帐使用情况。

海南省从重、中、轻度流行区中分别抽取东方市、白沙县和万宁市作为调查县，问卷调查了3县9个乡镇27个行政村的居民和18所中小学校的1 148名学生，入户调查了27个行政村的居民疟史、蚊帐使用情况，调查了9个乡镇卫生院和抽样村卫生室的病例登记和门诊日志。

（一）云南省25个项目县和海南省10个项目县疟疾调查推断发病率

云南省疟疾调查推断发病率为133.58/万（9 512/712 108）。海南省疟疾调查推断发病率为27.89/万（3 189/1 143 669）。由于云南地理环境以及其他条件的影响，特别是疟疾病例通过信息网络报告的比例较低的相关因素影响，使得相关数据的获得有一定的难度，也造成获得的数据存在一定的误差，但总体而言，云南省发病率相对去年而言有了一定的下降，海南省项目进展良好，该项指标已达到2006年的目标。

（二）海南省10个项目县恶性疟发病率

海南省恶性疟调查推断发病率为0.71/万（81/1 143 669）。从结果看海南省恶性疟发病率达到《监督评价（ME）计划与实施指南（第四年）》的≤2/万的标准。

（三）拥有杀虫剂浸泡蚊帐（ITNs）的家庭比例

项目地区拥有ITNs的居民家庭比例为30.40%（1 397/4 596）。其中云南省为16.45%（442/2 687），海南省为50.03%（955/1 909）。

（四）目标地区中小学生能够正确回答至少3个与疟疾相关问题的比例

目标地区能正确回答至少3个与疟疾相关问题的学生比例为75.83%（1 672/2 205），基本符合该项指标2006年目标的要求，其中云南省这一比例为72.56%（767/1 057），海南省为78.83%（905/1 148）。

（五）发热病人在症状出现两天内求诊的比例

目标地区发热病人在症状出现两天内求诊的比例为 85.25%（2 503/2 936），其中云南省为 82.85%（981/1 184），海南省为 86.87%（1 522/1 752），基本符合项目要求。

（六）疟疾病人通过信息网络报告的比例

项目地区疟疾病人通过疟疾监测网络报告的比例为 42.26%（202/478）。其中云南省为 25.82%（47/182），海南省为 52.36%（155/296）。云南省该指标比去年的调查数据有了较大的提高，但比例还是较低，这主要因为受云南山区大、人员居住分散、交通不便利、基层镜检能力相对薄弱、当地居民自诊自疗的现象普遍和部分地区受当地行政部门的干预等多方面的因素影响所致。

结论

全球基金第一轮疟疾项目实施以来，疟疾控制效果得到进一步提高，2006 年度各项指标基本达到了预期目标，但部分指标仍有待提高，需加强相关的项目工作。其中，2006 年度云南省项目各指标较 2005 年度均有了明显的改善，但部分指标还存在完成不足和执行不到位的情况，项目下阶段应采取有效措施，重点解决指标完成不足的问题。2006 年度海南省项目各指标除目标地区中小学生能够回答至少 3 个与疟疾相关问题的比例稍低于 2006 年规定的指标比例外，其余指标均达到或超过规定的指标比例，调查结果显示项目进展良好。

表 3–4　项目指标 2006 年度专项调查结果汇总表

	指标	云南			海南			合计		
		分子	分母	比例	分子	分母	比例	分子	分母	比例
1	云南省 25 个项目县和海南省 10 个项目县疟疾调查推断发病率	9 512	712 108	133.58/ 万	3 189	1 143 669	27.89/ 万	-	-	-
2	海南省恶性疟调查推断发病率	-	-	-	81	1 143 669	0.71/ 万	-	-	-

续表

3	拥有杀虫剂浸泡蚊帐(ITNs)的家庭比例	442	2 687	16.45%	955	1 909	50.03%	1 397	4 596	30.40%
4	目标地区中小学生能够回答至少3个与疟疾相关问题的比例	767	1 057	72.56%	905	1 148	78.83%	1 672	2 205	75.83%
5	发热病人在症状出现2天内求诊的比例	981	1 184	82.85%	1 522	1 752	86.87%	2 503	2 936	85.25%
6	疟疾病人通过信息网络报告的比例	47	182	25.82%	155	296	52.36%	202	478	42.26%

第五节　全球基金疟疾项目终期调查报告

为全面了解第一轮中国全球基金疟疾项目 5 年实施效果，根据项目监督与评价（M&E）计划要求，国家项目办组织云南省项目办和海南省项目办制定了终期专项调查具体实施方案，并开展了相关指标的年度专项调查。

一、调查内容与方法

（一）调查范围

在第一轮云南省全球基金疟疾项目的 25 个项目县（市）和第一轮海南省全球基金疟疾项目的所有 10 个项目县（市），经分层随机整群抽样，进行回顾性调查，时间涵盖 2007 年全年。

（二）调查时间

2008 年 1 月。

（三）调查指标与方法

1. 疟疾调查推断发病率

1.1 分母：被调查县（市）当年人口总数。

1.2 分子：项目县（市）当年疟疾推算实际病例数。

1.3 调查方法：分层随机整群抽样，回顾性调查。

1.3.1 抽样方法：采取分层随机整群抽样法。第一层：按近 3 年（2005—2007 年）的疟疾发病率，将全县（市）的各乡镇按发病率高、中、低分为 3 类。在每类乡镇中随机抽取 1 个乡镇为调查点。第二层：以抽取的乡镇为单位，按近 3 年的疟疾发病率，将全乡镇的各行政村按发病率高、中、低分为 3 类。在每类行政村中随机抽取 1 个行政村。第三层：在每个抽中的行政村中随机抽取 1—3 个自然村或村民组。即全县（市）共 3 个乡镇 9 个行政村 9—27 个自然村，每一行政村调查村民数不少于 300 人，总人数不少于 2 700 人。

1.3.2 调查对象：被调查县 CDC、乡镇卫生院、村诊所和被调查村民。

1.3.3 调查内容与实际疟疾发病率推算方法：(1) 采用捕获 - 再捕获方法（CMR）推算被调查乡镇实际疟疾发病例数。在被调查县（市）CDC 疫情网络直报系统上获得被调查村疟疾病例数（C 值）；符合“血检阳性、典型临床症状、药物试治有效”其中之一即为疟疾病例，挨户走访调查当年有疟史的居民数（R 值）；核对走访调查中发现的有疟史者名单和被调查村的上报疟疾病例名单，记录相符的疟疾病例数（M 值）；按公式 N=[（C+1）（R+1）/（M+1）]–1 推算各县（市）被调查村的疟疾实际发病数。(2) 推算项目县（市）实际疟疾病例数 = 项目县（市）报告疟疾病例总数 ÷（项目县（市）被调查村疟疾报告病例数 /N）。(3) 从统计局获得项目县（市）人口总数。(4) 推算项目县（市）实际疟疾发病率 = 推算项目县（市）实际疟疾病例数 / 项目县（市）当年人口总数 ×10 000/ 万。

1.3.4 汇总表

被调查县人口数(1)	被调查县上报疟疾病例数(2)	受调查人群中通过网络直报的疟疾病例数(C值)(3)	走访调查出的疟疾病例数(R值)(4)	走访调查出的疟疾病例中作为疫情网络直报的病例数(M值)(5)	推算被调查人群实际疟疾病例数(N值)(6)	推算被调查县(市)实际发病数(7)＝(2)/{(3)/(6)}	推算被调查县(市)实际发病率(1/万)(8)＝(7)/(1)×10000

填表人：　　　　　　　　填表日期：

2. 海南省 10 个项目县（市）的恶性疟发病率

2.1 分母：被调查项目县（市）当年人口总数。

2.2 分子：项目县（市）当年恶性疟推算实际病例数。

2.3 调查方法：分层随机抽样，回顾性调查。

2.3.1 抽样方法：采取分层随机整群抽样法。按近三年的恶性疟发病率将全县（市）的各乡镇分为恶性疟流行重、中、轻三类，每类中随机抽取 1 个乡镇。即全县（市）抽取 3 个乡镇。

2.3.2 调查对象：被调查县（市）CDC 和乡镇卫生院。

2.3.3 调查内容与实际恶性疟发病率推算方法：(1) 采用捕获 - 再捕获方法（CMR）

推算被调查乡镇实际恶性疟发病例数。在被调查县（市）CDC疫情网络直报系统上获得被调查乡镇恶性疟病例数（C值）；核查被调查乡镇卫生院恶性疟病例登记数（R值）；核对恶性疟病例登记名单和上报名单，记录相符的恶性疟病例数（M值）；按下列公式推算各县(市)被调查乡镇实际恶性疟病例数 N=[(C+1)(R+1)/(M+1)]–1。(2) 推算项目县（市）实际恶性疟病例数 = 项目县（市）报告恶性疟病例总数 ÷（项目县（市）被调查乡镇恶性疟报告病例数/N)。(3) 从统计局获得项目县（市）人口总数。(4) 推算项目县（市）实际恶性疟发病率 = 推算项目县（市）实际恶性疟病例数 / 项目县（市）当年人口总数 ×10 000/ 万。

2.3.4 汇总表

被调查县人口数(1)	被调查县上报恶性疟病例数(2)	被调查乡镇卫生院恶性疟疫情报告数 数(C值)(3)	被调查乡镇恶性疟病例登记数(R值)(4)	恶性疟名单相符的病例数(M值)(5)	推算被调查乡镇实际恶性疟病例数(N值)(6)	推算被调查县(市)实际恶性疟病例数(7)=(2)/{(3)/(6)}	推算被调查县(市)恶性疟实际发病率(1/万)(8)=(7)/(1)×10000

填表人：　　　　　　　　　　填表日期：

3. 目标地区中小学生能够回答至少3个与疟疾相关问题的比例

3.1 分母：抽查的中小学生数。

3.2 分子：调查出能正确回答3个疟疾相关问题的中小学生数。

3.3 调查方法：采取分层随机整群抽样法，全县（市）抽取3个项目乡镇（场），每个乡镇（场）抽取中、小学校各1所，每所学校各60名学生。即每县（市）3个乡镇（场）6所学校共360人（小学三年级到初中三年级）。通过问卷调查能够正确回答三个疟疾相关问题的人数。

3.4 汇总表

乡镇名 (1)	调查的中小学校数 (2)	调查的学生数 (3)	能正确回答三个疟疾相关问题的学生数(4)	能正确回答三个疟疾相关问题的学生的比例(%) (5) = (4) / (3) ×100
合计				

填表人：　　　　　　　　　　填表日期：

4. 发热病人在症状出现两天内求诊的比例

4.1 分母：调查的发热病人数。

4.2 分子：发热病人在症状出现两天内求诊的人数。

4.3 调查方法：采取分层随机整群抽样法，方法同（一），即每县（市）共 3 个乡镇（场）9 个行政村（作业区）9—27 个自然村（队）。入户走访调查村民中曾经发热病人数和 2 天内求诊的人数。

4.4 汇总表

乡镇名 (1)	调查的行政村数 (2)	自述有发热史的村民数 (3)	自述有发热史的村民中发热 2 天内求诊的人数(4)	发热病人在症状出现 2 天内求诊的比例(%) (5) = (4) / (3) ×100
合计				

填表人：　　　　　　　　　　填表日期：

5. 拥有杀虫剂浸泡蚊帐（ITNs）的家庭比例

5.1 分母：走访调查的户数。

5.2 分子：走访调查出的拥有药浸蚊帐（ITNs）户数。

5.3 调查方法：分层随机整群抽样，方法同（一），即每县（市）共 3 个乡镇（场）9 个行政村（作业区）9—27 个自然村（队），入户走访调查。

5.4 汇总表

乡镇名（1）	调查的行政村数（2）	调查户数（3）	拥有 ITNs 的户数（4）	拥有 ITNs 户数的比例（%）（5）=（4）/（3）×100
合计				

填表人：　　　　　　　　　　填表日期：

6. 网络直报疟疾病人比例

6.1 分母：走访调查出的疟疾病例

6.2 分子：走访调查出的疟疾病例中通过网络直报的人数

6.3 调查方法：采取分层随机整群抽样法，方法同（一），即全县（市）共 3 个乡镇（场）9 个行政村（作业区）9—27 个自然村（队）。入户走访调查，符合“血检阳性、典型临床症状、药物试治有效”其中之一即为疟疾病例（分母）。根据走访调查的疟疾病例名单，与县 CDC 网络直报疫情进行核对，相符者为分子。

6.4 汇总表

乡镇名（1）	调查的行政村数（2）	走访调查的疟疾病例数（3）	走访调查的疟疾病例中通过网络直报的病例数（4）	网络直报疟疾病人比例（%）（5）=（4）/（3）×100

二、调查结果

云南省将所有 25 个项目县（市）全部作为调查县，问卷调查了 25 县 75 个乡镇 225 个行政村的 16 784 户居民和 141 所中小学校的 9 961 名学生，入户调查了 225 个行政村的居民疟史、蚊帐使用情况。

海南省将所有 10 个项目县（市）全部作为调查县，问卷调查了 10 县 30 个乡镇 90 个行政村的 5 954 户居民和 60 所中小学校的 4 315 名学生，入户调查了 90 个行政村的居民疟史、蚊帐使用情况，调查了 30 个乡镇卫生院和抽样村卫生室的病例登记和门诊日志。

（一）云南省25个项目县和海南省10个项目县疟疾调查推断发病率

云南省疟疾调查推断发病率为65.88/万（40 795/6 192 565）。海南省疟疾调查推断发病率为31.13/万（10 120/3 251 196）。由于2007年来，受5方面因素的影响，云南省疟疾调查推断发病率有了较大的降低：(1) 国家、省、县项目办确实加强了第一轮全球基金项目执行力度，使辖区项目乡、村落实项目工作措施力度加强；(2) 项目执行以来，第一轮的25个项目县，相继得到了第五、第六轮全球基金疟疾项目的投入，疟疾防治工作的进一步得到了加强；(3) 25个边境县还相继有国家、省、县等的疟疾及其与蚊媒有关疾病（如登革热和乙型脑炎等）防治项目或工作加强投入；(4) 近几年来，云南省新型农村卫生合作医疗工作（新农合）在25个边境县得到了较好的开展，使得农村居民就医积极性和规范治疗率较大提高，对当地的疟疾防治工作起到了非常有效的促进作用，有效遏制了疟疾的传播和流行；(5) 2005年以来中缅边境管理加强，出入边境的流动人员减少，使得境外输入病例有所减少。总体而言，云南省、海南省项目进展良好，该项指标已达到2007年的目标。

（二）海南省10个项目县恶性疟发病率

海南省恶性疟调查推断发病率为0.40/万（129/3 251 196）。从结果看海南省恶性疟发病率达到《监督评价（ME）计划与实施指南（第四年）》的≤ 2/万的标准。

（三）目标地区中小学生能够正确回答至少3个与疟疾相关问题的比例

目标地区能正确回答至少3个与疟疾相关问题的学生比例为93.18%（13 303/14 276），基本符合该项指标2007年目标的要求，其中云南省这一比例为94.83%（9 446/9 961），海南省为89.39%（3 857/4 315）。

（四）发热病人在症状出现两天内求诊的比例

目标地区发热病人在症状出现2天内求诊的比例为89.95%（15 938/17 718），其中云南省为92.36%（10 816/11 711），海南省为85.27%（5 122/6 007），基本符合项目要求。

（五）拥有杀虫剂浸泡蚊帐（ITNs）的家庭比例

项目地区拥有ITNs的居民家庭比例为37.60%（8 550/22 738）。其中云南省为32.36%（5 431/16 784），海南省为52.38%（3 119/5 954）。

（六）疟疾病人通过信息网络报告的比例

项目地区疟疾病人通过疟疾监测网络报告的比例为 38.92%（534/1 372）。其中云南省为 45.30%（289/638），海南省为 33.38%（245/734）。

结论

第一轮全球基金疟疾项目实施以来，疟疾控制效果得到进一步提高，2007 年度各项指标基本达到了预期目标。其中，由于国家、省、县项目办加强了项目管理力度，通过各种方法加强基层的疟疾防治能力，随着第五、第六轮全球基金疟疾项目的相继执行，项目执行能力得到了较大的提高，有效地降低了当地疟疾的发病与传播，以及 2005 年以来中缅边境管理加强，出入边境的流动人员减少，使得境外输入病例有所减少，境内发病降低。2007 年度第一轮云南省全球基金疟疾项目各指标较 2006 年度均有了明显的改善，其中疟疾调查推算发病率为 65.88/ 万，比 2006 年的专项调查数据 133.58/ 万降低了 50.68%，比基线值 197/ 万降低了 66.56%；2007 年度第一轮海南省全球基金疟疾项目六项指标除发热病人在症状出现 2 天内求诊的比例稍低于 2007 年《监督评价（ME）计划与实施指南（第 5 年）》规定的指标，疟疾病例通过信息网络报告的比例这项指标由于部分县（市）乡镇级的疫情网络直报系统不够健全，致使病例漏报还比较严重，其余指标均达到或超过规定的指标比例，调查结果显示项目进展良好。

第一轮全球基金疟疾项目即将接近尾声，由于第一轮云南、海南省项目的项目县大多被第五、六轮全球基金疟疾项目覆盖，故第一轮疟疾项目结束后，项目地区的疟疾防治工作将在第五轮疟疾项目或常规疟防工作的管理下进一步得到巩固。

表 3–5　项目指标 2007 年度专项调查结果汇总表

	指标	云南			海南			合计		
		分子	分母	比例	分子	分母	比例	分子	分母	比例
1	云南省 25 个项目县和海南省 10 个项目县疟疾调查推断发病率	40 795	6 192 565	65.88/ 万	10 120	3 251 196	31.13/ 万	-	-	-

续表

2	海南省恶性疟调查推断发病率	-	-	-	129	3 251 196	0.40/ 万	-	-	-
3	目标地区中小学生能够回答至少3个与疟疾相关问题的比例	9 446	9 961	94.83%	3 857	4 315	89.39%	13 303	14 276	93.18%
4	发热病人在症状出现2天内求诊的比例	10 816	11 711	92.36%	5 122	6 007	85.27%	15 938	17 718	89.95%
5	拥有杀虫剂浸泡蚊帐(ITNs)的家庭比例	5 431	16 784	32.36%	3 119	5 954	52.38%	8 550	22 738	37.60%
6	疟疾病人通过信息网络报告的比例	289	638	45.30%	245	734	33.38%	534	1 372	38.92%

第四章

管理方案

第一节 项目管理方案

一、项目管理基本办法

（一）总则

第一条 为保证全球基金疟疾项目主要任务目标的实现，确保项目第二阶段计划中各项活动顺利实施，特制订本管理办法。

第二条 本办法适用于全球基金疟疾项目覆盖的云南、海南、安徽、湖北、河南、江苏、广东、广西、贵州、四川 10 个项目省（自治区）、县、乡各级项目执行单位。

第三条 此管理办法系对“全球基金项目管理与技术方案”、“全球基金财务管理手册”及“全球基金物资管理和使用规定”的补充。

（二）项目常规管理

第四条 项目实施以各级项目办公室为主体，采取主任负责制。项目报表、年度报告、计划方案、阶段总结及其他重要文件均由项目办主任或其委托人签字盖章方可作为有效文档上报。

第五条 各级项目执行机构应主动加强与卫生行政部门的协调和沟通，积极接受卫生行政部门的监督与检查。

第六条 国家、省、县项目办公室应确定专人分别负责项目常规管理、信息管理和财务管理，明确工作职责和管理程序，并采取每月例会制度加强项目办内部的沟通与合作。

第七条 各级项目办公室应加强沟通与联系，实行逐级请示制度。凡涉及项目计划和经费预算的调整、项目执行出现问题及其他重大情况等，应及时向上一级项目办公室报批和请示。

第八条 各级项目实施机构应积极发挥项目专家组或技术指导小组的作用，项目执行和管理中存在技术问题应及时组织专家进行论证。

第九条 加强资料管理和归档。各级项目执行单位视各自职责和工作范畴，以纸制文档和电子档案两种形式保留工作记录、原始数据、项目报表、计划方案、工作总结等各类资料。上一级执行机构应保留下一级机构上报的电子资料和纸制文档。

（三）项目季度报表管理

第十条　各级项目实施机构必须严格按照工作计划分季度开展项目活动，不得擅自调整计划任务和经费预算。

第十一条　季度报表依据工作计划中本季度包含的项目活动逐项对照填写“计划数”、“完成数”、“预算额”、“实际支出额”。同时填写督导与评价计划（M&E 计划）中本季度考核指标的完成情况。计划任务与实际完成情况、预算与实际支出出现较大差异时，应寻找原因并作出合理解释。

第十二条　项目季度报表应严格按照上级项目办要求按时、如实上报。县项目办应在季度结束后 15 日内将季度任务完成情况和经费开支情况上报省项目办；省项目办应在季度结束 30 日内将全省汇总数据上报国家项目办；国家项目办在季度结束 45 日内上报中央执行机构（PR）。

第十三条　省项目办在收到县项目办季度报表 10 日内对报表数据予以审核，确保季报数据真实、可信，同时抽查 1 至 2 个县进行证实，一旦发现弄虚作假或拖延报表现象，将通报批评或暂停拨款。

第十四条　各级季度报表应由项目管理人员和财务管理人员共同填写。工作报表和财务报表分别由项目主管和财务主管签字后，项目主任或其委托人签发盖章后上报，同时通过电子邮件逐级上报。

（四）项目重点业务活动执行管理

第十五条　省项目办负责发热病人血检工作的计划制订，按计划对县中心镜检站工作进行督导。按季度对血片进行抽查，每年应复检辖区内不少于 30% 的阳性血片，抽检不少于 0.5% 的阴性血片。

第十六条　县项目办专人负责血检器材的发放、人员培训、资料统计及血检工作的具体实施。每月对上月各镜检站的血检登记本、血片进行收集。抽查 10% 阴性血片和复检全部的阳性血片。对血片制作和染色进行质量控制，血片合格率和符合率应保持在 85% 以上。

第十七条　乡（镇）卫生院镜检站按计划完成每季度要求的血检数量，保留发热病人血检登记本，保存当月的阴性血片和全部阳性血片。

第十八条　乡镇卫生院应按时上送所有血片到县项目办。

第十九条　疟疾病例的治疗应依据《中国高传播区疟疾控制项目管理与技术方

案（试行）》的要求进行。

第二十条　在使用全球基金项目提供的药物治疗疟疾病人时，医生应开具处方并妥善保管。县项目办每月抽查部分乡镇卫生院 10% 的疟疾处方进行质量核查。

第二十一条　发放药物时，应有药物发放记录，病人或其监护者应在发放记录上签字。发放记录应妥善保管。

（五）经费使用管理

第二十二条　各级项目实施机构应严格遵守《全球基金财务管理手册》，按项目计划使用资金，确保专款专用，一旦发现财务违规现象，将影响下一季度的资金拨付。

第二十三条　各级项目机构不得截留资金，应按工作计划逐级下达季度任务和经费。确保乡镇卫生院有经费开展本季度的项目活动，不得采取“先工作，后报帐”机制。

第二十四条　发热病人血检和疟疾病人治疗补助应在预算范围内按统一标准、采取“双联单”按月定期发放。查病补助应依据血检记录、血片、送检单，治病补助应依据门诊记录、有效处方和病人治疗登记表。由县项目办验收后，由乡镇卫生院发放，本人签字领取并保留底联。

第二十五条　各级项目人员出差交通费和住宿费实报实销，相关标准由各省根据实际情况自行制定，上报国家项目办，经报批同意后方可执行。省级项目人员住宿标准项目主任、副主任、主管不超过 150 元 / 天，项目办其他人员不超过 100 元 / 天，出差补助不超过 30 元 / 天；县级项目人员住宿标准不超过 50 元 / 天，出差补助不超过 15 元 / 天。补助费从各级项目办管理预算和督导预算中列支，不得挤占其他工作经费，非项目出差不能领取补助。

第二十六条　结余经费转入下季度项目计划活动，不得擅自处理。

（六）物资管理

第二十七条　项目物资管理严格按照《全球基金物资管理和使用规定》执行，确保物资流向清楚、出入和库存物资数量与单据相符。

第二十八条　物资发放要有计划和方案，领用手续齐全，须项目主任或其委托人、领用人和物资发放人的签字。

第二十九条　项目提供的药品、杀虫剂、蚊帐是用于项目地区疟疾防治的免费物资，任何机构和个人不能挪用或倒卖，一旦发现将停止项目并追究当事人和项目负责人的责任。

第三十条 对于免费药品、蚊帐，各省应根据当地实际情况制订发放依据、标准和管理方法，各县项目办负责具体实施，切实保证免费物资用于病人和贫困家庭。

第三十一条 使用全球基金提供的免费药品和物资不得收费。

二、信息管理方案

（一）目的

为确保全球基金疟疾项目的顺利实施，应加强对项目地区的疟疾疫情资料和项目活动资料在收集、传递、处理和反馈过程的规范性管理，以便获得可靠、准确、完整的信息资料，为项目中期和终期的评估提供科学的依据。为此，制订了本信息管理方案。

（二）基本管理构架

1. 各级机构间的关系

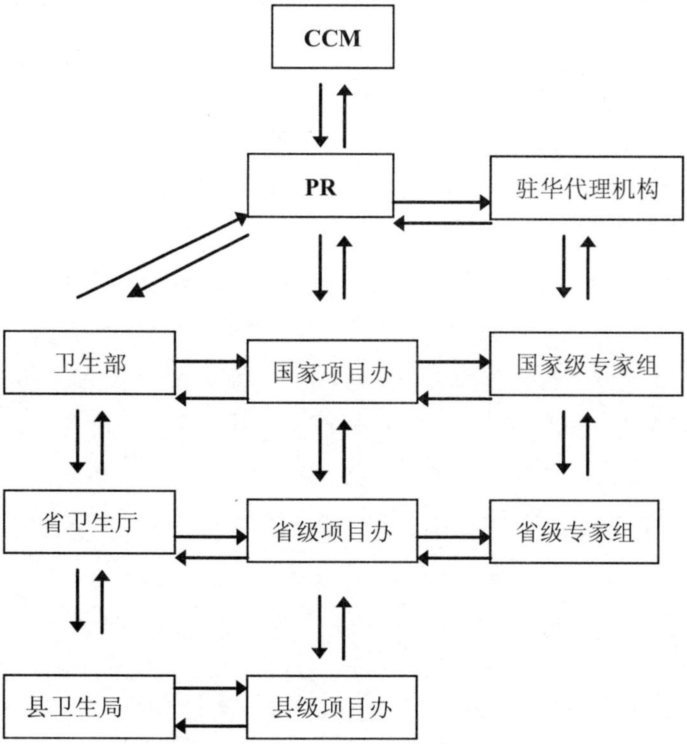

疟疾项目信息管理总体构架示意图

2. 以因特网为依托，逐步建立、健全项目地区的信息管理网络，承担与项目活动有关的信息上传、发布与反馈。

3. 国家级项目办负责对相关表格、技术标准、规范的制定；以及对省级、县级信息管理人员的培训与指导。

4. 国家级与省级项目办设置信息管理中心，县级项目办为资料收集的基本单位。

（三）管理范围

1. 各级项目办起草的相关文本，包括项目申请书、实施细则和方案等。
2. 疟疾疫情动态资料，包括月、旬的疟疾发病情况资料。
3. 项目活动的相关资料，包括各方案的实施情况与进度资料。
4. 各类相关会议资料、上传下达的文件和通知等。
5. 各级项目办对项目实施的阶段性督导和评估的结果资料。
6. 项目地区的基线调查资料。
7. 疟疾监测资料。
8. 传播媒介调查资料，等等。

（四）原则与要求

1. 各级项目办的信息管理，应有 1 至 2 名专人负责。

2. 各级项目办对管辖区内相关的调查资料进行分类、汇总、存储、建立数据库，并进行统计、分析，撰写分析报告，并逐级上报。

3. 项目地区的各级各类医疗机构发现疟疾病人、疑似疟疾病人，应按《传染病法》的有关规定，城镇于 12 小时内、农村于 24 小时内上报给县级项目办，县级项目办每季的 10 日前上报给省级项目办，省级项目办每季的 15 日前上报给国家级项目办。

4. 各级项目办对相关信息的上传或下达，须经项目办负责人审阅签字后，方可发出。

5. 各级项目办信息数据库应对外开放，实现资源共享，并提供不同权限的信息查询服务。

6. 各级项目办应逐步建立相关网页，介绍项目活动的最新动态，便于信息的传递和反馈。

7. 国家项目办不定期编辑出版一份项目活动《简报》，分发给各级项目办和有关领导机构。

8. 对与项目活动有关的文字材料和电子文件等载体资料进行归类、编目、集中保管。

（五）质量控制

1. 各类原始调查表和疟疾疫情报告卡应无错项、漏项，随时检查，发现问题及时补充或订正。

2. 信息传递和反馈，要及时、准确、无误，体现时效性。

3. 采取逐级督导和评估的方式，每年进行 1 至 2 次，具体指标如下：

（1）各类调查表原始数据的纠正率，调查人和负责人的签字率。

（2）调查资料分类、汇总、存储的合格率。

（3）疟疾报告卡填写合格率、报出及时率（或迟报率）。

（4）定期报表合格率、上报及时率。

（5）信息反馈应答率。

（6）资料归档率。

（7）上传下达文件，领导审核签字率，等等。

三、督导与评价方案

（一）目的

为了加强项目管理，提高实施质量，确保目标如期实现，特制订此督导考核评估方案，用于对各级项目执行单位的项目管理和执行情况进行督导和考核评估。

（二）督导考核评估内容

根据全球基金疟疾项目的需要，采用逐级、定期、抽样方式，对项目的管理和执行情况进行督导和考核评估。

1. 项目管理

主要考核各级项目办公室建设和运转情况，工作的计划和总结，项目信息管理、财务管理和物资管理，以及项目有关人员参加和组织培训的情况。

2. 项目执行

主要考核各级项目执行机构，按照项目年度和季度工作计划，各项项目活动的执行情况。考核指标为四个项目目标中具体活动的工作量。

（三）组织与实施

1. 督导考核组成员的组成

各级项目办公室负责组织对本级的自我评估和对下级的督导考核。督导考核组由卫生行政部门、项目办和专家组共同组成。国家级督导考核可邀请国际组织和合作伙伴等参加。

2. 督导考核方式

（1）自我评估：省、县项目办结合对下级项目执行机构的督导，并参照考核评估标准进行自我评估，并及时将自我评估结果报送上级项目办。

（2）督导考核：国家或省项目办在接到下级自我评估报告后，采用随机抽样和重点调查相结合的方法确定进行督导考核的项目省或县，按以下工作程序进行督导考核。

①听取该项目办自我评估报告，包括对项目实施、项目管理和经费使用情况的汇报。

②查阅项目活动、项目管理、经费使用和物资发放情况的工作记录、文件、资料等。

③采取随机抽样和重点抽查相结合的方法，每个项目省抽查 1 个项目县（市），每个项目县（市）抽查两个乡镇（农场）卫生院，4 个村诊所，对项目实施、项目管理、经费使用和物资发放情况进行实地督查，并对两个自然村进行走访调查。

④根据督导检查表（附件 1）对督导结果进行评估，并完成考核评估表（附件 2）。

⑤根据督导考核评估结果，与当地项目管理和实施机构进行反馈交流，并对存在的问题提出具体整改意见。

⑥撰写督导考核报告，报同级卫生行政部门并反馈给被督导考核单位。

3. 督导考核频度

按照工作计划，督导考核频度如下：

（1）国家项目办每年在第 3 和第 4 季度分别对两个项目省进行 1 次督导考核。

（2）云南和海南两省项目办对项目县的督导考核在第 2 至第 4 季度进行，每个季度对 1/3 项目县进行 1 次督导考核，每个项目县每年至少被督导考核 1 次；其他 8 个省在第 3 季度对项目县进行 1 次督导考核。

（3）县项目办对乡镇的督导在第 2 至第 4 季度进行，云南和海南两省每县每月对 3 个乡镇进行 1 次督导；其他 8 个省每县每季度对不少于 3 个乡镇进行 1 次督导。

4. 分析与报告

各级要做好督导考核记录，每次督导考核后应在 1 周内完成书面督导考核报告，报上级项目办和同级卫生行政部门，并反馈给被督导考核单位，同时可抄送相关部门。

（四）考核评估评分标准

项目考核评估主要分项目管理和项目执行两大部分，每个部分有多个考核项目，每个考核项目分若干考核指标，各个考核指标具有不同分值，总分为100分。考核评估时，考核组根据被考核单位各项指标的完成情况，参照以下评分标准对被考核单位的项目管理和执行情况进行评定（未达到要求的进行扣分，扣分最多不超过该指标的分值，扣完为止，扣分最小单位为1分）。

1. 项目管理（共60分）

（1）项目办公室建设和运转情况（共14分）

①项目办专人负责项目管理（3分）：无专人管理扣3分。

②卫生行政部门组织和支持项目活动（2分）：无相关文件扣2分，文件不全扣1分。

③合作伙伴按计划参与项目活动（2分）：无相关的方案和记录扣2分，方案和记录不全扣1分。

④各项目省按计划召开项目年会（2分）：未召开年会扣2分，未能按期召开扣1分。

⑤云南和海南各项目县按计划召开项目年会（2分）：未召开年会扣2分，未能按期召开扣1分。

⑥各级项目办按计划进行逐级督导和自我评估（3分）：未进行督导和自我评估扣3分，未能按期进行督导和自我评估扣2分。

（2）项目信息管理（共10分）

①按规定及时上报项目季度报表（包括工作报表和财务报表）(5分)：未上报季度报表扣5分，未及时上报扣3分。

②项目季度报表填写规范，数据准确可靠，有出处（3分）：季度报表填写不规范扣3分。

③档案资料管理专人负责、专柜保存（2分）：资料档案无专人专柜保存管理扣2分，资料保管不完整扣1分。

（3）项目工作计划和总结（共6分）

①项目年度和季度工作计划（4分）：无项目年度和季度工作计划扣4分，项目年度和季度工作计划不符合要求扣2分。

②本季度各项具体活动的实施方案和总结（2分）：无具体活动的实施方案和总结扣2分，各项具体活动实施方案和总结不完整扣1分。

（4）项目财务管理（共16分）

①全球基金项目专用账户（4分）：无全球基金项目专用账户扣4分。

②按规定及时下拨和支付各项经费（4分）：未按规定及时下拨和支付各项经费扣4分。

③按项目计划和活动专款专用（4分）：未按项目计划和活动专款专用扣4分。

④报销凭证规范、合理（4分）：每张不合格报销凭据扣1分。

（5）项目器材物资管理（共8分）

①物资管理制度、物品库存和出入库登记账册（2分）：无物资登记账册扣2分，账册登记不完整或账物不符扣1分。

②固定资产专人保管、能正常使用，有使用和维护记录（2分）：无使用维护记录扣2分，使用维护记录不完整扣1分。

③药品管理制度、药品库存和使用登记账册（2分）：无药品登记账册扣2分，账册登记不完整或账物不符扣1分。

④蚊帐和/或杀虫剂库存、领用和分发记录（2分）：无分发记录扣2分，记录不完整或账物不符扣1分。

（6）项目培训（共6分）

①当地项目管理和执行人员按要求参加有关的项目培训（2分）：缺席1人次培训扣1分。

②按计划完成当地的项目培训活动（有培训计划和方案、学员名单、授课内容和教材以及课程安排等培训记录）（4分）：培训活动未按计划进行的每次扣2分，记录不完整的培训班每个扣1分。

2. 项目执行（共40分）

（1）使云南省边境地区流动人口更好地获得疟疾诊断和合理治疗（共6分）

①边境流动人口中发热病人的血检（3分）：如未完成计划任务，且无合理解释，每10%扣1分。

②边境流动人口中的疟疾病人规范治疗（3分）：如未完成计划任务，且无合理解释，每10%扣1分。

（2）使目标地区当地居民得到更好的早期诊断和个人防护（共15分）

①项目地区发热病人的血检（3分）：如未完成计划任务，且无合理解释，每10%扣1分。

②项目地区疟疾病人规范治疗（3分）：如未完成计划任务，且无合理解释，每10%扣1分。

③项目地区乡、村医生/个体医生诊断和治疗培训（3分）：如未完成计划任务，且无合理解释，每10%扣1分。

④项目地区镜检员培训（3 分）：如未完成计划任务，且无合理解释，每 10%扣 1 分。

⑤项目地区药浸蚊帐（3 分）：如未完成计划任务，且无合理解释，每 10%扣 1 分。

（3）使云南省和海南省流行区居民更有效地采取疟疾预防措施，及时治疗（共 9 分）

①云南和海南项目县用广播进行疟疾知识宣传（3 分）：对照计划任务，每少完成 1 次扣 1 分。

②云南和海南项目县中小学生疟防知识课（3 分）：如未完成计划任务，且无合理解释，每 10%扣 1 分。

③云南和海南项目县在公共场所张贴疟疾知识宣传画（3 分）：如未完成计划任务，且无合理解释，每 10%扣 1 分。

（4）优化云南、海南及其他八个项目省的疟疾控制项目管理（共 10 分）

①项目地区哨点病例主动监测（2 分）：未按计划开展哨点病例主动监测工作扣 2 分，未按期上报病例主动监测结果扣 1 分。

②项目地区药物抗性监测（2 分）：未按计划开展药物抗性监测工作扣 2 分，未按期上报药物抗性监测结果扣 1 分。

③项目地区媒介监测（2 分）：未按计划开展媒介监测工作扣 2 分，未按期上报媒介监测结果扣 1 分。

④项目地区专项调查（4 分）：未按计划开展专项调查扣 4 分，专项调查存在较严重质量问题扣 3 分，专项调查不完全符合要求扣 2 分，未按期上报调查结果和报告扣 1 分。

（五）考核评估及奖惩

根据督导考核评分的总分对项目执行单位进行评估，分为“优秀、良好、合格、基本合格、不合格”五个等次，其中：90 及 90 分以上为“优秀”；80—89 分为“良好”；70—79 分为“合格”；60—69 分为“基本合格”；低于 60 分为“不合格”，如发现在督导考核评估中有弄虚作假行为，直接评为“不合格”。

每次督导考核结果在“全球基金项目简报”和项目例会或年会上公布。对督导考核成绩突出的项目办进行适当奖励（云南、海南 2 省 90 及 90 分以上，其他 8 个省 95 及 95 分以上）。对考核评估为“不合格”者进行通报批评并暂停拨款，进行整改，整改结果得到上级项目办考核认可后，方可继续得到拨款执行项目；评估为“基本合格”者进行通报批评，连续两次被“基本合格”者，暂停拨款，进行整改。

（六）项目评价

1. 评价的组织和人员

项目评价由全球基金（GF）牵头，组织专家或委托中央执行机构（PR）组织相关人员，对项目省、县进行评价。机构和人员由全球基金委托和选定。

2. 评价的形式

按照全球基金的要求，采取全球基金提议或认可的方式进行。

3. 评价的时间

中期评价：项目两年度结束后（2005 年 2 月 24 日），进行中期评价，具体时间由全球基金确定。

终期评价：项目 5 年结束后（2008 年 2 月 24 日），进行终期评价，具体时间由全球基金确定。

4. 评价内容与指标

（1）重点地区的疟疾控制

①提高项目重点地区疟疾诊治能力；

②增强当地居民自我防护意识和提高规范治疗的依从性；

③加强当地居民个人防护措施；

④加强对局部暴发流行的控制。

评价指标：

序号	评价指标	基线（2002 年）	目标				
			2003	2004	2005	2006	2007
1	拥有镜检站的乡镇比例						
2	镜检培训班的次数						
3	血检覆盖率						
4	血检率						
5	血片制作合格率						
6	血检误 / 漏检率						
7	血检复查率						
8	抗疟药集中采购 / 供应 / 销售比例						
9	规范治疗率						
10	乡医接受培训的比例						
11	收到健教材料的家庭比例						
12	居民疟防知识知晓率						

续表

13	中小学生疟防知识知晓率						
14	蚊帐拥有率						
15	浸帐率						
16	药浸蚊帐使用率						
17	发现暴发流行到应急措施的时间						

（2）重点人群的疟疾控制

①加强边境流动人口的疟疾控制。

②加强上山住宿高危人群的疟疾控制。

评价指标：

序号	评价指标	基线（2002 年）	目标				
			2003	2004	2005	2006	2007
1	边境口岸拥有镜检站的比例						
2	边境口岸医生接受培训的比例						
3	流动人口中发热病人血检率						
4	流动人口疟疾患者规范治疗比例						
5	边境口岸张贴指示牌的比例						
6	边境口岸医院 / 诊所张贴宣传画的比例						
7	上山住宿人群集中的乡镇拥有疟疾巡视员的比例						
8	上山住宿高危人群疟疾患者及时诊治的比例						
9	疟疾患者规范治疗的比例						

（3）建立监测系统与信息网络

①改进疫情报告系统，减少疫情漏报。

②加强疫情监测与抗药性监测。

③建立疟疾信息网络。

评价指标：

序号	评价内容与指标	基线（2002 年）	目标				
			2003	2004	2005	2006	2007
1	乡村卫生院发热病人血检登记的比例						
2	乡村卫生院疟疾疫情报告比例						
3	有无疟疾信息网络						

附件 1　全球基金疟疾项目督导检查表

表 1　乡村医生 / 镜检员培训

被督导单位			督导日期	
督导方式			被督导单位签收	
督导内容	是	否	备注	
1. 有书面计划、方案、安排				
2. 已开展				
3. 已完成				
4. 有学员名单表				
5. 有培训内容				
6. 有课程安排				
7. 有学习成绩				
8. 有书面小结				
建议：				
上次督导建议执行情况：				

督导单位：　　　　督导员：　　　　督导单位负责人：

注：此表一式两份，一份存被督导单位，一份存督导单位。

表 2 发热病人血检

<table>
<tr><td>被督导单位</td><td colspan="2"></td><td>督导日期</td><td></td></tr>
<tr><td>督导方式</td><td colspan="2"></td><td>被督导单位签收</td><td></td></tr>
<tr><td colspan="2">督导内容</td><td>是</td><td>否</td><td>备注</td></tr>
<tr><td colspan="2">1. 有书面计划、方案、安排</td><td></td><td></td><td></td></tr>
<tr><td colspan="2">2. 已开展</td><td></td><td></td><td></td></tr>
<tr><td colspan="2">3. 已完成</td><td></td><td></td><td></td></tr>
<tr><td colspan="2">4. 镜检站运转正常</td><td></td><td></td><td></td></tr>
<tr><td colspan="2">5. 血检登记齐全</td><td></td><td></td><td></td></tr>
<tr><td colspan="2">6. 血片制作规范</td><td></td><td></td><td></td></tr>
<tr><td colspan="2">7. 血片染色规范</td><td></td><td></td><td></td></tr>
<tr><td colspan="2">8. 有血片抽检、反馈记录</td><td></td><td></td><td></td></tr>
<tr><td colspan="2">9. 抽查发热病人与血检登记相符</td><td></td><td></td><td></td></tr>
<tr><td colspan="5">建议：</td></tr>
<tr><td colspan="5">上次督导建议执行情况：</td></tr>
</table>

督导单位：　　　　督导员：　　　　督导单位负责人：

注：此表一式两份，一份存被督导单位，一份存督导单位。

表 3 疟疾病人规范治疗

被督导单位			督导日期	
督导方式			被督导单位签收	
督导内容	是	否	备注	
1. 有书面计划、方案、安排				
2. 已开展				
3. 已完成				
4. 疟疾病人治疗记录、登记齐全				
5. 治疗及时				
6. 治疗用药、剂量规范				
7. 抽查疟疾病人与治疗记录相符				
建议：				
上次督导建议执行情况：				

督导单位：　　　　督导员：　　　督导单位负责人：

注：此表一式两份，一份存被督导单位，一份存督导单位。

表 4 中小学生疟疾知识课、张贴宣传画

<table>
<tr><td colspan="2">被督导单位</td><td colspan="2"></td><td>督导日期</td><td></td></tr>
<tr><td colspan="2">督导方式</td><td colspan="2"></td><td>被督导单位签收</td><td></td></tr>
<tr><td colspan="3">督导内容</td><td>是</td><td>否</td><td>备注</td></tr>
<tr><td rowspan="5">学生授课</td><td colspan="2">1. 有书面计划、方案、安排</td><td></td><td></td><td></td></tr>
<tr><td colspan="2">2. 已开展</td><td></td><td></td><td></td></tr>
<tr><td colspan="2">3. 已完成</td><td></td><td></td><td></td></tr>
<tr><td colspan="2">4. 讲课记录、登记齐全</td><td></td><td></td><td></td></tr>
<tr><td colspan="2">5. 有书面工作小结</td><td></td><td></td><td></td></tr>
<tr><td rowspan="5">张贴宣传画</td><td colspan="2">1. 有书面计划、方案、安排</td><td></td><td></td><td></td></tr>
<tr><td colspan="2">2. 已开展</td><td></td><td></td><td></td></tr>
<tr><td colspan="2">3. 已完成</td><td></td><td></td><td></td></tr>
<tr><td colspan="2">4. 记录、登记齐全</td><td></td><td></td><td></td></tr>
<tr><td colspan="2">5. 有书面工作小结</td><td></td><td></td><td></td></tr>
<tr><td colspan="6">建议：</td></tr>
<tr><td colspan="6">上次督导建议执行情况：</td></tr>
</table>

督导单位： 督导员： 督导单位负责人：

注：此表一式两份，一份存被督导单位，一份存督导单位。

表 5　广播电视节目、信息网络运行和维护

被督导单位			督导日期	
督导方式			被督导单位签收	
督导内容		是	否	备注
广播电视节目	1. 有广播电视节目计划、方案			
	2. 已开展			
	3. 已完成			
	4. 记录、登记齐全			
	5. 有书面工作小结			
信息网络	1. 电脑设备用于项目工作			
	2. 信息网络运行正常			
	3. 按要求从网络上报资料			
	4. 设备维护完好			
建议：				
上次督导建议执行情况：				

督导单位：　　　　督导员：　　　　督导单位负责人：

注：此表一式两份，一份存被督导单位，一份存督导单位。

表 6 监测工作

被督导单位			督导日期	
督导方式			被督导单位签收	

督导内容		是	否	备注
哨点监测	1. 有监测工作计划、方案			
	2. 已开展主动监测工作			
	3. 完成主动监测工作			
	4. 监测记录、登记齐全			
	5. 有书面工作报告			
抗性监测	1. 有抗性监测工作计划、方案			
	2. 已开展抗性监测工作			
	3. 完成抗性监测工作			
	4. 监测记录、登记齐全			
	5. 有书面工作报告			
媒介监测	1. 有媒介监测工作计划、方案			
	2. 已开展媒介监测工作			
	3. 完成媒介监测工作			
	4. 监测记录、登记齐全			
	5. 有书面工作报告			
建议：				
上次督导建议执行情况：				

督导单位：　　　　督导员：　　　　督导单位负责人：

注：此表一式二份，一份存被督导单位，一份存督导单位。

表 7　财务、物资管理

<table>
<tr><td colspan="2">被督导单位</td><td colspan="2"></td><td>督导日期</td><td></td></tr>
<tr><td colspan="2">督导方式</td><td colspan="2"></td><td>被督导单位签收</td><td></td></tr>
<tr><td colspan="2">督导内容</td><td>是</td><td>否</td><td colspan="2">备注</td></tr>
<tr><td rowspan="6">财务管理</td><td>1. 收到项目经费及数额</td><td></td><td></td><td colspan="2"></td></tr>
<tr><td>2. 是否明确用于哪项项目工作</td><td></td><td></td><td colspan="2"></td></tr>
<tr><td>3. 按任务下拨经费及数额</td><td></td><td></td><td colspan="2"></td></tr>
<tr><td>4. 经费按规定开支</td><td></td><td></td><td colspan="2"></td></tr>
<tr><td>5. 账目清楚</td><td></td><td></td><td colspan="2"></td></tr>
<tr><td>6. 作账符合项目管理要求</td><td></td><td></td><td colspan="2"></td></tr>
<tr><td rowspan="5">物资管理</td><td>1. 有药品、器材分配计划</td><td></td><td></td><td colspan="2"></td></tr>
<tr><td>2. 分配合理</td><td></td><td></td><td colspan="2"></td></tr>
<tr><td>3. 分发手续齐全</td><td></td><td></td><td colspan="2"></td></tr>
<tr><td>4. 使用记录齐全</td><td></td><td></td><td colspan="2"></td></tr>
<tr><td>5. 器材维护保养完好</td><td></td><td></td><td colspan="2"></td></tr>
<tr><td colspan="6">建议：</td></tr>
<tr><td colspan="6">上次督导建议执行情况：</td></tr>
</table>

督导单位：　　　　督导员：　　　　督导单位负责人：

注：此表一式两份，一份存被督导单位，一份存督导单位。

表 8 督导和资料管理

被督导单位				督导日期	
督导方式				被督导单位签收	
督导内容		是	否	备注	
督导工作	1. 有书面计划、方案、安排				
	2. 已开展				
	3. 已完成				
	4. 督导记录、登记齐全				
	5. 有督导反馈				
	6. 有书面工作小结				
资料管理	1. 项目资料有专人专柜保管				
	2. 资料分类清楚、保存完整				
	3. 项目资料上报、反馈及时				
	4. 资料填写规范				
	5. 资料数据真实准确				
	6. 资料有调查人、负责人签名				
建议：					
上次督导建议执行情况：					

督导单位： 督导员： 督导单位负责人：

注：此表一式两份，一份存被督导单位，一份存督导单位。

附件 2 全球基金疟疾项目考核评估表

被考核单位			
考核阶段	第___季度（200___年___月___日－200___年___月___日）		
考核方式	□自我评估　□督导考核	考核时间	200___年___月___日
项目管理情况			
考核项目	考核指标	分值	扣分
1. 项目办公室建设和运转情况（共 14 分）	（1）项目办专人负责项目管理	3	
	（2）卫生行政部门组织和支持项目活动	2	
	（3）合作伙伴按计划参与项目活动	2	
	（4）各项目省按计划召开项目年会	2	
	（5）云南和海南各项目县按计划召开项目年会	2	
	（6）各级项目办按计划进行逐级督导和自我评估	3	
2. 项目信息管理（共 10 分）	（1）按规定及时上报项目季度报表	5	
	（2）项目季度报表填写规范，数据准确可靠，有出处	3	
	（3）档案资料管理专人负责、专柜保存	2	
3. 项目工作计划和总结（共 6 分）	（1）项目年度和季度工作计划	4	
	（2）各项具体活动的实施方案和总结	2	
4. 项目财务管理（共 16 分）	（1）全球基金项目专用账户	4	
	（2）按规定及时下拨和支付经费	4	
	（3）按项目计划和活动专款专用	4	
	（4）报销凭证规范、合理	4	
5. 项目器材物资管理（共 8 分）	（1）物资管理制度、物品库存和出入库登记账册	2	
	（2）固定资产专人保管、能正常使用，有使用和维护记录	2	
	（3）药品管理制度、药品库存和使用登记账册	2	
	（4）蚊帐和 / 或杀虫剂库存、领用和分发记录	2	
6. 项目培训（共 6 分）	（1）当地项目管理和执行人员按要求参加有关的项目培训	2	
	（2）按计划完成当地的项目培训活动	4	
项目管理情况合计扣分（A）			
项目执行情况			
考核项目	考核指标	分值	扣分

续表

1. 使云南省边境地区流动人口更好地获得疟疾诊断和合理治疗(共6分)	(1) 边境流动人口中发热病人的血检	3	
	(2) 边境流动人口中的疟疾病人规范治疗	3	
2. 使目标地区当地居民得到更好的早期诊断和个人防护(共15分)	(1) 项目地区发热病人的血检	3	
	(2) 项目地区疟疾病人规范治疗	3	
	(3) 项目地区乡、村医生 / 个体医生诊断和治疗培训	3	
	(4) 项目地区镜检员培训	3	
	(5) 项目地区药浸蚊帐	3	
3. 使云南省和海南省流行区居民更有效地采取疟疾预防措施，及时治疗(共9分)	(1) 云南和海南项目县用广播进行疟疾知识宣传	3	
	(2) 云南和海南项目县中小学生疟防知识课	3	
	(3) 云南和海南项目县在公共场所张贴疟疾知识宣传画	3	
4. 优化云南、海南及其他八个项目省的疟疾控制项目管理(共10分)	(1) 项目地区哨点病例主动监测	2	
	(2) 项目地区药物抗性监测	2	
	(3) 项目地区媒介监测	2	
	(4) 项目地区专项调查	4	
项目执行情况合计扣分(B)			
考核评估合计得分(C) =100-（A）-（B）			
评估等次	□优秀　□良好　□合格　□基本合格　□不合格		
考核意见及建议			
考核单位			

续表

考核小组成员	
考核小组组长	(签字)
被考核单位 负责人签收	(签字)

注：此表一式两份，一份存被考核单位，一份存考核单位。

第二节　财务管理方案

一、财务管理手册

为加强全球基金的项目资金管理，保证项目资金安全、有效，专款专用，以顺利完成各项目的预期目标，特制定本财务管理手册。

本财务管理手册中“总项目负责人”是指国家级项目负责人；“分项目负责人”是指总项目下各病种项目负责人；“项目点负责人”是指各省、地、市、县项目负责人。

本财务管理手册适用于所有参与全球基金项目的单位。

（一）预算管理

1. 预算编制

（1）采取财务部门与业务部门相结合、自下而上的办法编制。分项目负责人根据全球基金的要求及中国的现状确定项目目标和工作任务，负责组织编制业务工作计划及基金支出计划，总项目负责人所在单位的财务部门负责编制汇总，经总项目负责人审核后确定。

（2）编制预算应本着提高资金使用效益的原则，以项目目标为依据，分清工作的轻重缓急，制定出预算及用款计划。

（3）预算的编制必须有财务部门参与。各项计划要严谨、周密，符合实际需求。

2. 预算审批

（1）项目总预算由总项目负责人签字审批并监督执行。

（2）项目的分预算由分项目负责人签字审批并监督执行。

3. 预算执行

（1）财务部门严格按照总项目负责人审批的预算及用款计划拨付项目资金；加强经济核算，建立健全财务制度。

（2）预算调整必须经总项目负责人同意并签字审批。

（3）支出管理（参见以下有关内容）。

（4）决算（参见以下有关内容）。

（二）货币资金管理

1. 本手册中的货币资金包括总项目、分项目及各项目点准备用于该项目的现金、银行存款。

2. 各级项目点应按以下要求管理现金。

（1）严格遵守中国人民银行颁布的《现金管理暂行条例》。

（2）为保证资金安全，现金当日库存不得超过人民币 5000 元，不得坐支现金；

（3）任何人未经批准不得借用现金。

（4）出纳人员必须将收、付的现金及时入账，并每日盘点库存现金，做到日清月结。

（5）超过 1000 元的支出，原则上使用支票结算。

（6）空白支票严禁提前加盖印鉴或提前填写密码。

（7）现金收、付由出纳员专人负责。

（8）出纳员支出现金前，必须仔细审核原始凭证，保证原始凭证的合法性、合规性。

（9）出纳员收、付现金后，必须立即在原始凭证上加盖“现金收讫”或“现金付讫”戳记。

（10）付出现金后必须取得有效票据入账，严禁发生“白条抵库”的现象。

（11）严禁出纳人员填制现金收、付款记账凭证。

（12）现金必须使用符合安全标准规定的保险柜保管。

（13）各项目点财务主管或各项目点项目负责人应经常或不定期地对库存现金进行抽查，并记录检查结果。

3. 银行存款的管理

（1）严格遵守中国人民银行颁布的《支付结算办法》。

（2）出纳人员必须及时登记银行存款日记账，做到日清月结。

（3）不得出租、出借账户，不开空头支票，不开远期支票。

（4）各项目财务主管或核算会计负责及时与银行对账，每月填制“银行存款余额调节表”，查明未达账项及原因。

（5）出纳人员不得签发盖有印鉴的空白支票，支票必须写明签发日期、用途、使用金额或限额（限额需用大写填列）。

（6）妥善保管支票、汇票、本票等重要票据。设置“全球基金项目空白票据购置、领用登记簿”（附表 1），及时登记空白票据的购入、使用、结存事项。

（7）财务印鉴与空白票据必须分人保管，严禁一人保管财务印鉴和空白票据。

（三）固定资产管理

1.“项目固定资产”是指使用本项目资金购置的使用年限在一年以上，办公设备单位价值在500元以上、专用设备单位价值在800元以上，并在使用过程中基本保持原来物质形态的资产；或单位价值虽不足规定标准，但耐用时间在一年以上，批量（5件以上，含5件）购置的同类物资，使用过程中基本保持原来物质形态的资产。

2. 固定资产的购置必须避免关联方交易。用项目资金购置固定资产必须在预算范围内进行。

3. 购置固定资产必须由两人以上的人员经办，严禁一人既从事固定资产的购置，又进行固定资产的报账工作。

4. 一次性购置固定资产在50万元人民币以上的（含50万元），必须进行招投标；采购工作必须保证不受关联方交易的侵害。

5. 各项目点的财务部门必须设置项目固定资产分类明细账，按照中华人民共和国财政部的要求进行固定资产的核算。

6. 项目固定资产的使用部门必须派出一人（可以是兼职）管理项目固定资产，填制“全球基金项目固定资产管理辅助账”（附表2）。

7. 各项目点财务部门与项目固定资产使用部门必须半年清查一次固定资产，进行账、实的核对。如果出现差异，必须查明原因，并由各项目点负责人签字批准后进行账务调整。

8. 根据国际惯例及中华人民共和国科技部的规定，由项目资金购置的固定资产，其产权在项目完成后属于项目依托单位。

9. 用项目资金购置的固定资产，在各项目点之间调拨时，使用“全球基金项目固定资产调拨单”（附表3），经交接双方项目负责人签字后，作为会计记账凭证。

10. 项目结束前，固定资产报废必须经固定资产管理人、使用固定资产部门负责人、财务负责人及项目点负责人审批签字。

（四）项目物品管理

1.“项目物品”是指用本项目资金购置的材料、药品、试剂等需要入库保管的物品。

2. 各项目点一次性购置50万元人民币以上（含50万元）的物品时，必须进行招投标；采购工作必须保证不受关联方交易的侵害。

3. 各项目点购置的材料物品必须由专人保管，并建立“全球基金项目物品辅助账”（附表4）。

4. 物品入库时，必须填写“全球基金项目物品入库清单”（附表5），并由项目负责人、项目财务负责人、物品管理人员（收货人）及购买人员（交货人）共同签字认可。

5. 物品领用时，必须填写“全球基金项目物品领用清单”（附表6），项目负责人签字后，由物品管理人员（出货人）及领用人员共同签字认可。

6. 物品管理人员不可从事物品采购工作。

7. 应按季度对库存物品进行盘点工作，并填制“全球基金项目物品盘点明细表”（附表7）。对盘点出现的物品盈、亏现象，必须查明原因，经各项目点项目负责人签字批准后进行账务调整。

（五）财务组织

1. 总项目的财务设在中国疾病预防控制中心规划财务处，由中国疾病预防控制中心规划财务处负责组织总项目的财务核算管理工作。

2. 分项目和各项目点的财务设在各项目依托单位的财务部门，由其负责财务核算。

3. 中国疾病预防控制中心规划财务处负责组织、指导、监督项目财务核算工作，省级项目财务负责组织、指导、监督本省各项目点的财务核算工作。

4. 中国疾病预防控制中心规划财务处负责组织项目财务人员的培训工作，省级项目财务负责本省各项目点财务人员的培训工作。

5. 资金核算必须设专户，分项目，按工作目标进行。

6. 项目核算使用统一的会计科目、财务报表。

（六）财务人员职责

1. 财务人员参与项目预算的编制。

2. 财务人员监督资金的使用，并及时向项目负责人汇报资金使用情况。

3. 随时关注项目资金的到账情况，并及时通知项目负责人，以保证资金的及时拨付和正常使用。

4. 按业务发生的时间，及时记账核算。

5. 按时编制、上报财务报表，认真编写报表说明。

6. 配合项目的年度审计工作。

7. 进行会计档案的整理、保管。

（七）财务支付程序

1. 各级项目的项目负责人必须将审批后的预算、用款计划及项目负责人签批权限报财务部门备案。

2. 各级项目负责人若有委托签字事项，必须将委托书交财务部门备案，口头通知无效。

3. 各项目点在支付项目费用时按以下程序办理。

（1）用款

①用款时，负责项目财务报账的人员需填制“全球基金项目用款申请书”（附表 8），写明款项用途、金额或限额、用款方式（现金或支票）等。

②各级项目负责人必须在报账人员所填制的“全球基金项目用款申请书”上，在权限以内签批意见并签名；总项目资金由总项目负责人签批后方可使用，分项目资金由分项目负责人签批后方可使用，项目点的项目资金由项目点负责人签批后使用。各级项目负责人可以用书面形式将签批权力进行委托，并将签批委托书提交财务部门备案。

③财务人员收到各级项目负责人签批的“全球基金项目用款申请书”后，必须将其用款金额与项目预算或用款计划书核对无误，并核查签字是否有效后方可付款。

（2）报账

①报账时，项目人员需填制“全球基金项目费用支出结算单”（附表 9），并提供有关合法、合规的原始单据，如发票、收据等各类费用票据。

②报账时，除停车费票、出租车票、过路过桥票等小额发票可由一名经办人在原始发票背面签字外，其余原始票据均需由经办人及证明人两人在发票背面签字。

③各级项目负责人必须在“全球基金项目费用支出结算单”上签署意见并签名。

④财务人员对各项目负责人签字后的“全球基金项目费用支出结算单”及原始单据进行审核。审核应依据财政部 1996 年颁布的《会计基础工作规范》第四十八条、第四十九条的规定进行。

⑤出纳人员对审核无误的“全球基金项目费用支出结算单”进行结算。

⑥结算后，出纳人员将“全球基金项目费用支出结算单”及所附单据交会计核算人员。

（3）用汇

①总项目单位用汇时，项目用汇部门填制“全球基金项目用汇申请书”（附表 10）进行外汇的结算工作。

②外汇用汇分别由总项目负责人及分项目负责人签字。

③财务人员接到“全球基金项目用汇申请书”审核无误后，立即办理用汇业务。

（4）拨款：

①项目资金向有关单位拨付时，必须由项目人员填制“全球基金项目用款申请书”，注明拨款用途、金额、收款单位名称、账号、开户行等。

②各分项目负责人签批拨付意见并签名。

③财务人员将“全球基金项目用款申请书”各项审核无误后，立即办理款项拨付业务。

④财务部门在拨款时，必须先由会计记账，再由出纳填制银行凭单并经会计审核后拨付，以免项目资金不足发生透支现象。

（八）会计核算

1. 本项目的会计年度按照公历年度确定，即自每年 1 月 1 日起至 12 月 31 日止。

2. 本项目以人民币作为记账本位币。

3. 本项目以权责发生制为记账原则。

4. 本项目采用借贷复式记账法。

5. 本项目的记账文字为中文。

6. 本项目的财产按实际成本核算。

7. 本项目会计核算应当以实际发生的经济业务为依据，做到记账准确、内容完整、方法正确、手续齐全、符合时限。

8. 本项目每发生一笔经济业务，都应当取得或填制原始凭证。原始凭证必须合法、合规，内容真实、完整，手续齐备，数字准确。原始凭证内容不得任意涂改，若有更改必须加盖原始凭证开具单位财务或发票专用章。

9. 按项目病种分别设置专户，专款专用。

10. 各级项目部门必须执行本财务管理手册，统一口径，使用统一的会计科目进行会计核算。

11. 各级项目单位就该项目编制统一的会计报表，提供财务分析资料。

12. 根据资助方的要求，提供有关财务资料。

13. 会计科目按中华人民共和国财政部《事业单位会计制度》设置，统一核算。本项目所涉及的会计科目及核算内容见下表：

全球基金项目会计科目表

类别	科目	核算方式	核算内容
资产类	现金	日记账	与本项目相关的收付款
	银行存款	日记账	与本项目相关的收付款
	其他应收款	按部门、人员核算	临时性借款
	固定资产	按设备类型、使用部门核算	用本项目资金购置的符合本手册规定的固定资产，包括调拨固定资产
	存货	按物品材料类别、使用部门核算	用本项目资金购置的符合本手册规定的物品材料，包括调拨物品材料
负债类	其他应付款	按部门、项目核算	核算本项目应付未付的款项
	待分发物品材料	按物品材料类别、使用部门核算	核算无偿调入，未发放的物品材料
收入类	合同预收款	按部门、项目核算	核算本项目的到账资金
	其他收入	按部门、项目核算	核算本项目资金的银行存款的利息收入等其他收入
支出类	合同预收款	按部门、项目核算	核算本项目拨出的资金
	科研成本	按部门、项目核算，并按核算内容设置二级、三级科目	核算本项目应支出的人员工资、病例报告管理费、信息监测费、印刷费、会议费、差旅费、设备购置费、物品材料费、培训费、咨询费、翻译费、宣传费、零星修缮费、交通费、财务培训监督检查费、项目监督检查评估费、外事活动费、其他支出等等
结存类	固定基金	按汇总数核算	用本项目资金购置的符合本手册规定的固定资产所形成的基金，包括调拨固定资产。
	合同预收款（专款结存）	按部门、项目核算	本项目年底可用资金结存

注“合同预收款”科目为负债类科目。为便于理解，从项目资金核算角度将“合同预收款”分别列示在上表“收入类”、“支出类”、“结存类”。“合同预收款”科目贷方核算本项目的到账资金，“合同预收款”科目借方核算本项目拨出的资金，“合同预收款”科目余额反映本项目可用的资金结存。

14. 账簿设置

（1）各级项目单位必须设立项目专户进行财务管理，专款专用；

（2）本项目涉及的账簿名称为：

现金日记账簿

银行存款日记账簿

其他应收款明细账簿

固定资产明细账簿

存货明细账簿

其他应付款明细账簿

待分发物品材料明细账簿

合同预收款明细账簿

其他收入明细账簿

科研成本明细账簿

固定基金明细账簿

总账账簿

（九）会计报表

1. 项目的财务管理部门必须就全球基金项目分病种编制统一的会计报表。

2. 项目财务季度报表。

（1）报送内容

①各省汇总的资金平衡和需求表。

②各省汇总的项目季度收支明细表。

③各省汇总的项目工作目标季度收支明细表。

（2）报送时间

每季度初 30 日内将上季度的报表报中央项目办财务部门。即 4 月 30 日、7 月 30 日、10 月 30 日、1 月 30 日前，分别将第一、二、三、四季度报表报送中央项目办财务部门。

3. 项目年度报表

（1）报送内容

①各省汇总的、各省本级的、各省以下所有项目点的项目资产负债表。

②各省汇总的、各省本级的、各省以下所有项目点的项目年度收支明细表。

③各省汇总的、各省本级的、各省以下所有项目点的项目工作目标年度收支明细表。

④报表编制说明。

⑤项目审计报告。

（2）报送时间

次年 4 月 30 日前，将审计后的本年度会计报表、报表说明及项目审计报告报中央项目办财务部门。

4. 中央项目办财务部门将审计后的年度各项目会计报表合并，并将全年度合并后的会计报表及相关财务分析资料，于次年 5 月 30 日以前报总项目负责人。

（十）会计报表编制说明

1. 季度报表编制说明

（1）资金平衡和需求表编制说明

①“项目资金期初结存”指上季度末项目资金期末结存。“项目资金期初结存”等于“现金”+“银行存款”+“其他应收款”-“其他应付款”。

②“项目资金银行利息收入”是指本季度收到的项目资金形成的银行存款利息收入。

③“项目资金拨款收入”是指本季度收到的上级拨入的项目资金。

④“项目资金收入合计”等于“项目资金银行利息收入”+“项目资金拨款收入”。

⑤“项目可用资金合计”等于“项目资金期初结存”+“项目资金收入合计”。

⑥“项目资金总支出”是指本季度各项目点资金实际支出数，不含上级对下级的项目资金拨款数。

⑦“项目资金期末结存”等于“项目可用资金合计”-“项目资金总支出”。

⑧“项目点下两个季度资金需求”是指下一个支出期及下下个支出期项目支出的总预算。

⑨“项目资金期末结存”是指本表第 5 部分第 5 行。

⑩“下两个季度申请总经费”等于“项目点下两个季度资金需求”-“项目资金期末结存”。

（2）季度收支明细表编制说明

①本表反映的是本项目每季度资金的使用情况。

②“专款收入”以总账中“合同预收款”科目的贷方累计发生额填列。

③“其他收入”以总账中“其他收入”科目的贷方累计发生额填列。

④“专款支出”以“科研成本”明细科目的借方累计发生额填列。

⑤“拨出专款”以总账中“合同预收款”科目的借方累计发生额填列。

⑥“本期”栏指本季度的发生额。

⑦“累计”栏指本年度内至本季度末的累计发生额。

（3）工作目标季度收支明细表编制说明

①本表以工作目标为统计对象，依据本季度实际发生业务，反映项目资金季度内的收入支出情况。

②“本期”栏指本季度的发生额；“累计”栏指本年度内至本季度末发生额的累计数。

③本期支出中含有本期自行采购未使用的用“存货”科目核算的物品材料，并把此项支出金额在备注栏中注明。

④“期末结存”=“期初结存”+“收入”-“支出”（表内平衡），“期末结存”=“现金”+“银行存款”+“其他应收款”-“其他应付款”（账表核对），“期末结存”与“资金平衡和需求表”中的“项目资金期末结存”数一致（表间平衡）。

2. 年度报表编制说明

（1）资产负债表编制说明

①本表反映的是项目（按病种）每年 12 月 31 日资金的占用及结存情况。

②“现金”以总账中“现金”科目期末借方余额填列。

③“银行存款”以总账中“银行存款”科目期末借方余额填列。

④“其他应收款”以总账中“其他应收款”科目期末借方余额及“其他应付款”科目期末借方余额合计填列。

⑤“存货”以总账中“存货”科目期末借方余额填列。

⑥“固定资产”以总账中“固定资产”科目期末借方余额填列。

⑦“其他应付款”以总账中“其他应付款”科目期末贷方余额及“其他应收款”科目期末贷方余额合计填列。

⑧“待分发物品材料”以总账中“待分发物品材料”科目期末贷方余额填列。

⑨“项目资金结存”以本表的“现金”+“银行存款”+“其他应收款”-“其他应付款”的余额计算填列；

⑩“项目物资结存”以本表的“存货”+“固定资产”-“待分发物品材料”的余额计算填列。

（2）工作目标年度收支明细表编制说明

①本表以工作目标为统计对象，依据本年度实际发生业务，反映项目资金年度内的收入支出情况。

②“本期”栏指本年度的发生额；“累计”栏指各年度发生额的累计数。

③本期支出中含有本期自行采购未使用的用“存货”科目核算的物品材料，并把此项支出金额在备注栏中注明。

④“期末结存”=“期初结存”+“收入”-“支出”(表内平衡),“期末结存”=“现金”+“银行存款”+“其他应收款”-“其他应付款”(账表核对),“期末结存”与“资产负债表”中的“项目资金期末结存”数一致(表间平衡).

(3)年度收支明细表编制说明

①本表反映的是本项目每年资金的使用情况。

②“专款收入”以总账中“合同预收款”科目的贷方累计发生额填列。

③“其他收入”以总账中“其他收入”科目的贷方累计发生额填列。

④“专款支出”以“科研成本”明细科目的借方累计发生额填列。

⑤“拨出专款”以总账中“合同预收款”科目的借方累计发生额填列。

⑥“本期”栏指本年度的发生额。

⑦“累计”栏指各年度发生额的累计数。

3. 对财务报表编制说明的要求

(1)各项目执行单位在编制季度报表时,如无特殊事项可不编制财务报表说明书。

(2)各项目执行单位在编制年度会计报表时,应同时编制财务情况说明书,对会计报表进行文字说明和必要的补充。

①项目资金的预算执行情况。

②项目实施过程中存在的问题及今后应采取的对策和措施。

③说明本会计期间在会计政策上有何重大变化及其影响。

④对其他应收款、其他应付款和科研成本中的其他支出进行详细地说明。

⑤其他需要说明的事项。

编制财务情况说明书时,应先说明情况,再分析原因并提出改进建议。

4. 报送要求

(1)严格按《全球基金项目财务管理手册》中的报表格式、大小报送,财务决算报表及说明统一采用A4纸打印,竖向装订,页码按顺序编排,加具封面,封面要反映出决算报表名称、编制单位名称、项目负责人、项目财务负责人、制表人、报送日期、单位公章。

(2)各类报表、编报说明及审计报告各一式一份。

(3)有关人员及单位签章必须齐全。

(十一)内部控制检查及财务评价

1. 本手册的内部控制是指为加强本项目的资金核算,提高会计信息质量,保护资产的安全、完整,确保本财务管理手册一系列控制方法、措施和程序的实施。

2. 内部控制方法

不相容职务相互分离控制；授权批准控制；会计系统控制；预算控制；财产保全控制；内部报告控制；电子信息技术控制。

3. 内部控制检查

（1）内部控制及财务评价的依据为中华人民共和国《会计法》、会计人员岗位责任制及本财务管理手册。

（2）中央项目办财务部门（可进行委托）对各省项目点的项目资金使用情况进行监督、检查和评估，并抽查县项目点的资金使用情况。

（3）各省级项目点财务对本省的各项目点的项目资金使用情况进行监督、检查和评估。

（4）对各级项目的检查和审计均需出具检查、评估报告，对涉及会计工作的各项经济业务、内部机构和岗位设置在内部控制方面存在的缺陷应提出切实可行的改进建议。

4. 内部控制及财务评价指标及检查内容

（1）是否进行了预算编制、执行、分析、考核等环节的管理。

（2）预算执行情况评价指标：

总预算执行率 = 一定时期预算实际支出总额 / 同期预算总额 ×100%

未执行预算支出率 = 一定时期非预算支出金额 / 同期预算总额 ×100%

预算调整率 = 一定时期预算调整金额 / 同期预算总额 ×100%

（3）会计凭证、会计账簿和财务会计报告的处理程序是否正确，会计档案保管是否合规，会计工作人员交接是否符合中华人民共和国《会计法》有关规定，会计人员岗位责任制是否健全，并被一贯、彻底地执行。

（4）会计核算情况分析

出纳核算差错率 = 一定时期出纳错款（长、短）总额 / 同期出纳收付款总额 ×100%

会计记账差错率 = 一定时期会计记账差错笔数 / 同期会计记账总笔数 ×100%

库存现金准确率 = 检查时库存现金余额 / 现金日记账账面余额 ×100%

银行存款准确率 = 检查日单位银行存款调节表余额 / 银行对账单调节表余额 ×100%

（5）不相容职务是否由财务人员分别负责。不相容职务包括：授权批准、业务经办、会计记录、财产保管、稽核检查等职务。

（6）财产保全措施的分析。是否限制未经授权的人员对财产的直接接触；是否采取定期盘点、财产记录、账实核对、财产保险等措施；是否坚持拨付款的签批支付程序。

存货完好率 = 检查日实际存货金额 / 存货账面金额 × 100%

固定资产完好率 = 检查日实际正常使用固定资产金额 / 固定资产账面金额 × 100%

（7）是否建立和完善了内部报告制度。

（8）是否注意并加强了财务电子信息系统的数据输入与输出、文件储存与保管、网络安全等方面的控制。

（十二）项目会计档案的管理

本项目的会计档案按中国会计档案管理的要求进行建立和保管。

本项目的账簿、会计凭证、报表及说明等会计档案的保管要求按中华人民共和国财政部的有关规定执行。不得伪造、变造或者擅自毁损会计档案。

（十三）项目审计

1. 这里的审计是指中国国家审计机构、中国会计师事务所或单位内部审计部门对本项目进行的财务状况的审计。

2. 项目审计工作一年一次。各省级项目点的本年度审计报告要求于次年 4 月 30 日以前，随年度报表一并报送中央项目办财务部门。各地、市、县级项目点的本年度审计报告要求于次年 3 月 30 日以前，随年度报表一并报送省级项目办财务部门。

3. 省级以上项目点必须由国家审计机构或会计师事务所进行外部审计，省级以下项目点审计可以是内部审计，也可以是外部审计。如为内部审计，审计机构（人员）必须是独立于项目财务的部门（人员），审计报告必须以法人单位文件形式上报省级项目办财务部门。

4. 各省级项目点可根据情况，在当地自行聘请国家审计机构或有资质的会计师事务所进行审计。各省对省级以下项目点的审计，可依据项目经费预算、项目经费使用情况以及上述要求，制定本省的审计方式和形式。

附表 1　全球基金 ________ 项目 ________ 空白票据购置、领用登记簿

购置			领用				结存		说明
时间	数量	票号	时间	数量	票号	领用人签字	数量	票号	

项目财务负责人签字：　　　　　　　　　　　　　　记录人签字：

附表 2　全球基金 ____________ 项目固定资产辅助账

单位：元

固定资产名称	固定资产型号	固定资产购置			使用人(单位)	固定资产调拨			固定资产报废时间	报废审批人	报废经手人	说明(调拨地点)
		时间	数量	总价		时间	数量	总价				

项目负责人签字：　　　　　　　　　　　　　　记录人签字：

附表 3　全球基金 ______________ 项目固定资产调拨单

年　　月　　日　　　　　　　　单位：元

调拨设备名称	调拨设备型号	调出单位名称	调入单位名称	调拨数量	调拨金额	说　明

拨出单位项目负责人签字：　　　　接收单位项目负责人签字：

拨出单位项目财务负责人签字：　　接收单位项目财务负责人签字：

拨出单位经办人签字：　　　　　　接收单位经办人签字：

备注：此表必须交存项目财务部门一联，以便入账。

附表 4　全球基金项目 ______________ 物品辅助账

物品名称：　　　　　　　　单位：元

物品购置				物品领用					物品库存		说　明
时间	数量	金额	购置人	时间	数量	金额	领用人	审批人	数量	金额	

项目负责人：　　　　　　　　　　　　记录人：

附表 5　全球基金 ______________ 项目物品入库清单

年　月　日　　　　　　单位：元

物品名称	物品型号	物品数量	物品单价	物品金额	说明

项目负责人签字：　　项目财务负责人签字：　　收货人签字：　　交货人签字：

备注：此表必须交存项目财务部门一联，以便入账。

附表 6　全球基金 ______________ 项目物品领用清单

年　月　日　　　　　　单位：元

物品名称	物品型号	物品数量	物品单价	物品金额	说明

项目负责人签字：　　领用人签字：　　出货人签字：

备注：此表必须交存项目财务部门一联，以便入账。

附表 7　全球基金 ______________ 项目物品盘点明细表

年　　月　　日　　　　　　　　单位：元

物品名称	物品型号	盈（亏）数量	盈（亏）金额	原因说明	处理意见

项目负责人签字：　　　　　　项目财务负责人签字：　　　　　　经办人签字：

备注：此表必须交存项目财务部门一联，以便入账。

附表 8　全球基金 ______________ 项目用款申请书

我在此确认，本申请书所述内容真实正确。
款项用途：
款项来源：
支付方式：现金、银行存款
收款单位全称： 收款单位邮编： 收款单位开户银行名称： 收款单位银行账号：
用款金额（或限额）：人民币（大写） （小写）￥

续表

项目负责人签字： 年　月　日
经手人签字： 年　月　日
报账情况说明：

财务审核人员签章：　　　　　　　　财务出纳员签章：

附表 9　全球基金 ____________ 项目费用支出结算单

我在此确认，本报销单所述内容真实正确。
款项用途：
款项来源：
报账金额：人民币（大写）： （小写）￥
项目负责人签字： 年　月　日
经手人签字： 年　月　日
报账单据　　张
备注：

财务审核人员签章：　　　　　　　　财务出纳员签章：

附表 10　全球基金 ______________ 项目用汇申请书

我在此确认，本申请书所述内容真实正确。
款项用途：
款项来源：
支付方式：结汇、电汇、汇票、旅行支票、现钞、内部转账
收款单位全称： 收款单位开户银行名称： 收款单位开户银行地址： 收款单位银行账号：
用汇金额：美元（大写） （小写）
项目负责人签字： 年　月　日
经手人签字： 年　月　日
报账情况说明：

财务审核人员签章：　　　　　　财务出纳员签章：

附件　全球基金项目主要会计事项分录举例

一、资产类核算

（一）货币资金

1. 提取现金
借：现金
贷：银行存款
2. 存现金
借：银行存款
贷：现金
3. 收取货币资金
借：现金（银行存款）
贷：合同预收款等有关科目
4. 支付货币资金
借：科研成本等有关科目
贷：现金（银行存款）

（二）临时性借款

1. 差旅费等临时性借款
借：其他应收款——差旅费等
贷：现金（银行存款）

（三）固定资产

1. 购建固定资产
借：科研成本—设备购置费
贷：银行存款
同时：
借：固定资产—专用设备等
贷：固定基金
2. 收到无偿拨入固定资产

借：固定资产—专用设备等
贷：固定基金
3. 无偿调拨固定资产
借：固定基金
贷：固定资产—专用设备等

（四）物品材料

1. 购入物品材料
借：存货—材料、药品等
贷：银行存款等
2. 领用自购物品材料
借：科研成本—物品材料费
贷：存货—材料、药品等

二、负债类核算

1. 代扣个人所得税
借：现金
贷：其他应付款— 个人所得税
2. 上缴个人所得税
借：其他应付款— 个人所得税
贷：现金等
3. 收到无偿拨入物品材料
借：存货—材料、药品等
贷：待分发物品材料
4. 分发或下拨无偿拨入的物品材料
借：待分发物品材料
贷：存货—材料、药品等

三、收入类核算

1. 收到项目拨入资金（不含配套资金）
借：银行存款
贷：合同预收款

2. 项目存款利息收入等
借：银行存款
贷：其他收入——利息收入等

四、支出类核算

1. 项目日常支出
借：科研成本——病例报告管理费等
贷：现金（银行存款）
2. 下拨项目资金
借：合同预收款
贷：银行存款

五、结存类核算

1. 固定基金参照固定资产中的有关核算
2. 年终转账
其他收入转入合同预收款贷方
借：其他收入——利息收入等（当年累计发生数）
贷：合同预收款
科研成本转入合同预收款借方
借：合同预收款
贷：科研成本—病例报告管理费等（当年累计发生数）

二、财务督导方案

（一）目的

为进一步促进全球基金疟疾项目工作的深入开展，督促保证资金安全、有效，专款专用，以顺利完成各项目的预期目标，特制定本财务督导计划。

（二）督导考评内容

1. 预算制订与预算执行情况

了解财务人员参与项目的情况。

了解项目财务与项目业务的沟通情况。

项目预算书是否交财务，即财务是否有项目预算。请财务人员提交。

支出是否按预算。将财务账上的支出与预算核对。

开支标准是否符合预算或规定。将财务账上的支出标准与预算标准或规定核对。

预算调整是否有批准。将财务账上的支出与预算比较，若有差异，检查是否有中央项目办审批的预算调整。

2. 银行账号设置情况

调阅相关资料，检查是否为本项目开设的独立银行账号。若末设置，写出出面原因。检查人员依旧必须要求独立开设账号。

3. 财务管理

根据业务处理程序，了解财务不相容职务是否分人担任。

调阅凭单，检查是否严格执行授权批准制度，签批手续是否齐全。

是否按照《全球基金财务管理手册》的要求，建立相应的辅助账册进行辅助核算（《全球基金财务管理手册》中要求建立的辅助账）。

是否使用《全球基金财务管理手册》中规定的全球基金专用凭证。

如独立设置全球基金银行账号的，检查是否使用“全球基金项目空白票据购置、领用登记簿”。重要空白凭证的保管是否符合要求，即重要空白凭证是否放入保险柜保管。

调阅以前年度会计资料，检查财务票据、账簿、报表的装订和保管情况。

财务工作交接是否有登记簿或交接清单。

4. 财务核算及资金使用

是否将全球基金资金按照《全球基金财务管理手册》要求单独建账管理，账簿设置情况。

是否已将全球基金资金按照病种、分工作目标进行财务核算。

省级项目点是否及时按预算下拨项目经费。注意所查县级项目点几天受到上级拨款。

调阅账簿及会计凭单，检查是否有挤占挪用全球基金项目资金的情况；若有，必须当时提出更改要求。

调阅账簿，检查是否使用《全球基金财务管理手册》规定的会计科目进行财务核算，科目使用是否合理。

财务人员是否及时查询项目资到账情况；是否按照业务发生日期及时记账。

会议、培训、采购等费用支出，是否有详细预算、结算清单。

如独立设置全球基金银行账号并有现金库的要进行库存盘点，核对库存中现金与现金账的现金节余数是否相等。

库存现金的保管是否符合要求，即是否放入保险柜保管。

(10) 应将单位银行存款账的银行账号余额与银行对账单的银行余额进行核对。

(11) 如单独为全球基金设账号，检查银行存款利息是否入账。

5. 固定资产的管理

调阅账簿及凭单，检查调拨的固定资产是否入账（调入调出），手续是否健全。

调阅账簿及凭单，检查报废固定资产的手续是否健全，若有残值，残值是否入账。

清点全球基金项目固定资产，检查账实是否相等。

6. 报表及审计情况

项目点当年期初数的项目资金结存是否与上年底项目资金结存一致。

调阅季报、年报、账簿，检查季报、年报与账簿数据是否相等。

地、市、县级项目是否进行了审计，是否有审计报告，审计报告的质量如何。

7. 培训及督导

省级项目点是否对县级项目财务人员进行了培训 .

省级项目点是否对县级项目点的财务进行了督导检查。是否有督导检查报告。若有，复印一份带回；若没有，提出该项工作的要求。

8. 其他需要检查的内容

各位财务督导人员 , 可根据项目点的具体情况 , 提出检查内容及要求。

（三）组织与实施

1. 省级督导自查：在国家级督导考核前，各省根据本方案组织对本省各县、乡、村工作进行自查。自查工作应在每年第三季度前完成，并将对县、乡、村的现场督导考评报告报国家疟疾项目办公室。

2. 国家级督导考评：财务督导与项目督导相结合，每年第四季度前对云南、海南及其他 8 省分别进行一次财务督导。

3. 财务现场督导工作步骤：

熟悉被督导地区的项目预算实施计划、各类信息、汇报等资料。

收集项目工作进展、项目活动情况、质量指标等情况。

督导小组成员填写财务督导检查工作底稿和督导评估。

督导小组讨论督导情况，汇总、整理督导反馈意见。

向被督导地区反馈意见，听取被督导区对督导意见的陈述。

15 天后完成现场督导报告，并将督导报告报被督导地区单位和上级主管部门 PR。

督导报告的内容：督导时间、地点、参加督导人员、督导内容、整改意见与建议。

4. 督导与考评的评价标准

以全球基金项目财务管理手册为准。

附表1 全球基金疟疾项目财务现场督导考评方案

（省级自查和国家级督导时填报）

督导区名称	省 县(区)	督导组长	
督导时间	200 年 月 日一 月 日	总 分	
项 目	内 容	100分	实得分
一、预算制订与预算执行情况(20分)	1．了解财务人员参与项目预算的情况	3分	
	2．了解项目财务与项目业务的沟通情况	4分	
	3．项目预算书是否交财务,即财务是否有项目预算。请财务人员提交。	3分	
	4．支出是否按预算。将财务账上的支出与预算核对。	4分	
	5．开支标准是否符合预算或规定。将支出标准与预算标准或规定核对。	4分	
	6．预算调整是否有批准。	2分	
二、银行账号设置情况(5分)	调阅相关资料,检查银行账户是否独立。若未设置,写出书面原因。检查人员依旧必须要求独立开设账户	5分	
三、财务管理(15分)	1．根据业务处理程序,了解财务不相容职务是否分人担任	2分	
	2. 调阅凭单,检查是否严格执行授权批准制度,签批手续是否齐全。	2分	
	3. 是否按照《全球基金财务管理手册》的要求,建立相应的辅助账册进行辅助核算(《全球基金财务管理手册》中要求建立的辅助账)。	2分	
	4. 是否使用《全球基金财务管理手册》中规定的全球基金专用凭证。	2分	
	5. 如独立设置全球基金银行账号的,检查是否使用“全球基金项目空白票据购置、领用登记簿”。重要空白凭证的保管是否符合要求,即重要空白凭证是否放入保险柜保管。	2分	
	6. 调阅以前年度会计资料,检查财务票据、账簿、报表的装订和保管情况。	3分	
	7. 财务工作交接是否有登记簿或交接清单。	2分	

续表

四、财务核算及资金使用(20分)	1. 是否将全球基金资金按照《全球基金财务管理手册》要求单独建账管理,账簿设置情况;	2分	
	2. 是否已将全球基金资金按照病种、分工作目标进行财务核算,如此次检查时,项目点尚未按工作目标核算,应督促其财务与项目办尽快解决此问题。	2分	
	3. 省级项目点是否及时按预算下拨项目经费。注意所查县级项目点几天受到上级拨款。	2分	
	4. 调阅账簿及会计凭单,检查是否有挤占挪用全球基金项目资金的情况;若有,必须当时提出更改要求。	2分	
	5. 调阅账簿,检查是否使用《全球基金财务管理手册》规定的会计科目进行财务核算,科目使用是否合理。	2分	
	6. 财务人员是否及时查询项目资到账情况;是否按照业务发生日期及时记账。	2分	
	7. 会议、培训、采购等费用支出,是否有详细预算、结算清单。	2分	
	8. 如独立设置全球基金银行账号并有现金库的要进行库存盘点,核对库存中现金与现金账的现金节余数是否相等。	2分	
	9 库存现金的保管是否符合要求,即是否放入保险柜保管。	2分	
	10. 应将单位银行存款账的银行账号余额与银行对账单的银行余额进行核对。	1分	
	11. 如单独为全球基金设账号,检查银行存款利息是否入账。	1分	
五、固定资产的管理(10分)	1. 调阅账簿及凭单,检查调拨的固定资产是否入账(调入调出),手续是否健全。	4分	
	2. 调阅账簿及凭单,检查报废固定资产的手续是否健全,若有残值,残值是否入账。	4分	
	3. 清点全球基金项目固定资产,检查账实是否相等。	2分	
六、报表及审计情况(10分)	1. 项目点当年期初数的项目资金结存是否与上年底项目资金结存一致。	3分	
	2. 调阅季报、年报、账簿,检查季报、年报与账簿数据是否相等。	3分	
	3. 地、市、县级项目是否进行了审计,是否有审计报告,审计报告的质量如何。	4分	

续表

七、培训及督导（10 分）	1. 省级项目点是否对下一级项目财务人员进行了培训。	4 分	
	2. 省级项目点是否对下一级项目点的财务进行了督导检查。是否有督导检查报告。若有，复印一份带回；若没有，提出该项工作的要求。	3 分	
	3. 省级项目点是否上缴对下一级项目财务督导的报告。	3 分	
八、其他（10 分）	根据项目点的具体情况，提出检查内容及要求。	10 分	

附表 2　全球基金项目财务督导检查工作底稿

督导项目：

督导检查情况记录：
附件：
被督导检查项目财务负责人或项目负责人对上述情况签字确认：

财务督导检查记录人：　　　　　　　　复核人：

三、中国全球基金审计指南

（一）选择会计师事务所采用的方式

1. 公开招标选择会计师事务所（适合省级或全省统一选择同一个会计师事务所的招标）。

2. 邀请招标选择会计师事务所（适合省、地市、县级）。

3. 指定审计（适合该县仅有一家会计师事务所）。

4. 内部审计（适合省级以下的地市、县级）。

省级以下项目点可以选择会计师事务所审计也可以委托内部审计机构进行审计，但委托内部审计的，必须有独立于财务部门之外的内审机构，审计报告必须以法人单位形式上报省级项目办财务部门。

（二）选择会计师事务所的招标程序

1. 发布招标公告（公开招标方式下）或发出投标邀请书（邀请招标方式下，需向 3 家以上会计师事务所发出投标邀请书）、编制招标文件、向潜在投标会计师事务所发出招标文件。

发出的招标文件或投标邀请书应明确审计项目的内容、报价、会计师事务所的资质、业绩要求等内容。

2. 开标（在规定时间统一开标）。

3. 评标（评标文件或报告必须有全体评标小组成员的手写签字）。

4. 确定中标会计师事务所，发中标通知书。

具体招标程序和评标标准应按照财政部关于印发《委托会计师事务所审计招标规范》的通知执行。

（三）招标档案的管理

项目点要保存选择会计师事务所的原始书面资料（包括招投标文件、评标报告、中标通知书、会计师事务所资质证明材料等）。

（四）签订审计业务约定书

与会计师事务所签定审计业务约定书应包括的主要内容有双方的名称、委托目的、委托审计的范围、出具审计报告的时间、双方责任、收费标准、有效期限、违约责任、其他事项和签订时间。

各项目点也可参照我部起草的审计业务约定书的要素格式，结合各项目点的实际情况增加或修改有关条款内容（业务约定书参考格式见附件）。

如果委托内部审计机构进行审计的，也应按照《中国全球基金项目审计工作指南》的要求执行，可以不签订审计业务约定书。

（五）审计经费来源

审计经费由项目经费列支，预算不足部分由配套经费负担。

（六）委托审计需向会计师事务所（或内审机构）提供的资料

1. 财务报表（包括资产负债表、收入支出明细表、工作目标收支明细表等）
2. 本项目涉及的会计账簿（含全球基金项目固定资产辅助账及全球基金项目物品辅助账）、会计凭证
3. 项目管理与会计核算等内部控制制度
4. 项目预算书及预算调整批文
5. 项目签订的相关合同
6. 上一期审计报告
7. 项目工作人员花名册
8. 会计师事务所要求的其他相关资料

（七）委托会计师事务所审计的主要内容

1. 项目单位内控制度的建立及执行情况
2. 项目预算资金的到位及下拨（限省级）情况
3. 项目资金的收、支、结余情况
4. 项目主要（核心）指标的进展情况
5. 项目往来款情况
6. 货币资金、存货、固定资产的情况

（八）重点审计领域

1. 项目内控制度的建立与执行情况

检查各项目点是否按照中华人民共和国《会计法》、《事业单位会计制度》、《全球基金财务管理手册》、《物资采购与资产管理手册》和国家项目办的有关规定，建

立了项目管理制度、财务管理及会计核算等制度。重点关注不相容职务相互分离控制、预算控制、授权批准控制和财产保全控制。

2. 预算安排情况

查阅下达预算的文件，了解安排预算情况，如有预算调整，是否经国家项目办审批。

3. 项目经费到位情况

审查项目资金拨入的总额，每次拨款具体时间及金额、拨入单位等具体情况，审查预算到位率。重点关注是否与预算一致。

4. 经费拨付情况

审核项目资金到位后，其下拨经费的时间、数额及拨入单位名称，如有调整，需要查阅专项经费调整的有关审批文件。重点关注的是通过调阅账簿及会计凭证，检查项目资金是否在到账后10个工作日内按批准预算足额及时下拨（仅限省级），有无挤占挪用项目资金的情况。

5. 货币资金

主要是确认货币资金是否存在；货币资金的收支记录是否完整；库存现金、银行存款账户的余额是否正确。

（1）库存现金，应当查看库存现金是否超过核定的限额，现金收支是否符合现金管理规定；核对库存现金实际金额与现金日记账户余额是否相符，如有差异，应说明原因；编制库存现金盘点表及现金倒轧表。

（2）银行存款，主要审查各项目点是否按规定在金融机构开立了独立的项目账户等的情况；检查各项目点期末在开户银行存款的账面余额与该单位财务账面余额是否相符；根据银行存款对账单、银行询证函核实银行存款金额；检查银行存款余额调节表中未达账项的真实性；检查银行存款的利息是否入账。

6. 固定资产

检查是否按规定建立了全球基金项目固定资产管理辅助账；检查账实是否相符；对于调拨和购入的固定资产是否及时入账，报废的固定资产检查其相关手续是否健全、合规；丢失的固定资产是否及时上报中央项目办。

7. 存货

检查是否按规定建立了全球基金项目物品辅助账；物品出入库时，手续是否健全；收到无偿拨入的物资是否及时入账；检查账实是否相符。

8. 往来款（其他应收款、其他应付款）

往来款内容主要包括项目点在业务活动中与其他单位和个人发生的待结算款项，是否按往来款项的类别或单位、个人列示明细；是否有长期挂账未及时清理结算的情况。

9. 项目经费的管理与使用情况

检查各项目点经费的管理与使用是否按《全球基金财务管理手册》、《物资采购与资产管理手册》和国家项目办的有关规定执行，主要包括：

经费的开支是否与项目有关；

经费的开支是否按批准计划或预算执行；

会议、培训、采购等费用支出，是否有签到册、详细预算、结算清单；

会议、培训、开展活动报账是否及时，手续是否齐全；

人员费支出是否符合规定标准，手续是否齐全；

委托经费、印刷、制作、广告宣传等费用是否与对方签订了合同或协议，其约定内容和产出指标是否明确；

检查是否按规定建立了工作目标辅助账，项目经费是否按工作目标核算，核对经费执行率与实际目标完成情况。通过相关的审计程序，对项目经费使用的真实性、合规性进行认定，并分别与预算和决算报表相核对，如有差异需说明原因。

10. 固定基金

结合固定资产的检查，判断固定基金形成的合理性以及真实性、完整性；是否账账相符、账表相符。

（九）审计报告包括的主要内容

1. 项目办基本情况
2. 项目概况
3. 项目内控制度建立及执行情况
4. 项目经费预算及执行情况

项目预算安排情况

项目经费到位情况

项目经费拨付情况（限省级）

配套经费到位情况

项目经费使用情况

项目经费结余情况

5. 项目经费管理和使用中存在的主要问题及建议
6. 其他需说明的事项
7. 审计意见
8. 附表

附件：审计业务约定书要素格式参考版

附件 1：

审计业务约定书
（要素参考格式）

甲方（委托人）：

乙方（受托人）：

甲乙双方经协商一致，就甲方委托乙方进行年度财务审计的有关事宜，特签订本业务约定书（以下简称协议），双方共同遵守：

一、业务约定内容

甲方委托乙方对______年______省/县全球基金第______轮______项目进行年度财务审计并出具审计报告。（具体审计内容见《中国全球基金项目审计工作指南》）

二、收费标准及付款方式

（一）收费标准：____

____

（二）审计费总金额为人民币（大写）____________元（________）。

（三）付款方式：（两种方式任选其一）

1. 本协议生效后____个工作日内，甲方向乙方确认账户内支付审计费总额___%的款项，计人民币（大写）____________________元（_______）；另___%的审计费尾款计人民币（大写）______________________元（_______），于乙方向甲方提交项目全部审计报告后 个工作日内付清。

2. 乙方提交甲方项目审计报告后_____个工作日内一次全额付清。

3. 乙方确认的开户银行为：____________________________

账号为：_________________________。

4. 乙方收到甲方支付的款项后，应为甲方开具等额有效发票。

三、甲方的权利与义务

（一）本协议生效后，乙方开始正式审计工作前 ____ 天，甲方应按乙方要求，提供与审计项目相关的文件及资料，并保证所提供资料的真实、合法、完整。

（二）甲方为乙方派出的审计人员提供必要的工作条件，并指定人员配合乙方开展年度项目财务审计工作。

（三）甲方应按本协议约定的时间按时支付审计费用。

（四）乙方对受托的审计事项不能保质保量或无故未按约定时间出具审计报告时，甲方有权解除本协议。协议解除后，甲方不支付任何费用，甲方已支付的费用乙方负有返还义务。

……

四、乙方的权利与义务

（一）乙方应按照《中国注册会计师独立审计准则》的要求和甲方委托审计的内容，出具真实、准确、合法的审计报告，并对审计报告所发表的意见负责。

（二）恪守职业道德、保守机密，未经甲方同意，不得将其所知悉的甲方文件、资料、信息等对外泄露。

（三）乙方应保证在 ____ 年 ____ 月 ____ 日前完成审计任务并出具本协议约定的正式审计报告　份交与甲方。

（四）若甲方未在约定的时间内向乙方提供所需要的审计资料，而影响了乙方的审计进度，乙方出具审计报告的时间可相应顺延。

（五）乙方项目审计人员如有变动时，应事先征得甲方的同意，以保证项目审计人员的相对稳定。

……

五、审计报告的使用责任

乙方向甲方出具的审计报告，因甲方使用不当的责任与乙方无关。

六、约定事项的变更

本协议履行过程中出现双方不可预见的情况，严重影响审计工作的完成；或甲方因特殊原因要求乙方加快出具审计报告；或甲方增加了审计内容等。届时，双方应就有关变更事项另行协商并在协商一致的基础上就变更事项签署补充协议或工作备忘录。

七、违约责任

（一）甲方无故迟延支付审计费用，每逾期一日，按合同总金额万分之 ___ 比例向乙方支付违约金。

（二）乙方无故迟延交付审计报告，每逾期一日，按合同总金额万分之 ___ 比例向甲方支付违约金。

（三）因乙方过失及违约给甲方造成损失的，根据乙方的过失及违约情形，在不低于合同总金额 ____%、不高于合同总金额 ____% 的范围内对甲方承担赔偿责任。

八、争议与解决方式

双方因履行本协议而发生的争议，应首先协商解决；协商未果，任何一方可向甲方所在地人民法院提起诉讼。

九、协议的有效期

（一）本协议自双方签字、盖章之日生效，至本协议项下双方的责任履行完毕时止。

（二）本协议一式 ____ 份，甲方 ____ 份，乙方 ____ 份，具有同等效力。

十、其他事项约定

（一）____

（二）____

（三）____

……____

甲方（公章）：	乙方（公章）：
项目负责人（签字）： 或委托代理人（签字）：	项目负责人（签字）： 或委托代理人（签字）：
_____ 年 _____ 月 _____ 日	_____ 年 _____ 月 _____ 日

附件 2：

审计业务约定书

（要素参考格式）

甲方（委托人）：

乙方（受托人）：

甲乙双方经协商一致，就甲方委托乙方进行年度财务审计的有关事宜，特签订本业务约定书（以下简称协议），双方共同遵守：

一、业务约定内容

甲方委托乙方对 ______ 年 ______ 省/县全球基金第 ______ 轮 ______ 项目进行年度财务审计并出具审计报告。（具体审计内容见《中国全球基金项目审计工作指南》）

二、收费标准及付款方式

（一）收费标准：____

____

（二）审计费总金额为人民币（大写）____________ 元（________）。

（三）付款方式：（两种方式任选其一）

1. 本协议生效后 ____ 个工作日内，甲方向乙方确认账户内支付审计费总额 ___% 的款项，计人民币（大写）____________________ 元（_______）；另 ___% 的审计费尾款计人民币（大写）____________________ 元（_______），于乙方向甲方提交项目全部审计报告后 个工作日内付清。

2. 乙方提交甲方项目审计报告后 _____ 个工作日内一次全额付清。

3. 乙方确认的开户银行为：____________________________

账号为：________________________。

4. 乙方收到甲方支付的款项后，应为甲方开具等额有效发票。

三、甲方的权利与义务

（一）本协议生效后，乙方开始正式审计工作前 ____ 天，甲方应按乙方要求，提供与审计项目相关的文件及资料，并保证所提供资料的真实、合法、完整。

（二）甲方为乙方派出的审计人员提供必要的工作条件，并指定人员配合乙方开展年度项目财务审计工作。

（三）甲方应按本协议约定的时间按时支付审计费用。

（四）乙方对受托的审计事项不能保质保量或无故未按约定时间出具审计报告时，甲方有权解除本协议。协议解除后，甲方不支付任何费用，甲方已支付的费用乙方负有返还义务。

……

四、乙方的权利与义务

（一）乙方应按照《中国注册会计师独立审计准则》的要求和甲方委托审计的内容，出具真实、准确、合法的审计报告，并对审计报告所发表的意见负责。

（二）恪守职业道德、保守机密，未经甲方同意，不得将其所知悉的甲方文件、资料、信息等对外泄露。

（三）乙方应保证在____年____月____日前完成审计任务并出具本协议约定的正式审计报告　份交与甲方。

（四）若甲方未在约定的时间内向乙方提供所需要的审计资料，而影响了乙方的审计进度，乙方出具审计报告的时间可相应顺延。

（五）乙方项目审计人员如有变动时，应事先征得甲方的同意，以保证项目审计人员的相对稳定。

……

五、审计报告的使用责任

乙方向甲方出具的审计报告，因甲方使用不当的责任与乙方无关。

六、约定事项的变更

本协议履行过程中出现双方不可预见的情况，严重影响审计工作的完成；或甲方因特殊原因要求乙方加快出具审计报告；或甲方增加了审计内容等。届时，双方应就有关变更事项另行协商并在协商一致的基础上就变更事项签署补充协议或工作备忘录。

七、违约责任

（一）甲方无故迟延支付审计费用，每逾期一日，按合同总金额万分之___比例向乙方支付违约金。

（二）乙方无故迟延交付审计报告，每逾期一日，按合同总金额万分之___比例向甲方支付违约金。

（三）因乙方过失及违约给甲方造成损失的，根据乙方的过失及违约情形，在不低于合同总金额 ____%、不高于合同总金额 ____% 的范围内对甲方承担赔偿责任。

八、争议与解决方式

双方因履行本协议而发生的争议，应首先协商解决；协商未果，任何一方可向甲方所在地人民法院提起诉讼。

九、协议的有效期

（一）本协议自双方签字、盖章之日生效，至本协议项下双方的责任履行完毕时止。

（二）本协议一式 ____ 份，甲方 ____ 份，乙方 ____ 份，具有同等效力。

十、其他事项约定

（一）____

（二）____

（三）____

……____

甲方（公章）： 乙方（公章）：

项目负责人（签字）： 项目负责人（签字）：

或委托代理人（签字）： 或委托代理人（签字）：

_____年_____月_____日 _____年_____月_____日

第三节　物资管理方案

一、设备采购管理手册

（一）全球基金物资采购实施指南

中国项目中央执行机构（简称 PR）为规范全球基金的物资采购行为，提高采购资金的经济效益，保证项目的顺利进行，特制定本实施指南。

1. 采购计划

(1) 计划制订、审批

由 PR 内设的各国家级项目管理办公室（简称国家级项目办）根据项目的计划要求和预算，制订相应的采购计划上报全球基金驻华代理机构（简称 LFA）和全球基金审批。

(2) 计划执行

采购计划通过 LFA，经全球基金批准后，由 PR 采购部依照《中华人民共和国采购法》（简称采购法）并按全球基金的相关要求组织实施采购计划。

2. 组织机构及职责

PR 内设采购部，专门负责全球基金中国项目的物资采购和管理事务。

PR 采购部根据全球基金批准的采购计划和要求，负责实施项目物资的采购和发放任务。

PR 采购部负责对物资供应商的资格及所提供产品的质量进行审核。

国家级项目办及省、地（市）、县级项目办需设专人，按全球基金规定程序负责项目物资的接收、点验、保管、发放等事项。

单价或批量价格在人民币 5 万元以下的采购由国家级或省级项目办负责实施。

3. 采购原则、方式及程序

(1) 采购原则

依照《中华人民共和国采购法》（简称采购法）及全球基金采购原则，在国家法律法规范围内，遵循公开、公平、公正、透明的原则，以竞争性的购买活动获得有质量保证且价格最低的产品。全部采购必须以透明的方式进行。

（2）采购方式：

①项目的物资采购采用公开或邀请招标方式。

②在特殊或紧急情况下，依照《采购法》采用询价或单一来源方式采购。

（3）采购程序（附采购程序图）

①公开或邀请招标：

采购部根据招标项目（经批准的采购计划）→选择招标代理机构，委托办理招标事宜→编制招标文件→公开发布招标信息（发投标邀请书）→投标（投标商不得少于 3 家）→组成评标委员会→开标、评标、发中标通知书→与中标商订立书面合同。

②单一来源采购：

采购部与供应商遵循《采购法》规定的原则，在保证采购物资质量和双方商定合理价格的基础上，与供应商签订书面采购合同。

③询价采购：

采购部负责成立询价小组→确定被询价的供应商名单（供应商不得少于 3 家）→询价→确定成交供应商，发成交通知书→与供应商签订书面采购合同。

（4）验收及退、换货

为保证全球基金采购物资的质量，所购物资到达指定现场后，各级项目办必须按规定进行验收。

①按照项目验收表要求验收，并填写验收表。

②验收时如发现外包装有破损，应对破损处进行拍照（存档），停止开封验货，并立即通知 PR 采购部与供货商进行联系，协商解决。

③验收中发现验收物品与所购物品不符时，马上对货物进行封存，并立即通知 PR 采购部与供货商联系退、换货事宜。

（5）采购结算

①付预付款：待合同生效后，按采购惯例付预付款（国外合同：L/C、国内合同：T/T）。

②结算：到货后并经验收无误，各类单据手续齐全后，与供应商进行结算

4. 采购资金使用及资产管理

为保证全球基金的物资采购工作顺利进行，采购资金专款专用；PR 采购部将严格依照 PR 制定的《全球基金项目财务管理手册》的规定执行。

5. 监督审计

PR 和各级项目办接受国家各级审计部门和 LFA 的监督审计。PR 和各级项目办接受国家各级审计部门和 LFA 的监督 .

采购程序图

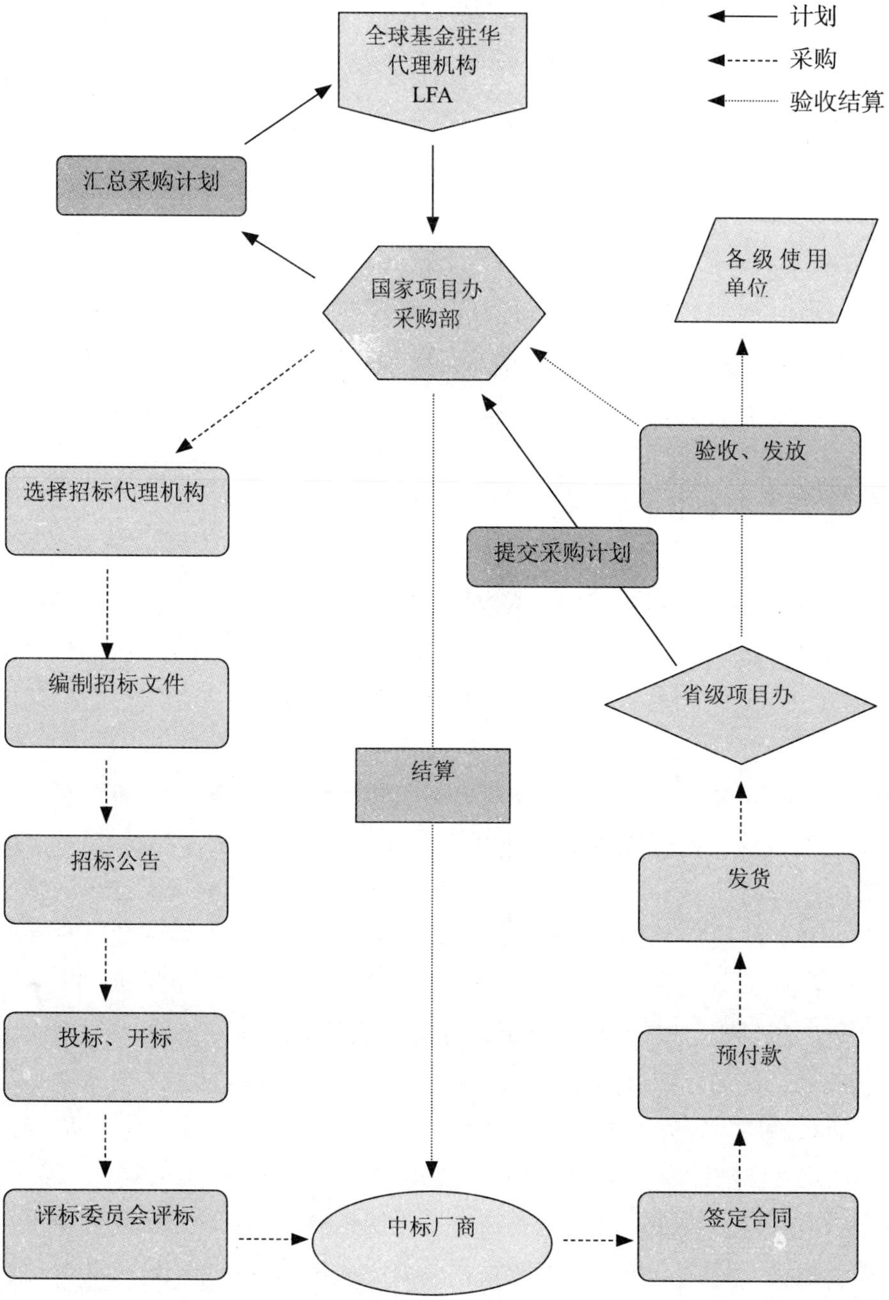
计划
采购
验收结算
全球基金驻华代理机构 LFA
汇总采购计划
国家项目办采购部
各级使用单位
验收、发放
选择招标代理机构
提交采购计划
省级项目办
编制招标文件
结算
招标公告
发货
投标、开标
预付款
评标委员会评标
中标厂商
签定合同

二、全球基金项目物资管理规定

第一条　全球基金中国项目中央执行机构（PR）为规范全球基金项目的物资管理，保证项目的顺利实施，特制定本规定。

第二条　本规定所指物资包括药品、试剂、医疗器械、办公设备、科研仪器及交通工具等。

第三条　PR 根据全球基金批准的采购计划要求，负责对项目物资进行统一招标采购，并按计划要求将采购物资发至各级项目执行单位。单价或批量价格在 5 万元人民币以下的物资采购由国家或省级项目办负责实施。

第四条　PR 负责对各级项目执行单位的项目物资管理工作进行监督、指导和协调。

第五条　PR 和各级项目办物资管理部门接受国家各级审计部门和全球基金驻华代理机构（LFA）的审计监督。

第六条　各级项目执行单位，应指定专人负责对全球基金项目的物资和固定资产进行管理。

第七条　全球基金物资不准挪做它用，发现后立即缴回，并停止下拨其剩余物资设备。

第八条　各级项目执行单位对物资的接收要严格按照 PR 采购部所发的固定资产调拨单上列明的物资调拨数量、型号和全球基金项目物资产品验收表（附表 3）的各项要求进行验收，并填写验收表。如发生与调拨单所列物资不符合的情况，应暂停接收，并立即通报 PR 采购部核查。验收结束后应及时将填好的验收表签字盖章后报 PR 采购部。

第九条　各级项目执行单位对项目所接收的各种物资设备，必须填写固定资产登记表或药品、试剂登记表（附表 1、2）；并严格依据 PR 制定的全球基金项目财务管理手册第三项固定资产的管理规定对项目所属固定资产进行管理，填制“全球基金项目固定资产辅助账”（附表 8）；单独建立完整的物资档案资料。

第十条　项目所属固定资产的调拨、处置依据 PR 制定的全球基金项目财务管理手册第三项规定执行。在对相关物资设备验收无误后，对 PR 采购部所发“全球基金项目固定资产调拨单”（附表 9），签字、盖章后，一份交当地项目财务部门存档，一份及时寄回 PR 采购部。

第十一条　各级项目执行单位要严格实行物资设备出入库登记制度。依据 PR 制定的全球基金项目财务管理手册第四项项目物品的管理规定，物资入库须填写“全球基金项目物品入库清单”（附表 5），出库须填写“全球基金项目物品领用清单”（附表 6）；对材料、药品、试剂等应填写“全球基金项目物品辅助账”（附表 7）。

第十二条 对库存物资，应每月定期进行核查，同时填写“全球基金项目物资定期库存检查表”（附表 4）根据有关项目管理规定上报上级项目主管部门。

第十三条 各级项目执行单位要保证物资储存的条件，项目物资应单独储存，不能同其他项目物资混放。对药品的储存根据“全球基金药品储存管理制度”；要建立完善的安全防盗及消防设施；对于可消耗品出库应遵循临近有效期物品优先出库的原则。

第十四条 进口物资管理：所有进口设备到货后应严格按照原分配计划分发，及时登记建账；严禁更改使用单位。各地项目单位须认真配合 PR 采购部及各级海关做好海关监管工作。

第十五条 车辆管理：车辆按计划分配后要按照国家有关规定及时办理车辆登记手续和固定资产的登记、建账。项目所分配车辆为项目专用，严禁挪做它用。按照随车使用手册要求，及时进行维护保养，确保车辆安全运行。车辆行驶必须遵照国家相关法律法规规定，无驾驶执照人员严禁驾驶。

第十六条 各级项目执行单位应根据本规定，制定具体设备管理制度，实行使用登记制度和定期检查制度，以保证仪器设备的正常使用。

第十七条 各级项目执行单位需要配备熟练的仪器设备操作人员，建立并健全各项操作规程，包括技术责任和岗位责任制，严禁违章操作和设备超负荷运行。

第十八条 各级项目执行单位应指定专人对设备进行经常性维护和保养，并定期检测，以保证其正常运转。维护、保养和检测应作好记录，并由相关负责人员签字。

第十九条 各级项目执行单位要重视对设备管理与技术操作人员的培训，提高技术和业务素质。

第二十条 使用特种设备要按照国家有关部门制定的规程，取得安全使用证或安全标志后方可使用；使用单位应在具有较大危险因素的设备上设置明显的安全警示标志。并定期进行安全检测，发现异常应停止使用，及时修理。

设备管理流程图

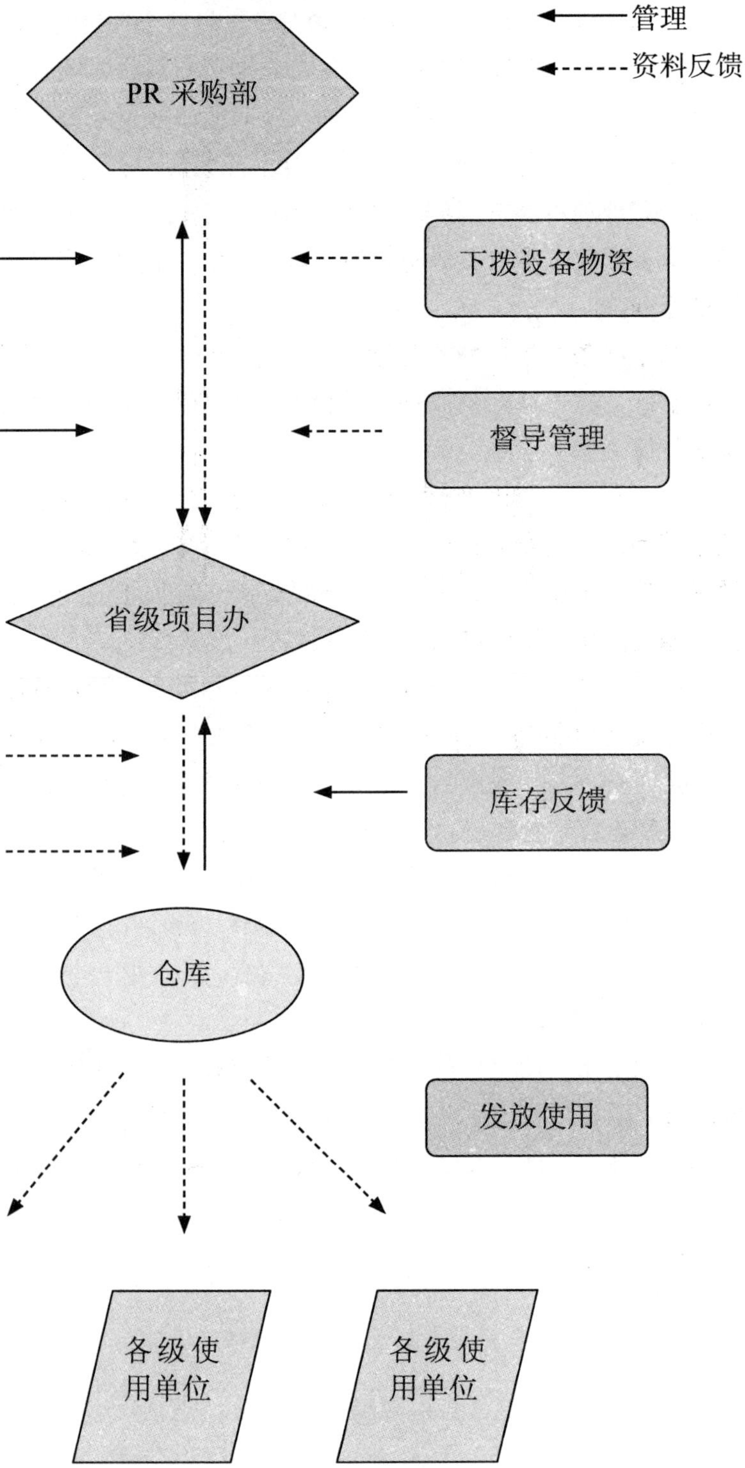
管理
资料反馈
PR 采购部
库存反馈
下拨设备物资
调拨单、验收单
督导管理
省级项目办
专人管理
验收入库
库存反馈
仓库
专人管理
发放使用
各级使
用单位
各级使
用单位
各级使
用单位

三、全球基金药品存储管理制度

1. 各项目执行单位要严格执行药品存储管理的规章制度，实行入库验收，在库养护，出库复核。

2. 项目执行单位的主管领导对所使用的药品负全部的法律责任和社会责任；

3. 药剂科或相关业务部门的负责人负责对药品质量进行判断、指导、监督和裁决；

4. 各项目执行单位要指定专人负责药品验收工作，对药品品名、规格、数量、批号、包装、效期按法律和合同规定进行验收；

5. 各项目执行单位要指定专人负责药品的保管。

6. 药品存储要按不同自然属性分类进行科学储存，防止差错、混淆、变质；做到账、卡、物相符。

7. 要建立入库验收台账，药品入库须填写“全球基金项目物品入库清单”（附表 5），建立出库台账，出库须填写“全球基金项目物品领用清单”（附表 6）；并建立“全球基金项目物品辅助账”（附表 7）等；要建立退货、养护记录。

8. 存贮场所应宽敞、明亮、洁净，按用途（剂型）分类摆放，有明显标志；按药品存贮温度要求，要有专用的冷库（2-10℃），阴凉库（≤ 20℃），常温库（0-30℃），库房内相对湿度一般应保持在 5% -75%内。

9. 存贮场所要有避光、通风和排水设施；要用适当材料做成的药品底垫，保持药品与地面、墙壁之间要有一定的距离；药品货架要有防尘设施；要有符合安全用电的照明设施；要有防鼠、防虫设施和完善的消防、安全、防盗等设施。

10. 对库存药品，应每月定期进行核查，同时填写“全球基金项目物资定期库存检查表”（附表 4），上报上级项目主管部门。

11. 注重库存的合理性、时效性，优化库存结构，控制库存总量，减少积压和损失；药品出库应遵循临近有效期药品优先出库的原则。

12. 对药品进、出流通应有按批号追踪的记录，原始记录应字迹清楚，项目填写完整，不能随意涂改，每个记录必须标明日期、记录人，以备检查，记录保存时间一般为 5 年；

13. 凡过期失效、霉烂变质的药品，一经发现应立即集中封存，不得再使用。同时做好不合格药品的处理记录；并逐级上报管理部门。对所有变质药品，应统一交当地药监部门按要求集中处理、销毁。

14. 凡发现重大药品质量问题要及时向当地药品监督管理部门报告、检验，并将药检所抽验情况及检验结果留单备查。同时将情况逐级上报中央 PR，以便及时联系药品生产商，商量退换货及索赔等相关事宜。

15. 以上制度同时适用于实验试剂的储存与管理。

附表 1　全球基金 ________ 项目固定资产登记表

<table>
<tr><td>项目单位</td><td colspan="3"></td><td colspan="3">设备编号</td><td colspan="2"></td></tr>
<tr><td>仪器设备名称</td><td colspan="8"></td></tr>
<tr><td>型 号</td><td colspan="8"></td></tr>
<tr><td>规 格</td><td colspan="8"></td></tr>
<tr><td>产品序列号</td><td colspan="2"></td><td colspan="3">数 量</td><td colspan="3"></td></tr>
<tr><td>生产厂商</td><td></td><td>国 别</td><td colspan="3"></td><td colspan="2">单 位</td><td></td></tr>
<tr><td>单价(元)</td><td colspan="2">¥：</td><td colspan="6">$：</td></tr>
<tr><td>总计(元)</td><td colspan="2">¥：</td><td colspan="6">$：</td></tr>
<tr><td>到货时间</td><td></td><td colspan="3">安装时间</td><td colspan="4"></td></tr>
<tr><td>验收安装情况</td><td colspan="8"></td></tr>
<tr><td>使用部门</td><td></td><td colspan="3">保 管 人</td><td colspan="4"></td></tr>
<tr><td>配件及附件</td><td colspan="8"></td></tr>
<tr><td>备 注</td><td colspan="8"></td></tr>
</table>

填表人：　　　　　　　　　　　　日期：

附表 2　全球基金 ________ 项目药品、试剂登记表

项目单位		药品编号	
药品名称			
批准文号		剂 型	
生产批号		规 格	
有 效 期		单 位	
生产厂商		数 量	
单价(元)	¥:	$:	
总计(元)	¥:	$:	
到货时间		验收情况	
保管部门		保 管 人	
贮藏条件			
注意事项			
备 注			

填表人:　　　　　　　　　　　　日期:

附表3　全球基金＿＿＿＿＿项目物资产品验收表

产品名称：

验收单位：　　　　　　　　　　　　　　　　　验收日期：

序号	验收项目	验收评价	说明
1	产品型号		
2	数量		
3	规格指标		
4	包装		完好 / 破损
5	装箱单		有 / 无
6	说明书		有 / 无
7	附件		是否齐全
8	产品合格证		有 / 无
9	生产日期		有 / 无
10	有效期		(药品或试剂类填)
11	到货日期		
12	产品情况		外观有无损坏 / 运行是否良好等
	验收结果		

验收人签字：

附表 4　全球基金 ________ 项目物资定期库存检查表

项目单位：　　　　　　　　　　　　　　　检查日期：

序号	物品名称	规格型号	有效期(批号)	库存数量	备注

填表人：

附表 5　全球基金 ________ 项目物品入库清单

年　月　日

单位：元

物品名称	物品型号	物品数量	物品单价	物品金额	说明

项目负责人签字：　　　　收货人签字：　　　　交货人签字：

注：药品需在“说明”栏内注明批号。

附表 6　全球基金 ________ 项目物品领用清单

年　月　日

单位：元

物品名称	物品型号	物品数量	物品单价	物品金额	说明

项目负责人签字：　　　　领用人签字：　　　　出货人签字：

注：药品需在“说明”栏内注明批号。

附表 7　全球基金 ________ 项目物品辅助账

物品名称：　　　　　　　　　　　　　　　　单位：元

物品购置				物品领用					物品库存		说明
时间	数量	金额	购置人	时间	数量	金额	领用人	审批人	数量	金额	

项目负责人：　　　　　　　　　　　　　　　　记录人：

注：药品需在“说明”栏内注明批号。

附表 8　全球基金 ________ 项目固定资产辅助账

单位：元

固定资产名称	固定资产型号	固定资产购置			使用人(单位)	固定资产调拨			固定资产报废时间	报废审批人	报废经手人	说明(调拨地点)
		时间	数量	总价		时间	数量	总价				

项目负责人签字：　　　　　　　　　　　　　　　　记录人签字：

附表 9　全球基金 ________ 项目固定资产调拨单

年　　月　　日

单位：元

调拨设备名称	调拨设备型号	调出单位名称	调入单位名称	调拨数量	调拨金额	说　明

拨出单位项目负责人签字：　　　　接收单位项目负责人签字：

拨出单位项目财务负责人签字：　　接收单位项目财务负责人签字：

拨出单位经办人签字：　　　　　　接收单位经办人签字：

第四节　M&E 管理方案

一、M&E 综合管理规定

（一）各级项目实施机构必须严格按照工作计划分季度开展项目活动，不得擅自调整计划任务和经费预算。每项活动的开展须有详细的实施方案、工作记录和工作总结。

（二）各级项目实施机构必须指定专人负责项目 M&E 计划的制定、培训、实施以及 M&E 数据的收集管理和分发利用。

（三）通过电话、电子邮件、报表、报告、会议、会展、简报、现场调查、现场督导评估等形式及时监督评价项目执行绩效，分享项目信息，为相关部门改进项目工作质量和制定疟防决策提供依据。

（四）国家项目办按项目季度和项目年度，评估项目省、项目县的季度、年度工作报表与总结报告。省级项目办按季度和年度评估项目县的工作报表与总结报告，项目县按月评估乡村报表与总结报告。

（五）需同时上报工作计划报表、M&E 报表和物资库存表。各级项目办应对下级的项目报表出具审核意见书并抄报上级项目办。当报表的计划目标与实际完成情况、预算与实际支出出现较大差异时，须明确偏差原因和改进计划。

（六）对通过年度专项调查获取数据的指标，项目省在组织每次调查时须根据本指南制定详细的实施方案，并报国家疟疾项目办审批。专项调查的数据资料在县级保管。实施专项调查的省、县在规定时限内上报指标结果的同时须上报专项调查报告。

（七）各级项目管理人员、财务管理人员和资产管理人员须保持良好沟通，完成的季度报表须项目主任或其委托人签发盖章后上报，同时通过电子邮件逐级上报。

（八）县项目办应每月上报县级月汇总表，并在季度结束后 15 日内上报季度报表；省项目办应在季度结束 30 日内将省级季度报表上报国家项目办；国家项目办在季度结束 45 日内将国家级季度报表上报中央执行机构（PR）。

（九）各级项目点须加强原始数据收集、整理、录入、统计、报告等管理，确保报表上报及时、填写规范、内容完整、数据准确、来源真实。各级的项目督导报告和整改报告要及时抄报上级项目办和同级卫生行政部门。

（十）上级项目办应组织必要的现场数据核实。对拖延报表、弄虚作假、工作敷衍和整改不力的项目机构进行通报批评或暂停拨款，直至项目执行质量得以改善。

二、监督评价（M&E）指标实施指南

（一）项目总目标与考核指标

总目标：遏制项目省疟疾流行，控制多重抗性恶性疟扩散。

指标 1：云南 25 个项目县和海南 10 个项目县的疟疾发病率

1. 分母：被调查项目县当年人口总数。

2. 分子：项目县当年疟疾推算实际病例数。

3. 数据来源：年度专项调查。

4. 负责机构：云南省寄生虫病防治所（寄防所）、海南省疾病预防控制中心（CDC）、两省被调查项目县 CDC。

5. 调查方法：分层随机整群抽样，回顾性调查。

抽样方法：分层随机整群抽样法。第一层：按近三年的疫情报告发病率将全省各项目县（市）分为疟疾流行重、中、轻三类，每类中随机抽取 1 个县（市）。第二层：按近三年的疫情报告发病率将抽样县（市）的各乡（镇、农、林场）分为疟疾流行重、中、轻三类，每类中随机抽取 1 个乡（镇、农、林场）。第三层：按近三年的疫情报告发病率将每个抽样乡（镇、农、林场）的各行政村（分场）分为疟疾流行重、中、轻三类，每类中随机抽取 1 个行政村（分场）。第四层：在每个抽中的行政村（分场）中随机抽取 1—3 个自然村（队）或村民组。即每县共 3 个乡 9 个行政村 9—27 个自然村，每一行政村调查村民数不少于 300 人。

调查对象：被调查县 CDC、乡镇卫生院、村诊所和被调查村民。

调查内容与实际疟疾发病率推算方法：（1）采用捕获 - 再捕获方法（CMR）推算被调查村实际疟疾发病例数。在被调查县（市）CDC 疫情网络直报系统上获得被调查村的疟疾病例数（C 值）；符合“血检阳性、典型临床症状、药物试治有效”其中之一即为疟疾病例，挨户走访调查当年有疟史的居民数（R 值）；核对走访调查中发现的有疟史者名单和被调查村的上报疟疾病例名单，记录相符的疟疾病例数（M 值）；按公式 $N=[(C+1)(R+1)/(M+1)]-1$ 推算各县被调查村的疟疾实际发病数。（2）推算项目县实际疟疾病例数 = 项目县报告疟疾病例总数 ÷（项目县被调查村疟疾报告病例数 /N）。（3）从统计局获得项目县人口总数。（4）推算项目县实

际疟疾发病率 = 推算项目县实际疟疾病例数 / 项目县当年人口总数 ×10 000。

6. 汇总表

县名（1）	被调查县人口数（2）	被调查县上报疟疾病例数（3）	受调查人群中通过网络直报的疟疾病例数（C 值）（4）	走访调查出的疟疾病例数（R 值）（5）	走访调查出的疟疾病例中作为疫情网络直报的病例数（M 值）（6）	推算被调查人群实际疟疾病例数（N）（7）	推算被调查县实际疟疾发病数（8）=（3）/{（4）/（7）}	推算被调查县实际发病率（/万）（9）=（8）/（2）×10 000

填表人：　　　　　　　　　　　　　　填表日期：

指标 2：海南 10 个项目县的恶性疟发病率

1. 分母：被调查项目县当年人口总数。

2. 分子：项目县当年恶性疟推算实际病例数。

3. 数据来源：年度专项调查。

4. 负责机构：海南省 CDC 及被调查项目县 CDC。

5. 调查方法：分层随机抽样，回顾性调查。

抽样方法：分层随机抽样法。第一层：按近 3 年的恶性疟疫情报告发病率将全省各项目县（市）分为恶性疟流行重、中、轻三类，每类中随机抽取 1 个县（市）。第二层：按近三年的恶性疟疫情报告发病率将抽样县（市）的各乡（镇、农、林场）分为恶性疟流行重、中、轻三类，每类中随机抽取 1 个乡（镇、农、林场）。即每县抽取 3 个乡镇，共 3 县 9 个乡镇。

调查对象：被调查县 CDC 和乡镇卫生院。

调查内容与实际恶性疟发病率推算方法：（1）采用捕获 - 再捕获方法（CMR）推算被调查乡镇实际恶性疟发病例数。在县（市）CDC 疫情网络直报系统上获得被调查乡镇恶性疟病例数（C 值）；核查被调查乡镇卫生院恶性疟病例登记数（R 值）；核对恶性疟病例登记名单和上报名单，记录相符的恶性疟病例数（M 值）；按下列公式推算被调查乡镇实际恶性疟病例数 N=[（C+1）（R+1）/（M+1）]–1。（2）推算项目县实际恶性疟病例数 = 项目县报告恶性疟病例总数 ÷（被调查乡镇恶性疟报告

病例数 /N)。(3) 从统计局获得项目县人口总数。(4) 推算项目县实际恶性疟发病率 = 推算项目县实际恶性疟病例数 / 项目县当年人口总数 ×10 000。

6. 汇总表

县名(1)	被调查县人口数(2)	被调查县上报恶性疟病例数(3)	被调查乡镇卫生院恶性疟疫情报告数(C 值)(4)	被调查乡镇恶性疟病例登记数(R 值)(5)	恶性疟名单相符病例数(M 值)(6)	推算被调查乡镇实际恶性疟病例数(N 值)(7)	推算被调查县实际恶性疟疾病例数(8) = (3)/{(4)/(7)}	推算被调查县恶性疟实际发病率(1/ 万)(9) = (8)/(2)×10 000

填表人:　　　　　　　　填表日期:

指标 3：云南和海南疟疾报告死亡人数

1. 数据来源：全省疫情年报数据。

2. 负责机构：云南省寄防所和海南省 CDC。

指标 4：拥有杀虫剂浸泡蚊帐(ITNs)的家庭比例

1. 分母：走访调查的户数。

2. 分子：走访调查出的拥有药浸蚊帐(ITNs)户数。

3. 数据来源：年度专项调查。

4. 负责机构：云南省寄防所、海南省 CDC、两省被调查项目县 CDC。

5. 调查方法：分层随机整群抽样，入户调查。

6. 汇总表

县名(1)	调查行政村数(2)	调查户数(3)	拥有 ITNs 的户数(4)	拥有 ITNs 户数的比例(5) = (4)/(3)

填表人:　　　　　　　　填表日期:

指标 5：目标地区中小学生能够正确回答至少 3 个与疟疾相关问题的比例

1. 分母：调查的中小学生数。

2. 分子：调查出能正确回答三个疟疾相关问题的中小学生数。

3. 数据来源：年度专项调查。

4. 负责机构：云南省寄防所、海南省 CDC、两省被调查项目县 CDC。

5. 调查方法：分层随机抽样，每省抽取 3 个项目县，每县抽取 3 个项目乡镇，每个乡镇抽取中、小学校各 1 所，每所学校各 60 名学生。即每县 3 个乡镇 6 所学校共 360 人（小学三年级到初中三年级）。通过问卷（由项目省统一确定），调查能够正确回答三个疟疾相关问题的人数。

6. 汇总表

县名 (1)	调查的 中小学校数 (2)	调查的 学生数 (3)	能正确回答三个 疟疾相关问题的 学生数(4)	能正确回答三个疟疾相关 问题的学生的比例(%) (5) = (4) / (3) ×100

填表人：　　　　　　　　　　　　　　填表日期：

指标 6：发热病人在症状出现 2 天内求诊的比例

1. 分母：调查的发热病人数。

2. 分子：发热病人在症状出现 2 天内求诊的人数。

3. 数据来源：年度专项调查。

4. 负责机构：云南省寄防所、海南省 CDC、两省被调查项目县 CDC。

5. 调查方法：分层随机整群抽样，入户调查村民中曾经发热病人数和 2 天内求诊的人数。

6. 汇总表

县名 (1)	调查的 行政村数 (2)	自述有发热 史的村民数 (3)	自述有发热史的 村民中发热 2 天 内求诊的人数 (4)	发热病人在症状出现 2 天内求诊的比例(%) (5) = (4) / (3) ×100

填表人：　　　　　　　　　　　　　　填表日期：

（二）项目具体目标与考核指标

目标 1：使云南省边境地区流动人口更好地获得疟疾诊断和规范治疗

指标 1：就诊的流动人口发热病人中得到镜检的人数和比例

1. 流动人口：指在当地居住时间小于 3 个月的外国、外省、外县人口。

2. 分母：就诊的流动人口发热病人总数。

3. 分子：就诊的流动人口发热病人中得到镜检的人数。

4. 数据来源：逐级报告。

5. 负责机构：云南省寄防所及其 25 个项目县 CDC。

6. 数据收集方法：从各级医疗机构门诊登记中收集就诊的流动人口发热病人资料，查阅血检登记，核对流动人口发热病人中的血检人数。

7. 汇总表：见附表 1.1–1.4。

8. 登记表：见附表 7。

指标 2：就诊的流动人口疟疾病人得到规范治疗的人数和比例

1. 流动人口：指在当地居住时间小于 3 个月的外国、外省、外县人口。

2. 分母：就诊的流动人口中疟疾病人总数。

3. 分子：就诊的流动人口疟疾病人中得到规范治疗（符合全球基金管理与技术规范中的治疗方案）的人数。

4. 数据来源：逐级报告。

5. 负责机构：云南省寄防所及其 25 个项目县 CDC。

6. 数据收集方法：从各级医疗机构门诊登记中收集就诊的流动人口发热病人资料，符合“血检阳性、典型临床症状、药物试治有效”其中之一即为疟疾病例，查阅门诊记录、血检登记和处方，核对疟疾病例数，统计诊断的疟疾病人中得到规范治疗的人数。

7. 汇总表：见附表 3.1–3.4。

8. 登记表：见附表 7。

目标 2：使云南和海南流行区居民得到更好的早期诊断和个人防护

指标 1：目标地区乡、村医生和镜检员接受疟疾早期诊断和规范治疗（EDAT）培训的人数和比例

1. 分母：目标地区乡、村医生和镜检员人数。

2. 分子：接受疟疾 EDAT 培训的目标地区乡、村医生和镜检员人数。

3. 数据来源：逐级报告。

4. 负责机构：云南省寄防所及其 25 个项目县 CDC，海南省 CDC 及其 10 个项

目县 CDC。

5. 数据收集方法：各省、县项目办统计项目地区乡、村医生和镜检员人数，并按工作计划开展情况，核对 EDAT 培训学员名单，统计培训人数。

6. 汇总表：见附表 5.1–5.3。

指标 2：云南和海南当地居民疟疾病人中接受规范治疗的人数和比例

1. 分母：各级医疗机构门诊的当地居民疟疾病例数。

2. 分子：接受规范治疗（符合全球基金管理与技术规范中的治疗方案）的疟疾病例数。

3. 数据来源：逐级报告。

4. 负责机构：云南省寄防所及其 25 个项目县 CDC，海南省 CDC 及其 10 个项目县 CDC。

5. 数据收集方法：核查各级医疗机构门诊记录，符合“血检阳性、典型临床症状、药物试治有效”其中之一即为疟疾病例，核查处方得到规范治疗的疟疾病例数。

6. 汇总表：见附表 3.1–3.4。

7. 登记表：见附表 7。

指标 3：接受规范治疗的疟疾病人中通过镜检确诊的人数和比例

1. 分母：接受规范治疗的当地居民疟疾病人总数。

2. 分子：接受规范治疗的当地居民疟疾病人中通过镜检确诊的人数。

3. 数据来源：逐级报告。

4. 负责机构：云南省寄防所及其 25 个项目县 CDC，海南省 CDC 及其 10 个项目县 CDC。

5. 方法：核查各级医疗机构处方，符合全球基金管理与技术规范中的治疗方案即为规范治疗，得到规范治疗的当地居民疟疾病例数，调查核对发热病人血检登记，统计分母中血检阳性人数。

6. 汇总表：见附表 2.1–2.4。

7. 登记表：见附表 7。

指标 4：杀虫剂浸泡蚊帐的数量

1. 数据来源：逐级报告。

2. 负责机构：云南省寄防所及其 25 个项目县 CDC，海南省 CDC 及其 10 个项目县 CDC。

3. 数据收集方法：各省、县项目办统计杀虫剂浸泡蚊帐的工作记录。

4. 汇总表：见附表 4.1–4.4；

5. 登记表：见附表 8。

目标 3：使云南和海南目标地区居民更有效地采取疟疾预防措施，及时治疗

指标 1：目标地区家庭收到“信息、教育和交流（IEC）”和健康教育（HE）材料的户数和比例

1. 分母：目标地区总户数。

2. 分子：目标地区收到 IEC 和 HE 材料的户数。

3. 数据来源：逐级报告。

4. 负责机构：云南省寄防所及其 25 个项目县 CDC，海南省 CDC 及其 10 个项目县 CDC。

5. 数据收集方法：各省、县项目办统计目标地区总户数和按工作计划开展 IEC 和 HE 活动覆盖的户数。

6. 汇总表：见附表 6.1–6.3。

目标 4: 优化云南、海南及其他八个项目省疟疾控制项目管理

指标 1：疟疾病例通过信息网络报告的比例

1. 分母：走访调查出的疟疾病例数。

2. 分子：走访调查出的疟疾病例中通过网络直报的人数。

3. 数据来源：年度专项调查。

4. 负责机构：云南省寄防所、海南省 CDC、两省被调查项目县 CDC。

5. 调查方法：分层随机整群抽样，入户调查，符合“血检阳性、典型临床症状、药物试治有效”其中之一即为疟疾病例；根据走访调查的疟疾病例名单，与县 CDC 网络直报疫情进行核对，相符者为分子。

6. 汇总表

县名 (1)	调查的 行政村数 (2)	走访调查的 疟疾病例数 (3)	走访调查的疟疾病例中通过网络直报的病例数 (4)	疟疾病例通过网络直报系统报告的比例(%) (5) = (4) / (3) ×100

填表人:　　　　　　　　　　　　　　　　　填表日期:

（三）形成 M&E 报表

根据数据汇总结果，形成县级和省级 M&E 季度报表。

第五章

技术规范

第一节　终期评估方案

一、背景

第一轮中国全球基金疟疾项目(2003 年 4 月 1 日至 2008 年 3 月 31 日)覆盖云南、海南等 10 省 47 个县，总预算 6 406 659.00 美元。项目旨在通过加强对项目地区疟疾的及时诊断、规范治疗和有效防护、加强云南边境地区流动人口疟疾管理、开展健康教育和健康促进、加强疟疾监测和项目管理能力等，遏制项目省疟疾流行，并有效控制多重抗性恶性疟的传播与扩散。

项目自 2003 年 4 月启动以来，已执行近 5 年，全球基金已拨付项目总预算 99.08% 的经费，各项目执行单位开展了大量的疟疾诊断、治疗、预防、培训、督导、药品和设备采购分发和管理、健康促进等工作，项目的顺利实施有力地推动了中国的疟疾防治。

为全面总结项目 5 年实施情况和了解项目实施效果，根据全球基金要求和项目计划安排，进行项目终期评估。主要评估项目计划和指标完成情况及工作质量，评估项目投入产出效果及对各级常规疟防的促进作用，并在此基础上提出各级更好落实国家疟疾防治规划和实施全球基金资助项目的建议。

二、评估目的

（一）评估项目计划和指标完成情况及工作质量。

（二）评估项目投入产出效果及对各级常规疟防的促进作用。

（三）为各级更好地落实国家疟疾防治规划和实施全球基金资助项目提供参考建议。

三、评估原则与组织实施办法

（一）坚持独立、科学、客观、公正的评估原则。

（二）终期评估由各级卫生行政部门领导，各级疾病控制中心、寄生虫病预防控制所负责具体的组织实施，各级项目办配合评估实施并提供相关支持。

1．各项目乡镇做好5年项目资料的收集、整理和总结工作。

2．各项目县抽查1/3的项目乡镇，核实和完善全县项目资料。

3．各项目省组织省级自评估，其中云南省抽查9个项目县，海南省抽查5个项目县，其他八省对其所有项目县进行检查评估。

4．国家级评估组对云南省、海南省和中部、南部各一省评估。

（1）在云南省抽查3个项目县，即两个自评估县和1个非自评估县，每县抽查两个项目乡镇，即1个县项目办核实过资料的乡镇和1个县项目办未核实过资料的乡镇。

（2）在海南省抽查两个项目县，即1个自评估县和1个非自评估县，每县抽查两个项目乡镇，即1个县项目办核实过资料的乡镇和1个县项目办未核实过资料的乡镇。

（3）在中部四个项目省中抽查1省、1县、1乡镇。

（4）在南部四个项目省中抽查1省、1县、1乡镇。

（三）评估组的组成。

1．国家级评估组应由以下部门、组织的代表组成，成员包含管理、技术、财务、物资等方面的专家。

（1）CCM疟疾专项工作组：卫生部、世界卫生组织（WHO）和其他非政府组织。

（2）中国疾病预防控制中心。

（3）卫生部寄生虫病专家咨询委员会。

2．省级评估组应由以下部门、组织的代表组成，成员包含管理、技术、财务、物资等方面的专家：

（1）省卫生厅。

（2）省级疾病预防控制中心或寄生虫病预防控制所。

（3）省级技术指导组。

（四）各地应按照本实施方案的统一部署，保证按时完成项目终期评估的各项工作。

四、评估内容与指标

（一）项目工作计划完成情况。（表2——详见附录，以下同）

按各级的项目工作计划内容进行计划完成率和预算执行率评估。

（二）项目考核指标达标情况。（表3）

云南省和海南省按终期专项调查方案（附件 2）调查评估以下 6 项指标，其他八省根据本省的项目协议书和工作计划制定本省的终期专项调查方案。

1．疟疾调查推断发病率。

2．海南省项目县恶性疟调查推断发病率。

3．中小学生能够正确回答至少 3 个与疟疾相关问题的比例。

4．发热病人在症状出现 2 天内求诊的比例。

5．拥有杀虫剂浸泡蚊帐的家庭比例。

6．网络直报疟疾病人比例。

（三）项目管理及监督与评估管理。

1．项目管理能力（表 4）

（1）项目办公室建设和运转情况；

①项目办机构健全、规章制度完善；

②各项目省、县按计划召开或参加项目年会、例会；

（2）项目工作计划和总结；

①制定项目年度和季度工作计划；

②制定各项具体活动的实施方案；

③项目工作记录规范；

④项目活动有总结；

⑤按规定及时上报项目报表和报告；

（3）项目培训；

①按计划开展项目培训活动；

②项目管理和执行人员按要求参加有关的项目培训。

2．M&E 管理能力（表 5）

（1）有专人负责项目数据报表的收集、审核、汇总和上报工作；

（2）项目季度报表上报及时、填写规范、数据准确；

（3）项目办有 M&E 工作指南和模板；

（4）组织开展或参加相关培训；

（5）项目督导规范、有成效。

（四）项目财务管理及物资管理（表 6-10）

1．项目财务管理能力

（1）财务人员队伍建设

①各级项目办财务人员配置是否齐全；

②各级项目办财务不相容职务是否分人担任；

③财务人员与项目人员是否经常沟通；

（2）预算制订与预算执行

①财务人员是否参与、了解项目预算；

②项目支出标准是否符合预算；

③项目资金的使用是否与工作计划相对应；

④预算调整是否有批准；

（3）项目资金管理

①银行账号是否独立设置；

②是否严格遵守中国人民银行颁布的《现金管理暂行条例》和《银行存款支付结算办法》；

③现金日记账和银行存款日记账是否账实相符；

④是否使用“全球基金项目空白票据购置、领用登记簿”，及时登记空白票据的购入、使用和结存；

（4）项目财务管理

①是否有项目财务管理、物资管理相关制度及实施情况；

②项目资金支出是否严格执行授权批准制度，是否使用全球基金专用凭证；

③项目资金使用是否合规；

④是否将全球基金资金按照病种建账管理、是否分工作目标进行财务核算；

⑤是否使用《全球基金财务管理手册》规定的会计科目进行财务核算，科目使用是否合理；

（5）财务报表及会计档案管理

①调阅财务季报、半年报和年报，是否账表相符；

②省、市、县级项目每年是否进行了审计，是否有审计报告；

③调阅项目开始至今的会计资料，检查财务票据、账簿、报表的装订和保管情况。

2．物资采购供应管理能力

（1）项目固定资产和药品的采购是否按工作计划完成，是否及时下拨给省、县级项目点；

（2）项目固定资产和药品的调拨、领用手续是否健全；

（3）是否按照《全球基金财务管理手册》的要求，建立相应的固定资产和项目物品辅助账；

（4）清点全球基金项目固定资产和药品，检查账实是否相符。

3．财务管理及物资管理评估的主要指标

（1）资金管理情况分析：项目资金到位率、项目资金使用率；

（2）预算执行情况分析：总预算执行率、未执行预算支出率、预算调整率；

（3）会计核算情况分析：出纳核算差错率、会计记账差错率、库存现金准确率、银行存款准确率；

（4）报表管理情况分析：财务报表上报及时率、财务报表上报准确率；

（5）物资管理情况分析：项目物资采购完成率、固定资产完好率、项目药品使用率、存货完好率。

（五）项目地区疟防投入（附表 11-12）

1. 卫生行政部门组织和支持项目活动

（1）卫生行政部门将本项目作为疟疾防治规划的重要部分；

（2）卫生行政部门对项目的支持与参与程度。

2. 疟疾防治资金投入

（六）受益人群对项目的满意度（表 13）

第一轮中国全球基金疟疾项目在云南省和海南省覆盖的疟疾病人及家属对项目提供的疟防服务的满意程度和建议。

五、评估方法

各级依照本方案制定终期评估实施计划，收集整理项目基线和 5 年实施资料，组织开展终期专项调查，并在规定时限内完成项目工作总结。各省按要求组成省级评估组，开展自评估。成立国家级评估组，开展国家级终期评估。具体评估方法如下：

（一）由被调查评估单位根据终期专项调查结果、项目资料的整理汇总和项目工作总结的结果填写附表中表 1、表 6、表 7、表 8、表 9、表 12 以及表 2、表 3 标有“A”的各列数据。

（二）评估组听取自评汇报，并与卫生行政部门、项目办、财政等相关部门主管人员座谈，了解卫生行政部门对项目的支持与参与程度及地方疟防投入的相关资讯。

（三）查阅文件、资料，包括项目办的工作计划、报表资料、活动记录、财务物资账目、终期评估专项调查的报告与数据资料，以及各相关部门制订的有关文件、工作规划、技术方案、工作总结等资料。

（四）实地调查，核对评估点附表填写内容的准确性和完整性。走访省、市、县、乡、村级各 1 名疟防业务人员，了解项目实施情况；走访了解村民、病人对项目服务措施的满意程度，填写表 13。

（五）根据终期专项调查结果、项目资料的整理汇总和项目工作总结的结果审核附表中表 1、表 6、表 7、表 8、表 9、表 12 以及表 2、表 3 标有“A”的各列数据，并据此在表4、表5、表10以及表2、表3标有“B”的各列中评分，填写表11。

（六）反馈交流。根据评估结果，评估组与当地项目管理与实施机构进行反馈交流。

（七）综合评价

1．评估组按附表的评分标准评分，并按以下办法进行综合评价。

（1）云南省和海南省项目：

①省级评价分=（表2得分×0.4）+（表3得分×0.2）+（表4得分×0.1）+（表5得分×0.1）+（表10得分×0.2）；

②县级评价分=（表2得分×0.4）+（表3得分×0.2）+（表4得分×0.1）+（表5得分×0.1）+（表10得分×0.2）；

③项目综合评价分=（省级评价分×0.4）+（县级评价分平均值×0.6）。

（2）其他八省项目：

①省级评价分=（表2得分×0.6）+（表4得分×0.1）+（表5得分×0.1）+（表10分×0.2）；

②县级评价分=（表2得分×0.6）+（表4得分×0.1）+（表5得分×0.1）+（表10得分×0.2）；

③项目综合评价分=（省级评价分×0.4）+（县级评价分平均值×0.6）。

2．综合评价分为“A、B、C、D、E”5个等级，综合评分在80分以上者为A，70—80分者为B，60—70分者为C，50—60分者为D，50分以下者为E。

六、评估报告

各项目省完成自评工作后，以项目省为单位，根据对各项目县评估结果起草自评报告，连同附表一并提交国家项目办。

国家级评估组根据各省自评报告和抽查评估情况完成终期评估报告，向有关部门及各省、自治区项目办通报评估结果。

七、质量控制

（一）采用统一的评估标准、方法和数据录入、汇总表格。

（二）组成专家组，认真设计、反复研讨实施方案。

（三）根据评估实施方案对国家评估小组和省、地、县级评估组成员和数据处理人员逐级进行培训。

（四）各级疾病预防控制机构负责调查表格填写、收集和数据录入的技术支持和资料完整性的审核。

（五）上级单位在下级单位终期评估结果的基础上进行抽查。

（六）对于抽查中发现自评结果与实际情况严重不符的单位，上报上级单位，要求其重新评估。

八、工作时间表

时间	工作内容
2007 年 10 月	制订终期评估方案初稿，并组织专家讨论修改。
2007 年 11 月	方案修订并进一步征求专家及各省意见。
2007 年 12 月	上报专项工作组审议，方案定稿并下发，项目终期评估动员培训。
2008 年 1 月	开展终期专项调查。
2008 年 3 月	省级自评估。
2008 年 4 月	各省上交自评报告，组成国家级评估组进行终期评估。
2008 年 5 月	完成终期评估报告中英文稿，并组织上报。

九、国家级评估组成员建议名单

共分三组进行国家级评估，建议每组由以下成员组成：

1. CCM 疟疾专项工作组成员单位代表 1 名；
2. 中国 CDC 财务与物资主管部门财务与物资方面的专家各 1 名；
3. 卫生部寄生虫病专家咨询委员会专家 1 名。

建议由 CCM 疟疾专项工作组成员单位代表担任评估组组长。

第二节　疟疾专项调查技术方案

一、目的

为全面了解和掌握项目地区实施前与标书有关的疟疾实际疫情、防治能力、疟防知识和流动人口等现状，并为项目实施的效果评价提供基线依据，故制订本方案，供项目地区实施。

二、方法

（一）调查范围为云南省25个项目实施县，海南省10个项目实施县以及广东、广西、贵州、四川、江苏、河南、安徽和湖北8个省（自治区）各1个项目实施县。

（二）调查采用回顾性调查方式，由各省（自治区）疾病预防控制中心（寄生虫病所）组织实施。

（三）调查实施时间安排在2003年的流行季节前（4～5月）。

（四）调查时段为2002年1～12月。

（五）以县为单位成立基线调查工作组。

三、内容

（一）当地实际疟疾疫情

1.抽样方法　采取分层随机不等比例抽样法。

第一层：以被调查县为单位，根据近3年的疫情报告，将全县的各乡镇分为疟疾流行重、中、轻3类。在每类乡镇中随机抽取1个乡镇为调查点。

第二层：以抽取的乡镇为单位，根据近3年的疫情报告，将全乡镇的各行政村按发病率高、中、低分为3类。在每类行政村中随机抽取1个行政村为调查点。

第三层：以抽取的行政村为单位，随机抽取1～3个自然村或村民组为调查点，云南和海南两省每一行政村调查村民数不少于300人，其他各省每一行政村调查不少于 500 人。

2. 调查对象

以被调查县疾控中心、乡镇卫生院、村诊所以及被调查村民为对象。

3. 基础数据调查

按上年度当地县统计局公布的人口数和县疾控中心的上报疟疾疫情数进行统计。

（1）调查县人口数、报告疟疾病例数、恶性疟病例数和死亡病例数。

（2）调查乡人口数、报告疟疾病例数、恶性疟病例数和死亡病例数。

（3）调查行政村人口数、报告疟疾病例数、恶性疟病例数和死亡病例数。

（4）疟疾间接荧光抗体调查，在流行季节末的 9 月，在各项目县抽到的 3 个调查乡镇，各选择 1 所小学，每所小学各采集 150 人份的滤纸干滴血，由省项目办集中组织抗体检测。

4. 捕获－再捕获方法（CMR）估算实际发病人数

（1）查阅县疾控中心疟疾疫情报告卡（或个案调查表），记录被调查乡镇卫生院上报的疟疾病例名单。

（2）查阅被调查乡镇卫生院疫情登记本，核对疟疾疫情登记名单和记录的上报疟疾病例名单，记录被调查村疟疾病例名单；查阅发热病人血检登记本，核对血检阳性病例名单和上报疟疾病例名单；阅查 7—9 月门诊抗疟药处方，核对使用抗疟药病例名单和上报疟疾病例名单。

（3）进行村民的疟史走访调查，核对走访调查中发现的有疟史者名单和被调查村的上报疟疾病例名单。

（4）按下列方法估算实际疫情数：

$N=[(C+1)(R+1)/(M+1)]-1$

N：估算实际疫情数；

C：第一来源数据（报告疫情数）

R：第二来源数据（核查疫情数）

M：重复捕获数（报告和核查相符病例数）

第一来源符合率（%）= C/ N ×100%

疫情漏报率（%）=1 －第一来源符合率（%）

注：第二来源数据 R（核查疫情数）依据不同核查对象和方式可分为 R 血检、R 处方和 R 走访等。因此，N 也可分为 N 血检、N 处方和 N 走访等，估算实际疫情数（N）可依据不同核查对象和方式确定范围并可进行比较和分析。

（二）当地的防治能力及现状调查

1. 抽样方法　同（一）中相应内容。

2. 调查对象　同（一）中相应内容。

3. 防治机构与能力调查

（1）统计被调查县的乡卫生院数、已开展发热病人血检的乡卫生院数和镜检设备完好的乡卫生院数。

(2)统计被调查乡镇卫生院镜检人员数,近3年受过镜检技能培训的镜检人员数。

（3）统计被调查村的村医及个体医生数，近3年受过疟防知识或技能培训的村医及个体医生数。

4. 疟防工作现状调查

（1）发热病人血检情况：

① 统计调查县发热病人血检数，血检阳性数和恶性疟病例数。

② 统计调查乡卫生院发热病人血检登记数，血检阳性数和恶性疟病例数。

（2）疟疾病人接受正规治疗情况（按我国抗疟药使用原则和用药方案的标准），统计被调查乡卫生院和村诊所抗疟药处方数（7—9月）和正规使用抗疟药处方数；抗疟药的品种和供应渠道。

（3）防蚊情况：在被调查村走访调查时，记录村民户数、人口数、蚊帐顶数、使用蚊帐顶数和使用药浸蚊帐顶数。计算蚊帐拥有率、人均蚊帐数、蚊帐使用率和药浸蚊帐使用率。

（三）当地的疟防知识知晓情况调查

1. 抽样方法　同（一）中相应内容。

2. 调查对象

（2）中小学生：在被调查乡选择一所中学和一所小学，每所学校各选择2—3个班级，不少于120名学生为调查对象。

（2）当地居民：与实际疫情调查、休止期根治情况调查和防蚊情况调查为同一人群。

3. 调查方法　采用问卷调查方式。

（1）以学生为对象，采取本人填写问卷调查表的方式进行问卷调查。

（2）以村民为对象，采取由调查人员提问，根据被调查村民的回答，由调查人员填写问卷调查表的方式进行问卷调查。

4. 判断标准　在5个疟疾基本知识问题中，被调查者能正确回答3个以上者，视为知晓疟疾防治知识。

（四）云南省边境流动人口的疟疾疫情和防治现状调查

1. 调查对象

（1）在云南省25个项目县中，以有边境线的县为调查县。

（2）在调查县中，以与边境线接壤的乡镇为调查点，每个调查县若与边境线接壤的乡镇超过3个时，采用随机抽样方法确定3个乡镇；否则，全部调查。可选择与当地疟疾疫情调查同一乡镇为调查点。

2. 基础数据调查

（1）正规出入境口岸数和非正规出入境口岸数。

（2）有边境口岸诊所的口岸数（包括正规和非正规出入境口岸）以及诊所总数。

（3）拥有完好镜检设备诊所的口岸数以及拥有完好镜检设备诊所的总数。

（4）有已开展发热病人血检诊所的口岸数以及已开展发热病人血检诊所的总数。

（5）各调查口岸每年的出入境人数（以当地边防或公安部门提供的数据为准）。

3. 边境流动人口疟疾疫情及防治现状调查

（1）查阅被调查口岸边境诊所的门诊登记本，记录就诊的出入境发热病人数、发热病人血检数、血检阳性数和恶性疟病例数。

（2）查阅被调查口岸边境诊所的门诊处方，记录使用抗疟药处方数和正规处方数。

（五）海南省上山流动人口的疟疾疫情和防治现状调查

1. 调查对象

（1）在海南省10个项目县中，以有上山住宿人群的县为调查县。

（2）每个被调查县，以有上山住宿人群的乡为调查点，若有上山住宿人群的乡超过3个时，采用随机抽样方法确定3个乡；否则，全部调查。 可选择与当地疟疾疫情调查同一乡镇为调查点。

（3）每个被调查乡以有上山住宿人群的行政村为调查点，若有上山住宿人群的行政村超过3个时，采用随机抽样方法确定3个行政村；否则，全部调查。可选择与疟疾疫情调查同一个乡（镇）为调查点。

（4）在每个被调查行政村中，选择上山住宿人群较多的1—3个自然村或村民组为调查点，每一行政村调查的人数不少于300人。

2. 上山住宿人群的疟疾疫情及防治现状调查

（1）调查上山住宿村民数、上山住宿村民中的发病数、恶性疟病例数、死亡病例数和报告病例数。

（2）调查上山住宿人群中有发热史的村民数、能得到血检的村民数和能得到正规治疗的村民数。

（六）南方4省流动人口集中地区的疟疾监测及其防治现状调查

1. 调查对象

（1）在广东、广西、四川和贵州四个省流动人口较集中地区，各选1个项目县为调查县。

（2）每个被调查县，选以流动人口较集中的乡或大型工地为调查点，若流动人口较集中的乡或大型工地超过3个时，采用随机抽样方法确定3个，否则，全部调查。

（3）每个被调查乡以流动人口较多的行政村或工矿企业为调查点，每个调查点调查2—3调查单位，每个调查单位的调查人数不少于500人。

2. 基础数据调查

（1）流动人口的来源和数量：调查点总人口数和流动人口数，从海南、云南和邻国疟疾高发区来的流动人口数。

（2）流动人口中的疟疾疫情：调查点报告疟疾病例数、恶性疟病例数、死亡病例数，流动人口病例数、流动人口恶性疟病例数、流动人口死亡病例数。

3. 流动人口疟疾的防治现状的调查

（1）发热病人血检情况：调查点的有发热史人数、就诊人数、血检人数、流动人口中的有发热史人数、就诊人数和血检人数。

（2）疟疾病人接受正规治疗情况：调查点发热病人使用抗疟药人数、得到正规治疗人数；流动人口中发热病人使用抗疟药人数、得到正规治疗人数。

四、质量控制

（一）收集报告疫情数据的质量控制

1. 报告疫情数　以被调查县2002年1—12月疟疾疫情报告资料为依据。

2. 用捕获—再捕获方法　疟疾疫情以被调查县保存的2002年1—12月法定传染病报告卡（或个案调查表）为依据。

（二）村民走访调查的质量控制

1. 以2002年1—12月在当地居住的、神智清楚且能正确回答问题的、调查时未外出的当地居民为调查对象。

2. 每一户被调查的村民，可以为同一户内的家庭成员回答问题，但不能为未居住在同一户内其他的家庭成员或邻居回答问题。

3. 12 岁以下的儿童的疟史情况，由其父母代答。

4. 调查员在进行村民走访调查前应进行统一的培训，提问时应注意避免使用提示性语言。

5. 在走访调查结束前，须对调查表核对无误后方可离开。

（三）数据分析的质量控制

1. 由基线调查组负责对各基线调查数据表进行复核，发现未按要求填写或原始数据填写缺漏或填写不清楚时，应重新调查。

2. 由各级项目办的专业人员负责对收集的原始数据进行统一整理、汇总和上报。

第三节　疟疾监测技术方案

一、目的

监测项目实施地区与疟疾流行有关的因素变动情况和疟疾的流行状况，预测流行趋势、修订防治措施、评估项目实施效果。

二、监测范围

云南省 25 个项目县和海南 10 个项目县，广东、广西、贵州、四川、江苏、河南、安徽和湖北 8 个省各选择 2 个县，其中 1 个县为疫情监测县，另 1 个县为广东、广西、贵州和四川 4 省为实施流动人口疟疾管理和监测的项目县；江苏、河南、安徽和湖北 4 个省为控制疟疾爆发流行的项目县。

三、监测内容及方法

（一）当地居民的疟疾监测

1．疫情报告

各监测县，按法定传染病报告系统和新建的疟疾疫情报告系统同时收集疟疾疫情。

2．发热病人血检

（1）血检范围：各监测县的所有乡镇均应开展发热病人血检。血检对象为典型疟疾、疑似疟疾、及原因不明发热的门诊发热病人，简称“三热”，以县为单位年血检率不低于 2%。

（2）血检时间：各监测县全年均应开展发热病人血检，在有传播休止期地区，以 6—10 月传播季节为血检重点时期。

3．IFA 检测

（1）采样范围

① 各监测县按基线调查抽样方式选择 3 个乡镇，每个乡镇选择 1—2 所小学；

② 每所小学在9月份采集2—4年级小学生滤纸血样本150—300人份（每个乡不少于300人份）。

（2）采样方法：推荐使用一次性使用的采血针。若使用可重复使用的采血针，在每次使用后都应清洗，并经高压或干热灭菌处理。采用耳垂或手指末端采血方式，先用75%乙醇棉球消毒取血部位，待干后，以左手拇指和食指轻轻捻转耳垂边缘或夹住被检者手指尖稍下方，右手持消毒刺针，迅速刺入取血部位1—2毫米深，然后用左手大拇指、食指和右手中指协同挤出血滴，滴于干净的滤纸条上，血滴大小应完全湿润滤纸1cm左右。

（3）保存和检测方法：待滤纸血完全干后，按编号装入塑料袋，送省级实验室统一按《疟疾防治手册》的方法进行IFA检测。

（二）流动人口的疟疾监测

1．云南省边境流动人口的疟疾监测

（1）疫情报告：各监测县按法定传染病报告系统和新建的疟疾疫情报告系统，同时收集边境流动人口中的疟疾疫情。

（2）发热病人血检：各监测县的所有边境口岸诊所全年均应开展发热病人血检，对前来就诊的出入境流动人员中的发热病人，均应进行血检和登记。对在乡镇卫生院血检的“三热”病人中的出入境流动人员，应进行分类血检登记。

2．海南省上山住宿人群的疟疾监测

（1）疫情报告：各监测县按法定传染病报告系统和新建的疟疾疫情报告系统，同时收集上山住宿人群的疟疾疫情。

（2）发热病人血检：各监测县的乡镇卫生院全年均应开展发热病人血检，对前来就诊的上山住宿人群中的发热病人，均应进行血检和分类登记。

3．广东、广西、贵州和四川4省流动人口的疟疾监测

（1）疫情报告：各监测县按法定传染病报告系统和新建的疟疾疫情报告系统，同时收集流动人口中的疟疾疫情。

（2）发热病人血检：各监测县的所有乡镇卫生院和大型工地诊所，全年均应开展发热病人血检，对前来就诊的来自高疟区的流动人员中的发热病人，均应进行血检和分类登记。

（三）恶性疟原虫对抗疟药的敏感性监测

1．监测点

（1）海南省：选择3个恶性疟发病率较高的县，并从中再选择恶性疟发病率较

高的1—2个乡进行监测。

（2）云南省：在滇东、滇西、滇南及滇中各选1个恶性疟发病率较高的县，并从中选择恶性疟发病率较高的1—2个乡进行监测。

2. 时间与方法

各监测点每2年1次，每次用体外微量法测定40—50例；体内4周法测定20—30例。此项监测在疟疾发病高峰季节的7—11月进行，测定方法均按《疟疾防治手册》的方案进行。

3. 测定药物

（1）体外微量法：测定对氯喹、哌喹、咯萘啶及青蒿琥酯的敏感性。所需测定板和培养基由中国疾病预防控制中心寄生虫病预防控制所统一提供。

（2）体内4周法：第1次测定对哌喹的敏感性；第2次测定对氯喹的敏感性。

（四）媒介按蚊监测

1. 媒介种群比例

（1）监测范围：江苏、河南、安徽和湖北4个省控制疟疾爆发流行的项目县，各选择发病率较高的2—3个乡镇，每个乡镇各选择3—5个行政村，每个行政村选择1个自然村为媒介种群比例监测村。

（2）监测时间和方法：在6月中、下旬采用清晨室内捕蚊的方法，一次性捕获自然村所有人房内（包括帐内和室内）的按蚊，同时采用形态学（成蚊和卵）基因鉴别方法，进行蚊种鉴别。

2. 媒介密度

（1）监测范围：江苏、河南、安徽和湖北4个省控制疟疾爆发流行的项目县进行的媒介种群比例监测的自然村中，选择1个自然村为媒介密度监测村。

（2）监测时间和方法：从6月下旬至10月上旬，每旬1次，采用19—22点室外人诱加清晨室内50顶居民帐内捕蚊的方法捕蚊。采用成蚊形态鉴别方法，进行蚊种鉴别。（居民帐内捕蚊的密度应为50顶帐内捕蚊数 / 夜间帐内人数）。

第四节　抗疟药应用技术方案

一、目的

为了在项目地区更有效地治愈病人，阻断传播，尽可能地有利于延缓恶性疟原虫对抗疟药产生抗药性，必须做到合理用药，对疟疾病人进行规范治疗。因此，根据实施地区疟原虫的虫种、株和抗药性恶性疟原虫的抗性程度，按照《我国抗疟药使用原则和用药方案》的规定，选择相应的用药方案，在项目地区参照实施。

二、使用原则

抗疟药物的应用，将遵循以下原则：

（一）云南、海南项目地区的恶性疟原虫对氯喹、哌喹等抗疟药呈现中、高度抗药性（抗性率高于30%），并由抗氯喹恶性疟已发展为多重抗性恶性疟。因此应选用蒿甲醚、青蒿琥酯、双氢青蒿素和磷酸咯萘啶（简称咯萘啶）等第二线或由第二线药物与其他抗疟药配伍联用的第三线药物进行治疗。当地的间日疟病例，仍应选用氯喹加服磷酸伯氨喹（简称伯氨喹）的根治疗法进行根治。

（二）在与云南、海南相邻的省份和中部地区的项目县（市）均为间日疟流行区，应选用磷酸氯喹（简称氯喹）、磷酸哌喹（简称哌喹）等第一线药物，按照《我国抗疟药使用原则和用药方案》中的有关疗法实施间日疟的治疗。

（三）第二、三线药物不得用于常规的集体预防服药，也不得用于间日疟流行区当地人口疑似疟疾病例的假定性治疗。

三、用药方案

氯喹、伯氨喹和咯萘啶的下列剂量均为其基质量和成人剂量，儿童剂量按常规法递减。

（一）间日疟的治疗（选用以下一种疗法），也可用于卵形疟和三日疟的治疗

1．8天疗法（氯喹加伯氨喹8天疗法）

氯喹：口服总剂量1.5g（常用于恶性疟或恶性疟与间日疟混合流行区），第1天0.6g，顿服或分2次服，每次0.3g；第2、3天各服1次，每次0.45g；或口服总剂量1.2g（常用于间日疟流行区），第1天0.6g，顿服或分2次服，每次0.3g；第2、3天各服1次，每次0.3g。

伯氨喹：口服总剂量180mg，在服用氯喹的第1天起，同时服用伯氨喹，每天服1次，每次22.5mg，连服8天。

2．双四天疗法（氯喹加伯氨喹双四天疗法）

氯喹：剂量和服法均同8天疗法。

伯氨喹：前4天的剂量和服法均同8天疗法的前4天，间隔1—4周后，再单服伯氨喹，每天服1次，每次22.5mg，连服4天。

（二）抗药性恶性疟的治疗（选用以下一种疗法）

1．青蒿琥酯5天或7天疗法

口服总剂量600mg，分5天服，每天服1次，每次100mg，首剂加倍；需增加剂量时，总剂量不超过800mg，应分7天服，每天服1次，每次100mg，首剂加倍。

2．蒿甲醚5天或7天疗法

口服总剂量600mg，分5天服，每天服1次，每次100mg，首剂加倍；需增加剂量时，总剂量不超过800mg，应分7天服，每天服1次，每次100mg，首剂加倍。

3．双氢青蒿素7天疗法

口服总剂量640mg，7天分服，每天服1次，每次80mg，首剂加倍。

4．咯萘啶3天疗法

口服总剂量1.2g或1.6g,，分3天服，第1天服2次，间隔8小时，第2、3天各服1次，每次均为0.3g或0.4g。

5．复方蒿甲醚片3天疗法

口服总剂量16片（每片含蒿甲醚20mg和本芴醇120mg），分3天服，第1天服2次，第2、3天各服1次，每次均为4片。

6．咯萘啶与磺胺多辛、伯氨喹联用（3种药同时口服）

咯萘啶口服总剂量1.2g，分2天服，第1天服2次，间隔8小时，第2天服1次，每次均为0.4g；

磺胺多辛口服总剂量1g，分2天服，每天服1次，每次0.5g；

伯氨喹总剂量45mg，分2天服，每天服1次，每次22.5mg。

7．蒿甲醚肌内注射与复方乙胺嘧啶（防疟片2号）联用

肌内注射蒿甲醚1剂300mg，同时顿服复方乙胺嘧啶4片（每片含磺胺多辛250mg及乙胺嘧啶为17.5mg）。

8．双氢青蒿素、蒿甲醚、青蒿琥酯分别与咯萘啶联用

双氢青蒿素或蒿甲醚或青蒿琥酯口服总剂量均为300mg，咯萘啶口服总剂量800mg，均分2天服，每天服1次，每次均服青蒿素类药物150mg及咯萘定400mg。或将上述总剂量分3天服，每天服1次，第1天服青蒿素类药物100mg和咯萘啶400mg，第2、3天各服青蒿素类药物100mg和咯萘啶200mg。

在治疗抗药性恶性疟的上述疗法中，除疗法6无需再加服伯氨喹外，选用其他疗法，用药后均需加服伯氨喹总剂量45mg，分2天服，1天服1次，每次22.5mg。

（三）恶性疟与间日疟混合感染的治疗

选用上述“（二）抗药性恶性疟的治疗”的药物治疗，将其中加服伯氨喹的剂量，改用总剂量180mg，每天服1次，每次22.5mg，连服8天；也可连服4天，间隔1—4周，再连服4天。

（四）重症疟疾的治疗（选用以下一种疗法）

1．蒿甲醚　肌内注射总剂量480mg，每天肌注1次，每次80mg，连续5天，首剂加倍。

2．咯萘啶　（1）肌内注射：每天肌注1次，每次160mg，连续2或3天。（2）静脉滴注：每天静滴1次，每次160mg，连续2或3天。静滴需加大剂量时，总剂量不超过640mg。

3．青蒿琥酯钠　静脉注射青蒿琥酯总剂量360mg—480mg，分5—7天静脉注射，每天静注1次，每次60mg，首剂加倍。每次静注临用时，将60mg青蒿琥酯粉针剂配制成其钠盐溶液，再经稀释后注射。

（五）间日疟抗复发治疗

乙胺嘧啶加伯氨喹疗法（第1、2天两药同时口服）：（1）乙胺嘧啶：口服总剂量100mg，分2天服，每天服1次，每次50mg；（2）伯氨喹：口服总剂量90mg，分4天服，每天服1次，每次22.5mg。

注：

1．对 G6PD 缺陷地区的人群，必须在医护人员的监护下服用伯氨喹；有溶血史者及孕妇禁用。

2．应用青蒿素类药物时，孕妇慎用，妊娠期在 3 个月以内的孕妇禁用。

3．有磺胺过敏史者，对含有磺胺药物的治疗方案应慎用或禁用。

4．在恶性疟流行区，不推荐集体预防服药，对进入高疟区的高危人群应采用适当的预防措施。

第五节　健康教育与健康促进技术方案

一、目的

为提高目标人群相关卫生知识的知晓率、对疟疾诊治及预防措施的理解和依从性，促进部门间的协作及相关政策与制度的形成、以实施，实现全球基金疟疾项目的总目标。

二、目标

（一）以大众传播结合人际传播方法，对不同目标人群开展健康教育与健康促进行动，开展相关疟疾防治基本知识的传播与普及，提高目标人群相关卫生知识的知晓率。

（二）用健康教育及相关措施，提高目标人群对诊断、治疗及预防手段的理解和依从性，形成正确的卫生行为。

（三）加强有关部门间的支持与协作，建立和改善相关的政策与规章制度。

三、目标人群

第一目标人群：中小学生、进山劳动力（海南），广大村民、流动人口。

第二目标人群：乡、村卫生院（所）有关医务人员。

四、工作内容与方法

各地区的条件和情况有较多差异，本栏中的某些内容可以有所选择。

（一）调查

1．调查内容

包括基线问卷调查中的疟疾防治知识知晓率，社区组织机构、相关政策、服务与环境，目标人群相关的知识、态度、行为指标等。

为便于在中期和终期对健康教育与健康促进行动作出评估，对疟疾发病和预防以及存在问题等相关资料也应予兼顾。

调查抽样和时间同项目总安排，不另设。

2．调查方法

定性：个案访谈、专题小组讨论。对目标人群和社区组织的需求以及符合当地民族、文化习俗及适宜于目标人群的传播方式应有清楚的了解。

定量：基线调查和中、终期评估问卷调查。

（二）材料制作

1．收集与疟防相关的音像片、公益广告片、张贴画与折页、培训教材等现有材料，针对需求进行选择或修改。

2．补充制作为目标人群喜闻乐见的健康教育材料。

(1) 张贴画和宣传画

(2) 折页、传单（乡村医生、学生用）

(3) 中小学生使用的健康教育材料

(4) 电视宣传片（VCD）、公益广告（PSAs）

(5) 广播：录音带，谈话节目等

3．新制作的健康教育材料要求内容通俗易懂、简单易记、少用科学术语、提倡使用少数民族语言等。

（三）培训

对项目人员，实施国家、项目省、项目县三级培训，且与项目专业技能培训结合进行。

基本培训内容（三级培训活动应有区别）：

(1) 健康教育与健康促进的基本概念及其与疟疾防治的关系。

(2) 常用的传播策略、人际传播技巧、材料制作。

(3) 疟疾传播和预防的基本知识、疟疾的诊断与规范治疗。

(4) 流动人口疟防工作的组织、管理。

(5) 怎样为流动人群、上山劳动力人群提供防护用品。

(6) 开展农村社区健康教育、建立村疟疾预防制度（如纳入村规民约），增进人群对使用蚊帐、发现病例的认知度，提高对规范服药的依从性。

（四）传播活动（视当地条件而定）

1．大众媒体传播

对家庭妇女和广大居民，选择以大众传播方式为主的干预模式。

（1）省、县级电视、广播电台义务为疟疾预防宣传教育提供免费宣传。部分电视覆盖率低的地区，采用县级电视台 VCD 光盘播放、差转台方式播放。流行季节每 1—2 周在黄金时段播放一次。

（2）广播站：在农闲期间，播放相关节目与采访，每 1—2 周播放一次。

2. 小媒介传播和小型咨询活动

适合于流动人口相对集中的场合：在边境口岸、工地、村委会、街道以及就近的诊室。组织流动人员、民工进行集中宣讲或观看 VCD，使之对疟疾及其防治有基本认识，并配合疟防活动。

在乡卫生院、商场集市、乡镇政府等地点以及少数民族节日，以科普展览和招贴画等形式进行宣传，提供咨询服务。

要争取乡、村两级干部的支持和领导，积极参加项目活动。

3. 人际传播

（1）学校

① 与教育部门合作，利用中小学常规的健康教育课（或与体育、生理课结合）对中小学生采用集中式人际传播，开展参与式、渗透式教育，辅以发放小折页和传单等健康教育材料，增加学生有关疟疾传播与防治的知识，每学期二次。

② 鼓励学生之间的同伴教育，如主题班会等。

③ 利用学校广播站、黑板报等，由学生自己组织活动。

④ 小手拉大手活动：通过学生影响家长。学生通过带回招贴画、折页等方式，向父母宣传预防疟疾知识，保护家庭安康。

（2）妇女团体：通过街道妇联、村妇女主任向妇女开展宣传，呼吁邻里间相互关爱，及时发现和治疗病人。

（3）乡村医生：应利用诊所或出诊机会随时宣传疟疾预防知识，保证病人完成全程服药。

（五）政策与协调发展政策和建立部门间的良好合作环境是健康促进的关键内容

1. 针对流动人口的疟疾管理，在流动人员及民工集中的地区应形成一个管理、协调委员会，由卫生、公安、社区 / 工地、民政、妇联、教育等部门的代表组成。

2. 在民工较集中地区的临时户口等管理制度中，应加入疟疾病例或可疑病例的登记报告要求。

2. 在有疟疾流行的乡、村，鼓励村委会将防蚊灭蚊、发热病人及时就诊与报告等列入村规民约。

4．在有疟疾爆发流行的乡、村，尤其对进山劳动力，要提供防护用品（蚊帐或药物浸泡蚊帐、特殊吊床、杀虫剂/驱避剂等）。对贫困家庭应予特别照顾。

五、评价

（一）过程评价

每年要根据项目需要评估健康教育与健康促进的实施情况，包括计划、干预方法、传播方式的选择、传播效果、存在问题等。

（二）效果评价

以基线调查为基础，比较目标人群相关知识、态度、行为的改变情况，可与第二年底的中期评价结合进行。

（三）评价方法

问卷调查、访谈、小组座谈等，并参考防治活动中有关技术指标的变化。

（四）主要的评价内容与指标

1．教育目标

(1) 中小学开展相关健康教育的比例；

(2) 中小学生疟防卫生知识的知晓率；

(3) 项目地区家庭收到相关健康教育材料的比例；

(4) 其他目标人群疟防卫生知识的知晓率；

(5) 流动人口中接受过疟防健康教育的覆盖率；

(6) 项目地区的广播电视媒体播放疟疾相关节目覆盖率；

(7) 乡村医生得到一次以上疟防知识、技能培训的比例。

2．行为目标

(1) 发热病人的就诊率、规范治疗率；

(2) 乡村医生正确诊断疟疾、规范处方的比例及病例报告情况的改善；

(3) 村民户外露宿的比例、蚊帐或药浸蚊帐拥有率及使用率；

(4) 有关流动人口疟疾管理的规章制度的执行情况；

(5) 流动人口疟疾管理（协调）委员会的建立、活动次数及合作效果。

第六节　杀虫剂浸泡蚊帐技术方案

一、目的

应用杀虫剂浸泡处理蚊帐是一项重要的疟疾防治措施，能迅速降低媒介密度，防止蚊虫叮咬，减少人蚊接触，保护健康人群，控制疟疾流行。因此，浸泡蚊帐的质量直接关系到疟疾控制的成效，必须加强和规范蚊帐浸泡工作，以确保质量。故制订本方案供项目地区实施。

二、浸帐前准备工作

（一）组织准备

1．成立浸帐专业组

各级项目办应有专人主管，具体负责杀虫剂浸帐工作的组织管理、技术培训，实施监督，质量控制和考核评价。由各乡镇卫生院或防保机构组织实施。以乡镇为单位，以乡村医生为实施主体，每个行政村2—3人参加组织一支浸帐专业队。具体负责蚊帐登记、浸帐记录、药液配制和实施浸帐工作。

2．技术培训

逐级做好培训：省要对县（区）技术骨干进行培训，县（区）对乡镇技术人员和专业队员进行培训。培训内容为专业队成员要能熟练掌握药品用量，浸帐药液配制方法，蚊帐浸泡标准，资料登记和统计等项技术。

3．宣传发动

在浸帐实施地区结合健康教育、宣传普及疟疾防治知识的基础上，向浸帐实施地区的居民大力宣传浸帐灭蚊的目的意义，讲清道理，提高认识，动员群众积极参与配合。

（二）技术准备

1　杀虫剂和器材的准备

浸帐杀虫剂由上级统一采购，逐级下拨。

2　登记与测量

逐户登记与测量蚊帐。蚊帐按大小（双人、单人）、质地（纯棉、尼龙）分别统计数量，并测量大小蚊帐的面积和测算不同大小、不同质地蚊帐的吸水量。

（1）测量大小蚊帐面积，包括四周及顶的面积，按下列公式计算：

蚊帐面积平方米（M^2）＝正面（宽 × 高 ×2）＋两侧（宽 × 高 ×2）＋顶部（宽 × 长）；

（2）测量不同质地及其大小蚊帐的吸水量

按下列步骤测量：

① 在一水桶中放入一定量的水，应测量其水量（Vi）。

② 取 3 顶同样大小，同一质地的蚊帐浸入水桶中，用手揉绞，将蚊帐浸湿浸透，取出略加力绞干，以不滴水为宜。

③ 再测量水桶中剩余的水量（Vr）。

④ 按下列公式计算每顶蚊帐的吸水量：

吸水量＝（Vi － Vr）/ 3

根据蚊帐大小、质地蚊帐的不同，列出面积与吸水量，以供参考。

蚊帐（不同大小、质地）的面积与吸水量

蚊帐种类		面积（m^2）	吸水量（ml）
双人（大）	尼龙	20	1 000
	纯棉	20	2 000
单人（小）	尼龙	10	600
	纯棉	10	1 400

3. 计算杀虫剂用量

本项目选用氟氯氰菊酯（cyfluthrin）进行蚊帐浸泡。目前常用的剂型产品有德国拜耳（Bayer）公司生产的 5% 杀飞克水乳剂（solfac EW 050），包装规格为 1 升 / 瓶和 12.5% 拜虫杀悬浮剂（responsar SC 125），包装规格为 1 升 / 瓶。

若用 5%杀飞克水乳剂，推荐剂量为每平方米蚊帐面积需用 30mg 氟氯氰菊酯。假定每顶双人蚊帐的总面积为 20 平方米，每顶蚊帐的用量为 30mg ×20 =600mg，即需用药量。按 5% 杀飞克水乳剂的包装规格每瓶 1 升含氟氯氰菊酯 50g(50 000mg）计算，50 000÷600 = 83 顶蚊帐，即 5% 杀飞克水乳剂 1 瓶（1 升）可浸泡双人蚊帐 83 顶或单人蚊帐 166 顶（面积以 10 平方米计算）。

若用 12.5%拜虫杀悬浮剂，推荐剂量为每平方米蚊帐面积需用 15mg 氟氯氰菊酯。假定每顶双人蚊帐的总面积为 20 平方米，每顶蚊帐的用量为 15mg ×20 =300mg，即需用药量。按 12.5%拜虫杀悬浮剂的包装规格每瓶 1L 含氟氯氰菊酯 125g（125 000mg）计算，125 000÷ 300 = 416 顶蚊帐，即可浸泡双人蚊帐 416 顶或单人蚊帐 832 顶（面积以 10 平方米计算）。

三、浸帐操作

（一）浸帐时间：杀虫剂浸泡处理蚊帐应安排在疟疾流行高峰季节前，1 年进行 1 次。

（二）浸帐方式：采取以自然村或居民组为单位，由专业队集中定点浸泡。

（三）计量工具：专业队应准备好能浸泡不同大小、质地蚊帐的 4 只大水桶和配制浸帐药液相应的计量工具。

（四）浸帐药液的配制：按上述计算的杀虫剂使用量，以自然村或居民组实际的蚊帐拥有情况，分开不同大小、质地 4 只水桶。按照实际蚊帐数量取不同剂量的杀虫剂倒入不同的水桶中，再加入不同的吸水量与之充分混匀。例如，若浸泡 83 顶尼龙双人蚊帐，则取 5%杀飞克水乳剂 1L（1 瓶）倒入水桶中，按尼龙双人蚊帐的吸水量（1 000ml/ 顶），加清水 83 升充分混匀浸泡。

（五）将洗净晒干的蚊帐，逐一放入现配制的浸帐药液水桶中，使蚊帐全部浸湿，拧起不滴水为准，在阴凉处晾干挂起使用。

（六）浸泡注意事项

1．为确保质量，浸帐药液必须现用现配。

2．必须在浸泡前要求居民先将蚊帐洗净晒干后待泡。

3．在浸泡揉搓蚊帐时操作人员应用橡皮手套，作业结束时要用清水洗净手、脸及其他身体暴露部分。

4．蚊帐浸泡后应放在阴凉处晾干，不可暴晒。

5．本年度疟疾流行季节内不要洗涤蚊帐，以免影响效果。

四、质量控制

（一）在杀虫剂浸帐实施前，各级项目办应对辖区内的计划安排、人员组织、药物器材和技术培训等各项准备工作认真检查、核实、督导，发现问题应立即改进和补充。

（二）在实施过程中，各级项目办及专业防治机构应派出专人到实施现场进行督导，严格控制杀虫剂的用量，配制浓度、浸帐程序。

（三）杀虫剂浸帐实施后，除专业防治机构定期进行效果考核外，各级项目办应对杀虫剂浸帐实施是否已达到质量指标进行考核，作出评估，未达标者应立即返工补浸。

（四）质量指标为村浸帐覆盖率、蚊帐浸泡率房间和居民药浸蚊帐使用率等。

第七节　发热病人血检操作规范

一、目的

血涂片显微镜检查，是疟疾诊断和虫种鉴别的主要方法。发热病人血涂片显微镜检查（简称发热病人血检），是疟疾控制和监测的重要手段。为规范全球基金疟疾项目实施地区的发热病人血检技术方法，加强对发热病人血检质量控制和管理，制订本操作规范供实施。

二、血检操作技术

（一）血涂片的制作

1．所需设备

（1）载玻片：玻片在使用前应清洗。新玻片应浸入有液态洗涤剂的清水中10—20分钟，用干净棉巾逐个擦拭，再放入盛有清水的容器中换水3—4次，晾干，最后用干净、柔软的棉巾将玻片擦亮。已用过的玻片应先浸泡于洗涤剂溶液中1—2天，或浸泡于煮沸的5%肥皂水1—2小时，逐个擦去玻片上的旧血膜痕迹，用清水漂洗3—4次，再玻片擦干和擦亮。洗净的玻片每10—20张用白纸包好后放入塑料袋内，保存于干燥环境中备用。

（2）采血针：推荐使用一次性使用的采血针。若使用可重复使用的采血针，在每次使用后都应清洗，并经高压或干热灭菌处理。

（3）75%乙醇棉球：用于采血前后的消毒。

2．采血部位及取血方法

采血部位以耳垂较为合适，也可在手指末端采血，婴儿可从拇趾或足跟取血。先用75%乙醇棉球消毒取血部位，待干后，以左手拇指和食指轻轻捻转耳垂边缘或夹住被检者手指尖稍下方，右手持消毒刺针，迅速刺入取血部位1—2毫米深，然后用左手大拇指、食指和右手中指协同挤出血滴。

3．涂制血膜

取玻片 2 张，1 张做载片，1 张作推片（具有光滑边缘），用右手大拇指和食指夹持推片侧缘中部，用推片的左下角刮取血液 4—5μl（约火柴头大小），再用该端中部刮取血液 1—1.5μl。将左下角的血滴涂于载片的中央偏右，由里向外划圈涂成直径为 0.8—1cm 的圆形厚血膜（厚血膜的厚度以一个油镜视野内可见到 5—10 个白细胞为宜）。用干棉球抹净角上的血渍，然后将推片下缘平抵载玻片的中线，当血液在载玻片与推片之间向两侧扩展至约 2cm 宽时，使两张玻片保持 25°—35°角，从右向左迅速向前推成舌状薄血膜。推制时速度要均匀，血滴大小、推片与载片之间夹角大小及展开血膜的速度快慢等常影响血膜的厚薄。制成的薄血膜应在玻片上形成平铺的血细胞，细胞之间互相接触而不相互重叠。每张载玻片上分别做 1 个薄血膜，1 个厚血膜。标准血膜的位置如下图所示。

标准血膜示意图

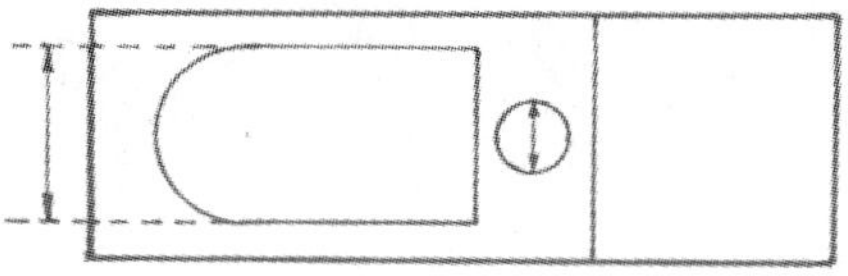

4．血膜染色前的处理

待血膜自然干燥后，用铅笔将受检者号码写在薄血膜上，然后用甲醇固定薄血膜并对厚血膜进行溶血处理。未处理血膜的放置时间夏天不宜超过 48 小时，冬天不宜超过 72 小时，否则厚血膜会自然固定且不能溶血，影响镜检。

（二）血膜的染色

1．吉姆萨（Giemsa）染液配制

吉姆萨粉 10g

甘油 500ml

甲醇加至 1 000ml

将吉姆萨粉 10g 置于研钵中，加入少量甘油小心充分研磨，溶解缓慢，边加边磨，至 500ml 甘油加完研磨均匀为止，然后倒入 1 000ml 容量瓶中。每次加入少量甲醇至研钵中，多次洗涤研钵中的残留液，洗净为止，洗液均并入容量瓶中，再加入部分甲醇，塞紧瓶塞，摇匀，再加甲醇稀释至 1 000ml 的刻度，塞紧瓶塞，充分摇匀，室温放置。每天用力摇动此溶液 5 分钟，3 天后即可储存至玻璃瓶中塞紧备用。

2. 缓冲液配制

溶液 I：无水磷酸氢二钠 9.5g

蒸馏水加至 1 000ml

溶液 II ：磷酸二氢钾 9.07g

蒸馏水加至 1 000ml

将上述两种磷酸盐分别置于 1000ml 容量瓶中，分别加入部分蒸馏水摇匀使溶解后，再加入蒸馏水稀释至 1000ml，充分摇匀。此配就的溶液 I 和溶液 II 分别装入玻璃瓶中塞紧备用。临用时，根据选用 pH 的不同，按下表用量，再配制成不同 pH 的缓冲溶液用于染液的稀释和染色后的冲洗。

配制不同 pH 缓冲溶液的用量表

pH	溶液 I 用量（ml）	溶液 II 用量（ml）	稀释成总数（ml）
6.6	37	63	1 000
6.8	49	51	1 000
7.0	63	37	1 000
7.2	73	27	1 000
7.4	81	19	1 000

根据选用的不同 pH，将上述表中溶液 I 和溶液的相应用量倒入 1 000ml 容量瓶中，加入部分蒸馏水，混合摇匀后，再加入蒸馏水稀释至 1 000ml 的刻度，塞紧瓶塞反复摇匀后，即配制成不同 pH 的缓冲溶液。

3. 染色用水

常用的染液的稀释用水和染色的冲洗用水，是中性的蒸馏水或经煮沸过滤的冷开水。在没有蒸馏水的情况下，也可用井水、河水、泉水或雨水。因稀释和冲洗用水的 pH 在 7.0—7.2 时，染色的效果最佳。因此，也可选用临时配制的缓冲蒸馏水溶液，以取得较好的染色效果。

4. 染色方法

（1）单张血膜片染色：取蒸馏水或 pH7.0—7.2 缓冲液 1ml 加入吉氏染液 1 滴，混合均匀后，滴在厚、薄血膜上，染色 20—30 分钟，然后水洗、晾干。

（2）成批血膜染色：将血膜片朝一个方向插入染色缸中，或每对玻片血膜朝外，背靠背插入染色缸中，倒入新配的 2% 吉氏染液（2ml 吉氏原液加入蒸馏水或 pH7.0—7.2 缓冲液至 100ml，摇匀），浸没厚薄血膜，染色 30 分钟后，向染色缸中注入缓冲液或自来水，直到溢出，除掉染液表面上的浮渣，将染色缸中残余的染液倾出，加入新水，反复冲洗 2—3 次，然后取出玻片，将血膜朝下插在晾片板上干燥。

染色较好的血膜，红细胞呈淡红色，嗜酸性细胞的颗粒呈鲜红色，淋巴细胞及疟原虫胞浆呈蓝色或淡蓝色，白细胞的核呈紫蓝色，疟原虫的核呈红色。

三、血检质量控制

（一）血片制作和染色质量规范

			好	中	差
血片制作质量	厚血膜	血量 位置 直径 外观	4.0—5.0mm^3 玻片右 1/3 0.8—1.0cm 圆形厚膜均匀，边缘整齐	略多或略少 稍偏右 0.7—0.8 或 1.0—1.2cm 圆形稍不均不整齐	过多或过少 偏右过多 ＜ 0.7 或＞ 1.2cm 厚薄不匀影响着色
	薄血膜	血量 位置 长宽 外观	1.5—2.0 mm^3 玻片 1/2—1/3 处 1.5 × 2.0cm 舌状厚薄均匀	略多或略少 稍偏右或偏左 稍大或稍小 舌状稍不匀	过多或过少 偏右或偏左过多 过大或过小 厚薄不匀呈波浪形
染色质量		外观 镜下	蓝紫色 白细胞疟原虫胞浆呈蓝色，核深红	深蓝色 胞浆淡蓝或深蓝，核红色	红色或灰白色 胞浆不易见，核淡红或蓝色
清洁度		外观 镜下	光洁无油灰 无沉渣	稍有油污 稍有沉渣	油灰粘连 沉渣多或有杂菌

（二）血片制作和染色质量判定标准

1. 血片制作质量判定标准

好：厚薄血膜均好，或薄血膜好，厚血膜中。

中：薄血膜中，厚血膜好或中。

差：薄血膜差，或厚薄血膜均差。

2. 血片制作和染色合格率要求

分别以血片制作、染色和清洁度的好、中，合并计算合格率。

（1）片制作合格率应在 85% 以上。

（2）染色合格率应在 85% 以上。

（3）清洁度合格率应在 80% 以上。

四、血检工作管理

（一）镜检站工作的管理

1．发热病人血检工作，应列入项目地区各级各类医疗机构常规检验工作的内容之一，至少有1人专职或兼职负责发热病人血检工作。

2．项目地区各级各类医疗机构的门诊镜检站（检验科），应全年对就诊的“三热”病人（临床初诊疟疾、疑似疟疾和原因不明发热）进行血检，所有外来流动人口和从高疟区回归的当地居民中的发热病人均应进行血检。以县为单位，年血检率不低于2%。

3．所有血检对象应及时登记，发现阳性应立即报告临床医生和同级防保组织。

4．每月血片应保留至下月底，以备上级中心镜检站抽片检查。

5．在全年工作结束后，应将血检登记表交给同级或上级防保机构归档保存。

6．做好镜检站器材日常养护及常用试剂的配备。

7．参加相关的业务例会和业务培训。

（二）各级中心镜检站的职责和管理

1．中心镜检站的建设和管理

（1）项目地区各省应建立省级、市级和县级中心镜检站，构成省、市、县和乡镇四级镜检网络，以承担项目地区的发热病人血检工作和管理。

（2）项目地区各省应依据《传染病防治法》加强对发热病人血检工作的管理。各省可根据各地的实际情况，制订发热病人血检工作的奖惩条例。对在血片涂制和镜检中发现的弄虚作假、严重的质量问题等，应进行通报批评，造成严重后果的应由当地行政部门追究当事人的责任，并进行经济处罚。后果特别严重的，应同时追究当事人的法律责任。

2．市、县中心镜检站的职责和管理

（1）负责制订本辖区的发热病人血检年度工作计划。

（2）定期举办镜检培训班，有计划地对门诊镜检站（检验科）镜检人员进行业务培训。

（3）对辖区内各医疗机构门诊镜检站（检验科）的发热病人血检工作进行检查、督导和业务指导。

（4）定期抽检门诊镜检站（检验科）的发热病人血片，并负责完成省疟疾中心镜检站下达的血片抽检或复检任务。

3．省疟疾中心镜检站的职责和管理

(1) 制订全省发热病人血检工作年度计划，负责全省发热病人血检管理工作。

(2) 定期举办镜检培训班，负责对市、县级镜检专业人员及重点地区门诊镜检站（检验科）镜检人员的培训。

(3) 负责对全省发热病人血检工作的检查和督导，定期抽检或复检门诊镜检站（检验科）已检血片，并及时反馈结果。

(4) 负责全省镜检网络的质量控制。

4．各级中心镜检站发热病人血检工作的质量控制

(1) 县级中心镜检站每年应复检辖区内门诊镜检站（检验科）的所有阳性血片，并抽检不少于 3% 的已检阴性血片。

(2) 省级中心镜检站每年应复检辖区内门诊镜检站（检验科）的所有阳性血片，并抽检不少于 0.5% 的已检阴性血片。

(3) 漏检率和错检率按每年复检和抽检总数分别计算，阳性血片错检率以县为单位，全年不应超过 10%；阴性血片漏检率以县为单位，全年不应超过 0.1%。

第八节　成本—效果分析方案

一、目的

为评价全球基金疟疾项目人力、物力和财力的投入和产出以及对项目执行结果进行效果评价，分析项目活动和疟疾防治措施在不同地区间是否需要适当调整或改善，使资源投入获得最佳的效率，特制订成本 - 效果分析方案，以便在项目中期和结束时进行卫生经济学评价。

二、总体说明

（一）成本—效果分析作为卫生经济学评价方法之一，基本前提是“多方案的比较选择”。由于全球基金疟疾项目为单一项目，不存在项目间的比较和优选，因此，在本方案中，成本—效果分析仅作为项目评价的形式之一，评价项目 2 年度阶段性和 5 年项目结束后投入与产出的关系，为项目总体评价服务，并不作为方案优选的决策依据。

（二）成本分析和效果分析以成本资料和效果资料的可计量、可获得为基本前提，在难以“求全”的情况下，重点收集和分析关键指标。

（三）本方案的成本—效果分析涉及两个层次，整个项目投入、产出的总体评价和云南、海南两个项目重点地区选点进行的详细分析。两个层次的成本 - 效果分析方法学上一致，但目的不同，前者旨在总体分析项目资源投入与总体目标的实现程度；后者着重分析资金在不同项目活动的分配结构，评价项目资源配置的效果与合理性。

三、时间与执行单位

（一）项目 2 年度结束

总体成本—效果分析，由国家项目办公室负责执行，目的是为全球基金阶段性评估提供卫生经济学评价结果，为争取下一阶段（后 3 年）经费资助提供有力依据；

两省点上的成本-效果分析，分别由两省项目办公室负责执行，主要分析前2年项目经费与人力投入在不同项目活动与不同地区间的效果与合理性，以利后阶段资源的合理使用与分配。

（二）项目5年结束

仅由国家项目办公室负责进行项目总体卫生经济学分析，为项目总体评价服务，以考核整个项目的效果和目标的完成情况。

四、内容

（一）成本分析

成本包括直接成本和间接成本，在本方案中，为了衡量和计算方便，直接成本指全球基金拨付的项目资金和购置的器材、设备等；间接成本主要指全球基金资助外的人力、物力与资金投入，包括地方配套资金、机构人力资源、车辆与房屋折旧等。

1．直接成本

(1) 全球基金支付的货币资金；

(2) 全球基金购置的药品、消耗器材等折算的费用；

(3) 全球基金购置的仪器、设备折旧费。

2．间接成本

政府或其他机构配套资金；

人员工资成本；

房屋与办公用房折旧费；

车辆折旧费；

燃料动力费用；

水电等维持费。

3．成本测量

(1) 资金复利或贴现

各项费用均以项目实施年限内平均年银行利率为复利系数或贴现率，复利到项目实施初或贴现到分析时的价值，以剔除年度间物价水平不同对成本的影响。经复利或贴现的费用为成本现值，公式为：

$$C = \sum_{t}^{n} C_t\ (1+i)^{t}$$

C 成本现值，n 实施年限，t 实施第 t 年，C_t 第 t 年的费用，i 复利系数或贴现率

(2) 人员费用的计算

专职人员：以月工资核算，包括津贴、补助等。

兼职人员：按实际工作天数计算工资成本，其他补助同专职人员。

临时工作人员：包括乡村干部协助工作的人员，按实际支付金额计算。

乡村医生采血、送检、取结果和送药观察等的疟防补助。

(3) 维护与折旧费

办公用房维修与折旧：根据实际情况按一定比例折旧。

设备维护与折旧：显微镜、计算机、冰箱等均按 20% 折旧率计算年使用成本。

车辆维护与折旧：根据车辆寿命估算折旧率进行折旧，计入成本；维护费用按实际支付计算。

(4) 药品、消耗器材等折算的费用：依据采购清单价格与数量进行成本核算。

(5) 单位成本计算：每一项项目活动的单位成本均由上述成本要素构成。如：

每镜检 1 例发热病人的费用涉及人员工资成本、玻片与染色液等消耗材料费、显微镜折旧费、办公用房折旧、水电维持费、送检血片的交通费等。

每治疗 1 例疟疾病人的费用包括医生工资成本、药品费、交通费、水电维持费、办公用房折旧等。

药物浸泡蚊帐（ITNs）的单位费用涉及蚊帐材料费、杀虫剂费用、人员工资成本、培训费、场地费等。

(二)效果分析

效果指标的选择与考核是成本 - 效果分析的难点和关键，卫生资源投入的产出往往多方位、多指标的，有短期结果（output)、中期效果（effectiveness）和远期影响（impact）；有直接效果和间接效果；有发病率、死亡率下降等生物学效果，也有改善旅游环境、提高生产率等社会学效益。因此，成本 - 效果分析中的效果界定和指标选择至关重要。

1．效果指标的选择原则

本方案的效果特指与投入直接相关的有用产出，选择与项目活动和目标密切相关、可考核、可收集的主要指标，剔除无法满足成本 - 效果分析条件、难以考核和获得的次要指标。当同一项目活动工作指标与效果指标均可考核时，采取效果指标优选的原则，而效果指标难以考核时则选择工作指标。

2．效果指标

(1) 疟疾总发病率下降幅度 (%)

（2）恶性疟发病率下降比例（%）

（3）疟疾死亡减少的比例（%）

（4）疟防知识普及率提高的比例（%）

（5）输入性恶性疟下降的比例（%）

（6）恶性疟抗药性降低程度（%）

（7）乡村医生正确处方率提高的比例（%）

（8）药浸蚊帐使用率提高的比例（%）

（9）疟疾漏报率下降的比例（%）

（10）血检覆盖率提高的比例（%）

（11）血片抽查合格率提高的比例（%）

3．效果分析

上述单个指标仅反映某一项目活动的效果，进行单一项目活动的经济学评价时，可以选用单一指标与该项目活动的投入进行成本 - 效果分析；而在评价整个项目时，需要一个能概括地反映整个项目实施效果的综合指标，与项目总体成本进行投入\产出比较，本方案推荐德尔菲（Delphi）综合指标法。

（1）德尔菲法基本原理：通过多轮信访专家的形式，对上述指标的重要程度进行评价，集中专家意见，筛选更为重要的指标；将第一轮结果反馈专家，进行第二轮指标体系的评价，确定每一指标的权重，根据专家确定的指标体系及其权重，建立综合效果指标。

（2）德尔菲法调查：调查内容包括：本项目的背景材料、德尔菲法简介、专家简况、对指标的了解程度调查表（表 1）、指标的重要程度调查表（表 2）。请专家对各项指标的了解程度和重要程度作出各自独立的判断。

（3）指标权重的确定：确定专家权威系数（Ai）：先给出专家的职称系数（Si）和对指标的了解程度系数（Ki）（表 3），处理后得专家权威系数，计算公式为：

$$Ai = Ki \cdot Si / \sum_{i=1}^{n} (Ki \cdot Si)$$

i 为某一专家，n 为专家总数

确定指标的权重：专家对每个指标的评分为 1，2，…… 10，共 10 个等级，假定 Qin 为第 i 个专家对第 n 个指标的评分，Win 为经专家权威系数调整后的第 i 个专家给予第 n 个指标的权重，则满足：

$$Win = \sum_{i=1}^{n} (Qin \cdot Ai) / n$$

归一化处理后，Win 即为第 n 项指标的实际权重。经过上述处理，得到各分指标在综合指标体系中的实际权重。

（4）合指标的建立：将每一个指标变化一个百分点作为一个变化单位，按下列公式计算即得综合指标：

$$综合指标 = \sum_{i=1}^{n} Xi \cdot Wi$$

n 为指标个数，i 为某一指标，Xi 为指标变化的单位数，Wi 为某指标的权重。

（三）成本－效果分析

1．总体成本－效果分析

总成本 / 综合效果指标（成本 / 效果比）。

2．单项成本－效果分析

每一效果指标均对应相应的投入，反映和评价某一项目活动的效率和资源配置的合理性，如：

（1）疟疾总发病率每下降一个百分点的成本；

（2）恶性疟发病率每下降一个百分点的成本；

（3）每减少一例疟疾死亡的成本；

（4）知识普及率每提高一个百分点的成本；

（5）输入性恶性疟下降一个百分点的成本，等。

第六章

第一轮中国全球基金疟疾项目标书

第一节　中文标书

抗艾滋病、结核和疟疾全球基金临时秘书处

日内瓦，2002 年 1 月 31 日

GFATM/B1/6　　附件

建议指南

建议表格

建议指南确定了资助的详细条件和审评建议的标准。此表提及原则的有关章节。

供全球基金秘书处使用：

收悉日期：

参考号：

本表格分为三部分：

A 部分询问总体建议的简明信息，要求的资金总额和有关一般资格标准的信息，包括国家协调机构的详情；

B 部分询问整体建议的进一步详情，其目的，如何对它进行检查并证实其补充性；

C 部分询问详情，包括建议每一部分的预算信息。

在增添页面上请明确标明 A、B 或 C 部分。

A 部分：总体信息

A.1. 国家（或区域）： 中华人民共和国

A.2. 建议标题：

中国疟疾高传播区疟疾控制项目

A.3. 详细说明这项建议旨在解决三个卫生问题的哪一个或包括全部（HIV/ 艾滋病、结核和 / 或疟疾）（指南第 4 段）：

疟疾

A.4. 这项建议预期产生什么其他成果？（指南，第 8 段和附件 1，II3）

1. 改善中国南方地区的卫生状况和当地居民的生活质量。
2. 改善中国南方地区的旅游环境，促进当地农民脱贫和经济发展。
3. 加强边境地区农村的传染病监测。

A.5. 要求全球基金提供的总金额：(以美元计，按年)

组成部分（C 部分有解释）	第 1 年	第 2 年	第 3 年	第 4 年	第 5 年	合计
	（预算）	（预计）				
第 1 部分	470 732	392 277	313 822	235 366	156 911	1 569 108
第 2 部分	816 000	680 000	544 000	408 000	272 000	2 720 000
第 3 部分	300 000	250 000	200 000	150 000	100 000	1 000 000
第 4 部分	335 265	279 388	223 510	167 633	111 755	1 117 550
总计（B 部分有概述）	1 921 997	1 601 665	1 281 332	960 999	640 666	6 406 658

A.6. 疾病负担（提及有关国家 / 区域 / 地区 HIV/ 艾滋病、结核和 / 或疟疾的流行和程度的官方文件或流行病资料出处）或可能的疾病负担（如发生新感染的指标等）（指南第 6 段）

尽管中国大部分地区疟疾已基本得到控制，但南部和中部地区疟疾形势仍相当严峻。云南和海南两省为中国疟疾流行最严重地区，两地疟疾发病占全国病例的 70% 以上。据 2000 年疟疾疫情分析，云南、海南两省的实际疟疾发病数分别为 14 万和 7 万病例，其中恶性疟分别占 17% 和 32.5%。2000 年云南省疟疾发病占传染病报告总数的 12.45%。大多数疟疾病例集中在

26个边境县，约占全省的66.8%。在海南，主要是10个山区县人群中的恶性疟流行问题，这10个县的恶性疟病例数占全省恶性疟病例的97% 。令人担忧的是，两地儿童疟疾问题日益严重。导致如此严重的疟疾负担主要由于：

1. 流动人口频繁。云南省位于中国南部边境，南部、西部有26个疟疾流行较为严重的县(市)分别与越南、老挝、缅甸为邻，边境全长4061公里。随着边境的开放和经济的发展，近年来每年约有1千万边境流动人员，出入境人员使传染源相互交换，互相输入和输出，加剧了疟疾在边境两侧的传播和流行。而边境地区由于流动人员的不稳定性，使疟疾的及时诊断和治疗相当困难，防治措施难以落实。海南为中国改革开放较早、内地流动人口较多的地区，内地每年流入海南的人口约2百万。除两省本身疟疾发病率较高外，国内其他地区恶性疟病人均为两省的输入病例。

2. 恶性疟多重抗性。根据恶性疟原虫对各类抗疟药敏感性测定，两省恶性疟原虫除对氯喹有抗性外，对哌喹、法西达、阿莫地喹等多种抗疟药均产生了抗性，对青蒿素类药物及咯萘啶的敏感性明显下降。当地基层对抗疟药使用不规范，药物滥用现象相当普遍，更加剧了抗性的产生。

3. 缺乏有效的媒介控制对策。边境地区多数存在2种以上的传疟媒介。在云南和海南，微小按蚊和大劣按蚊为主要传疟媒介，目前尚缺乏对这两种媒介的有效防制对策。

4. 因病致贫、因贫致病。云南边境地区和海南山区多为少数民族居住地，经济落后，文化水平较低，对疟疾的防护意识较差，疟疾控制措施受到极大的限制。疟疾不仅使当地居民贫困，而且严重阻碍了社会经济的发展。

5. 疫情漏报严重。据2000年在云南和海南进行的疟疾疫情漏报调查，两省疟疾漏报率分别为88.8%和94.6%，实际疟疾发病数是疫情报告数的18—25倍。

潜在的疟疾负担：

由于云南、海南两省流动人口问题突出，疟疾传播对中国其他地区构成潜在危险：1）中国中部地区曾经有恶性疟流行，目前已基本消灭，但致病因素和传疟媒介依然存在。近年其他地区的恶性疟均为两省输入病例，这对人口密集的中部地区构成极大威胁。2）恶性疟对中部省份的输入将导致恶性疟抗药性大范围扩散。

A.7. 经济情况：(提及诸如人均国民生产总值，人发指数的官方指数或资料可得性的其他信息)(指南第6段)

中国是一个发展中国家，有约13亿人口，其中超过80%的人口居住在农村。2000年人均国民生产总值为790美元。人发指数为0.718，2001年居世界第87位。中国各地区经济发展不均衡。中西部和南部地区人口受教育程度较低，人均生产总值也较低。云南和海南属中国经济不发达省（区）之一，云南省总人口数约4100万，其中三分之一为少数民族，2000年人均国民生产总值为488美元，全省农民人均纯收入仅为人民币1387.25元（约153美元），远低于中国其他发达省（区）。边境地区人均生产总值低于100美元（云南省2000年统计报告）。海南省2000年总人口约780万，人均生产总值（GDP）仅为808美元；恶性疟流行的山区主要为少数民族居住区，农民人均纯收入仅为人民币835元（约100美元）(海南省2000年统计报告)。

A.8. 政策承诺:(政府对资助建议的贡献,或公共卫生开支,或具有国家支持政策,或在建议方面具有一个国家对应单位,或其他指标)(指南第6段)。 1. 中国政府将积极支持和促进本项目在各部门间的合作。 2. 如果项目资金得到批准,中国政府将给予相应的支持,保证所有资金全部用于本项目的实施。中国政府和两省政府也将把这一疟疾控制项目作为疾病控制规划的重要组成部分。 4. 在项目执行中,国家卫生部和中国疾病预防控制中心寄生虫病预防控制所将承担组织、协调、实施、管理和督导等职能,以保证项目的顺利实施。
A.9. 与现有活动的联系:(这项建议例如通过国家卫生战略、减贫战略和部门范围途径与其他当前的支持性活动有哪些联系?提供这些情况的副本作为支持性文件,在附件1中注明) 1. 世界卫生组织遏制疟疾项目 本项目的目标与世界卫生组织遏制疟疾项目的目标一致,均旨在加强中国南部地区,特别是云南和海南省的疟疾控制。 2. 湄公河流域疾病监测项目 疟疾监测是湄公河流域疾病监测项目4个分项目之一,本项目不仅加强云南、海南两省的疟疾监测,而且为其他传染病监测提供可行的模式。 3. 中国"十五"疟疾防治规划和两省"十五"疟疾控制规划 本项目疟疾控制和监测两大内容为中国"十五"疟疾防治规划及两省疾病控制规划的重要组成部分。 4. 中国中西部脱贫规划 当前中国正在进行西部开发和开展中西部脱贫规划,这为减少中西部地区少数民族因病致贫,改善投资环境和经济发展提供了条件。云南省属于西部开发地区,因此当前西部脱贫规划为本项目的实施提供了契机。
A.10. 国家协调机制的情况(CCM)- 如果不通过国家协调机构提交,请直接填写A.12.(指南第9-14段) 支持这项建议的各种机构和合作伙伴(包括非政府组织和研究机构)均由本文件所称为CCM的一个国家协调机构予以协调和组织。 1. 国际协调机构的名称: 国家控制疟疾协调机制 2. 目前国家协调机制建立的日期:2002年2月 3. 组织机构(例如秘书处、小组委员会、独立存在): 为了适应全球艾滋病、结核和疟疾基金的要求,国家控制疟疾协调机制于2002年2月正式成立,部分国际组织、非政府组织和政府部门成为该机制的成员,主要负责国家"全球艾滋病、结核和疟疾基金"疟疾项目的申请、协调和管理。协调机制已经召开2次会议讨论向全球基金提交的项目申请书。 4. 会议频率(例如每月、每季度): 国家控制疟疾协调机制每年召开两次会议。 5. 国家协调机构的主要功能和职责: (1)审议、通过项目申请后,上报全球基金。 (2)在项目实施过程中,负责部门间的协调工作。

（3）对项目实施情况进行监测和评估。

6. 在今后 12 个月中加强国家协调机构作用和功能的主要战略：

（1）成立 CCM 秘书处。

（2）加强对全球基金的宣传，提高大众对全球基金项目的了解和参与。

（3）组织 CCM 会议，讨论项目实施计划。

（4）总结和了解国内、国际疟疾防治工作的最佳实践及存在问题。

（5）组织国家和地方项目管理和执行人员的培训，提高实施能力。

A.11. 请提供国家协调机构成员的总数和组成：

HIV/ 结核 / 疟疾患者 ....

非政府组织 / 以社区为基础的组织 .... .2 . . .

私立部门 ....

宗教 / 信仰组织 ....

学术 / 教育部门 ....

政府部门 .... 7 . . . .

其他（解释）.. . . . . . .10 . . . .

总数 .... 19. . . .

A.12. 签字：

国家协调机构的成员（CCM – 见下页）在下方签字认可这项建议。认可这项建议对伙伴机构或个人不产生任何财政（或法律）义务：

签字，

国家协调机制主席： 马晓伟 博士

主席姓名和联络信息： 马晓伟 中国 卫生部副部长
北京市西直门外南路 1 号 100044

____

CCM 成员签字

机构 / 组织	姓名 / 职称	日期	签字

A.13. 如果全球基金秘书处对这份提交的建议有问题，请联络： 姓名：　郝阳 职称 / 地址：　处长，中国国家卫生部疾病控制司地方病与寄生虫病处 电话号码：　86-10-68792376 传真号码：　86-10-68792514 电子邮件：　haoyang@chsi3.moh.gov.cn
A.14. 如果不是通过一个国家协调机构提交，而是作为个人或非政府组织（NGOs）或私立部门的一个合作伙伴提交建议，请阐明不能通过国家协调机构提交的情况、条件和 / 或原因。

B 部分：总体建议

B.1 总体建议概况：[建议大纲，说明总体目标，涉及的人员、受益者，列示主要的卫生部分以及各部分之间的协同作用。(各部分的更多详情见 C 部分)]。

尽管中国大部分地区疟疾已得到基本控制，但南部云南和海南省疟疾形势依然严峻，两省疟疾病例占全国发病总数的 70% 以上。随着社会经济的发展，这些地区流动人口日益增多，使疟疾传播显著增加，尤其云南边境和海南山区抗药性恶性疟大量扩散。本项目旨在加强中国南部疟疾高度流行区的疟疾控制，以遏制抗药性恶性疟向中部恶性疟已消除的省份扩散。

为了减少抗药性恶性疟在当地传播和限制其向中部地区扩散，最近中国卫生部制订了“十五”疟疾防治规划，将云南、海南两省列为疟疾防治重点省份；两省政府也将疟疾控制作为本省“十五”疾病控制规划优先内容。世界卫生组织湄公河流域遏制疟疾项目也把中国南部地区云南和海南省的疟疾控制纳入需加强重点控制的地区之一。尽管中央和地方政府加大了疟疾防治的投入，世界卫生组织湄公河流域遏制疟疾项目也提供了部分防治试点经费，但需要更多的资金以加快南部疟疾高度流行地区的疟疾控制进程。

本项目的总体目标是：通过 5 年项目的实施，云南省的疟疾发病率下降 50%，减少多重抗药性恶性疟在项目地区的传播和限制其向中部地区扩散，并在海南省阻断多重抗药性恶性疟的传播。

项目的目标人群为云南 26 个边境县约 580 万人口、海南 10 个恶性疟传播的山区县约 350 万人口，以及两省约 1200 万流动人口，因此项目的直接受益人群为 930 万当地居民和 1200 万流动人口；云南，海南两省与项目地区毗邻的受威胁地区的约 2000 万人口和中国中部地区已得到控制的原恶性疟流行区的约 5000 万人口共 7000 万人口将成为项目的间接受益人群。

本项目拟包括以下 4 个部分：

1. 流动人口的疟疾管理：通过改善边境地区对流动人口疟疾早期诊断及时正规治疗的可及性和加强对流动人口的健康教育，降低流动人口疟疾发病率和云南省边境地区及海南省山区的疟疾流行特别是多重抗药性恶性疟的传播和扩散。

2. 加强中国南方高传播地区的疟疾控制：通过提高疟疾快速诊断和正规治疗的能力，加强对抗疟药品供应和规范使用的管理，提高村民的自我保护和全程足量服药意识，并通过加强对传染源和局部暴发流行的控制，以降低当地的疟疾发病率并限制多重抗性恶性疟在当地的传播和向其他地区的扩散。

3. 健康教育和健康促进：通过加强项目地区居民和中小学生的健康教育，提高健康保护意识；加强乡村和个体医生的培训，提高疟疾诊断和正规治疗的能力。

4. 加强疟疾疫情和抗性监测和建立疟疾疫情信息网络：通过建立哨点监测，改进疫情报告和建立疟疾疫情信息网，加强该地区的疟疾疫情和对恶性疟原虫抗药性的监测，以减少当地疟疾暴发流行，降低多重抗药性恶性疟的传播和扩散。

项目的 4 个组成部分彼此联系，有机结合，通过在不同的目标人群中开展不同的项目活动达到共同的目标。为了有效控制云南、海南两省的疟疾疫情和遏制抗药性恶性疟通过流动人口向中部省份扩散，首先要加强云南 26 个边境县和海南有恶性疟流行的 10 个山区县的流动人口疟疾管理。为减少当地疟疾负担和限制流动人口所导致的恶性疟扩散，当地疟疾控制和监测工作必不可少。由于项目地区经济比较落后，居民的文化水平和健康防护意识较为低下，尤其基层乡村医生和个体医生缺少必要的疟疾诊断和正规治疗的知识和技能，因此本项目将加强当地居民和流动人口的健康教育以及乡村医生专业培训作为专题，以提高当地居民和流动人口的健康防护意识，以及基层医生的疟疾诊治能力，确保整个项目的顺利实施，达到预期的目标。

B.2 规划性检查和评价：[（指南第 34—37 段）（建议需要包括一项检查和评价程序的概况，它置于总体建议之后，包括活动时间表，和基线数据，收集数据的职责，建议 / 预期对收集信息的使用，以及目标人群对检查和评价的参与。(C 部分要求有关主要部分检查和评价方面的信息）]

项目的常规督导和评估

1. 项目领导小组将在项目开始后每年召开一次会议，研究讨论项目的进展、结果、效益和财务情况，制定下一步工作计划，组织协调各有关方面开展工作；

2. 每年国家项目技术指导组将开展一次督导，2 到 3 名小组成员将对项目地区进行检查；

3. 项目办公室每年召开一次会议研究讨论过去一年的项目的进展、结果、效益、存在的问题、财务情况；提出解决办法，确定工作方向，协调有关部门并对下一年工作作出安排；

4. 项目办公室将制定或修订督导标准并派出 2 到 3 名工作人员到项目省或县开展督导，每年一到两次。

5. 每季度项目办公室将负责制定项目实施计划，每年两次上报详细的项目进展报告。

支持性督导

支持性督导的目的是确保项目活动按计划及时和有效地开展。在督导过程中，不能简单地指责项目执行部门单位不应该做什么，而是应告诉他们应该如何去做。作为督导人员，要尽最大努力去及时发现问题，找原因并帮助执行单位尽快寻求解决办法。

项目的督导工作将逐级进行，GFATM 督导项目国卫生部，项目国卫生部分别督导云南和海南省卫生厅。而上述卫生部门将督导项目执行机构，如云南寄生虫病防治所和海南省热带病防治所。进而，上述机构应督导县级机构，县级机构督导乡级和村级医务人员（VHW），乡医院负责村级医务人员的管理和督导工作。

（1）GFATM 的支持性督导（方法、时间和地点需根据 GFATM 的安排）

（2）卫生部和国家 CDC 的支持性督导

卫生部和国家 CDC 主管官员将深入项目地区开展督导。首先，将在中国的昆明或思茅协调召开 GFATM 年度工作会议，并进入现场检查项目进展情况。

（3）省级和地区级支持性督导

云南和海南省寄生虫病防治机构其地区级相应业务机构将定期开展一年两次的督导工作。

评估

评估的目的在于系统地收集和使用现有资料以改进项目的实施、指导卫生资源的分配使用和确保项目及时有效的实施。通过提供有关项目的运作及所取得的成果等方面的信息，评估活动将对项目所产生的效果进行评价。

GFATM 评估（方法、时间、地点应根据 GFATM 的安排决定）

卫生部评估（方法、时间和地点应根据卫生部的安排决定）

省级或地区级评估

技术或专业机构如云南省寄生虫病防治所将派遣四个工作组赴项目县考评项目的实施、产出和效果。

以下为具体评估内容。

技术性督导和评估的参考工作框架

为提高项目实施的质量，需要在项目实施的各个阶段开展技术性督导和评估工作并在项目的起步阶段做好详尽的计划。具体步骤如下：

在评估框架文件中，确认方法一栏指出了如何收集所需的资料，如何对一些指标开展一个特别调查，这些指标应该根据流行病学的原则和方法进行设计。在调查中，对所列出的指标可根据不同地区不同情况有选择性地使用。如果需要也可加入其他指标。

B.3. 财政管理（指南第 19—22, 38—40 段）（说明现有的财务管理安排，包括建议的开支方法和计划）资金分配机制：

为了对全球艾滋病、结核和疟疾基金项目进行有效的管理和监督，充分体现基金使用的透明度，在国家协调机制的领导下，成立国家艾滋病、结核和疟疾项目管理办公室（以下简称“项目办公室”）。该项目办公室的职责不仅协调与管理全球基金，而且负责财务的管理与监督，包括制定资金分配计划、程序及其财务，并且通过国家协调机制向全球基金报告财务及项目执行情况。项目办将特选聘 2 名财务管理人员，主要工作任务如下：

1. 协调制定和批准项目的程序，包括向项目执行合作伙伴分配基金的标准和申请程序。
2. 提供基金项目的技术管理和监督。
3. 财务管理和监督，包括制定财务报告，并通过国家协调机制交至全球基金秘书处。
4. 安排项目的外部审计，及其资金分配程序。

资金分配计划和程序：

1. 项目办公室将制定年度计划，报交国家协调机制，以兹批准。
2. 根据年度总计划，要求执行合作伙伴提供具体的年度工作计划。这些工作计划包括可测量的用于监测的指标。执行合作伙伴的工作计划将递交到技术工作小组，以兹回顾、修改和批准。
3. 执行合作伙伴的具体工作计划批准后，项目办公室将向执行合作伙伴划拨 60% 的经费；在收到中期报告后，将划拨另外的 30% 经费；在收到终期技术和财务报告后，剩余 10% 的经费将拨至执行合作伙伴。
4. 项目办将与技术工作小组开展监测与监督，包括财务监督和技术支持。项目办将要求外部审计对执行合作伙伴进行独立审计。

审计：

国家审计署对项目办和执行合作伙伴进行审计。

B.4 陈述 2002 年的预算要求、财务承诺和未满足的需求

（指南第 8 段，附件 III.2）（说明建议的可补充性）

	预算类目（请按计划填写）							
	人力资源	后勤和供应	培训和指导	扩大的服务范围	商品或产品 *	数据和信息系统	其他（解释）	总计
预算需求	2 067 930	1 043 407	912 424	424 278	1 161 494	477 603		6 087 134
按来源的财务承诺								
政府	1 137 697	334 963	307 937	125 822	373 982	166 307		2 446 707
民间社会	699 531	66 346	48 844	35 026	73 785	26 546		950 077
私立部门	105 103	74 338	63 293	36 260	75 377	30 052		384 421
援助方	64 100	36 560	30 906	15 216	44 624	13 661		205 067
其他	61 500	32 240	25 120	9 064	38 296	12 645		178 865
总承诺	2 067 930	544 447	476 100	221 387	606 064	249 211		4 165 137
未满足的需求	0	498 960	436 324	202 891	555 430	228 392		1 921 997

B.5　时期（估计期限）：

开始和结束日期：

自：2002　至：2006

这项资助要求所覆盖的时期

自：2002　至：2006

C 部分：主要部分 C–1

（应为建议的每一主要部分准备另份 C 部分页篇，即如需要时提供更多的复制件。）

建议部分 1—流动人口的疟疾控制（以数码分别标识各部分：1– 4）

C.1 说明:(描述建议的这一部分(例如针对疾病的干预措施),建议所要实现的目标,受益者,执行伙伴和实施战略)。

理由

云南和海南省是中国疟疾流行最严重的地区。云南省与老挝、缅甸和越南三国有 4100 公里长的边境线，62 个正式边境口岸。边界两侧地区是东南亚，也是全球多重抗药性恶性疟传播和扩散最严重的地区之一。目前，每年约有 1000 万跨边界流动人口。随着改革开放，每年有 200 多万流动人口涌入海南。由于流动人口的流动性大，加之边境地区缺乏镜检设备和有经验医生，大量的流动人口不仅导致了大量疟疾传染源，特别是多重抗药性恶性疟的输入，而且加剧了云南省边境地区的疟疾流行和多重抗药性恶性疟的传播和扩散。对中国其他地区，特别是中国中部恶性疟流行已得到控制的地区构成严重的威胁。

本项目重点加强对流动人口疟疾的控制，以降低云南省边境地区及海南省山区的疟疾流行，特别是多重抗药性恶性疟的传播和扩散。

受益人群

1．入境的外国人，出境回归的中国人，外省到边境的流动人口和本省流动人口。

云南边境地区每年约 1 千万出入境的流动人口，边境地区的 580 万当地居民以及每年海南省疟疾流行区的 350 当地居民和 200 万流动人口将成为本项目的直接受益人群。

2．云南和海南两省高传播地区毗邻地区的近 2 千万居民和中国中部恶性疟流行已得到控制地区近 5 千万居民将成为本项目的间接受益人群。

策略和措施

由疟疾防治机构在边境口岸各医院和诊所以及流动人口密集的临时居住点建立镜检站或提供快速诊断试纸条。

流动人口中发热病人及时诊断和治疗。

流动人口通过边境口岸时，提供健康教育材料。

向不同级别疟疾防治机构提供显微镜和快速诊断试纸条。对流动人口中的发热病人血检，防止疟疾病人、带虫者，特别是恶性疟病例的输出。

中国预防医学会、红十字会和无国界卫生组织共同参与对流动人口进行健康教育。

C.2 目标和指标（提供有关这一部分的目标信息。）

主要目标（说明结束时预计的情况）

降低流动人口疟疾发病率和云南省边境地区及海南省山区的疟疾流行特别是多重抗药性恶性疟的传播和扩散。

具体目标：（与指标有关，包括基线数据，目前形势和全年指标）（指南第 34-37 段）

1. 改善边境地区流动人口疟疾早期诊断及时正规治疗的可及性。
2. 加强对流动人口的健康教育，提高流动人口的自我防护意识和就诊率。

* 为估计数

指标	基线	目标				
	2001*	2002	2003	2004	2005	2006
拥有镜检站的边境口岸比例(%)		50	100	100	100	100
流动人口发热病人血镜率(%)		50	60	60	70	80
流动人口接受健康教育的比率(%)		50	60	70	80	90
流动人口疟疾病人接受正规治疗的比率(%)	30	40	45	55	65	80

C.3 监测和评估计划

成立由卫生部门和 NGO（红十字会和无国界卫生组织）成员组成的督导组负责每年督导执行和评价

验证指标	验证方法	评价者
快速诊断试纸条和显微镜分配到公立和私立卫生机构	记录表	督导者
IEC 材料的分配	记录表	督导者
早期诊断和及时治疗的疟疾病例的比例	记录表	督导者
举办乡医和私立医生的培训班	报告	督导者
流动人口增加疟疾的知识	专题调查	专业人员

C.4 时期:(估计期限) 开始和结束日期: 自: 2002 至: 2006 这项资助要求所覆盖的时期: 自: 2002 至: 2006

C.5 实施计划，包括向合作伙伴的资源分配(指南第 40 段)

(美元)

	预算类目(请根据你的计划填写)							
实施合作伙伴	人力资源	后勤和供应	培训和指导	扩大的服务范围	商品或产品 *	数据和信息系统	其他(解释)	总计
政府	329 513	215 752	275 378	109 838	54 919	28 244	0	1 013 644
民间社会 **	23 537	58 842	33 893	15 691	7 846	4 707	0	144 515
私立部门	117 683	117 683	63 549	31 382	15 691	9 415	0	355 403
援助方	0	0	50 839	0	0	941	0	51 781
其他	0	0	0	0	0	3 766	0	3 766
总计	470 732	392 277	423 659	156 911	78 455	47 073	0	1 569 108
* 包括药物								

** 包括防治机构，预防医学会和无国界卫生组织

在项目开始时，由疟疾防治机构进行抽样调查了解有关流动人口疟疾阳性率，自我防护意识的基线资料。

由当地疟疾防治机构负责培训边境疟疾诊所和镜检站的工作人员，中国预防医学会、红十字会和无国界卫生组织将参与部分工作。将培训 130 人。

由疟疾防治机构负责在边境口岸建疟疾诊所和镜检站，提供必要的镜检设备。第 1 年将建立至少 31 个。对所有出入境的发热病人进行检查，阳性者给予治疗并对出境者分发健康教育手册。

红十字会和无国界组织将参与流动人口的健康教育工作。

流动疟疾诊所和镜检站将每月追踪流动人口密集的临时居住地，检查发热病人阳性者给与治疗。

C 部分：主要部分 C–2

（应为建议的每一主要部分准备另份 C 部分页篇，即如需要时提供更多的复制件。）

建议部分　2—加强中国南方高传播地区的疟疾控制（以数码分别标记各部分：2/4）

C.1 说明：(描述建议的这一部分(例如针对疾病的干预措施)，建议所要实现的目标，受益者，执行伙伴和实施战略)。

云南和海南两省是中国疟疾流行最严重的地区，也是多重抗性恶性疟传播和扩散最严重的地区。由于对当地的主要传播媒介—大劣按蚊的控制存在困难，病人的早期诊断和及时、正规的治疗以及加强人群的自我保护意识是控制当地疟疾流行最经济、有效的途径，也是降低由流动人口输入所导致多重抗性恶性疟在当地的传播和减少多重抗性恶性疟向其他地区扩散的重要方法之一。云南和海南两省的疟疾流行地区多为少数民族居住的边境地区或山区，经济不发达，村民文化水平较低和交通不便，当地农村地区缺少镜检条件和有经验的医生，村民也缺少自我保护的意识。因此本项目的重点是通过加强对抗疟药品供应和规范使用的管理，提高村民的自我保护和全程足量服药意识，并通过加强对传染源和局部暴发流行的控制，以降低当地的疟疾发病率并限制多重抗性恶性疟在当地的传播和向其他地区的扩散。

本项目的内容包括：

1．加强对传染源的控制

改善项目地区乡村医院，诊所对疟疾的诊断设备和条件。

提高乡村医生、农场医生和个体医生对疟疾的诊治技能。

加强对抗药性恶性疟的防治

（1）加强对恶性疟抗性的检测，停止使用已有明显抗性的抗疟药。

（2）制订抗疟药使用原则和用药方案，按标准剂量和方案治疗病人。

（3）加强对抗疟药品供应和规范使用的管理和监督。

（4）推广以青蒿素类衍生物为主和其他抗疟药的联合用药

（5）加强健康教育和培训，提高乡村医生、农场医生和个体医生的职业道德和疟疾诊治技能，以及提高村民接受诊治的依从性和全程足量服药的自觉性。(见健康教育一章)

2．加强人群的自我保护：

（1）推广杀虫剂浸泡蚊帐的使用，并向无蚊帐者提供蚊帐

（2）对当地居民和小学生进行疟疾防治知识的健康教育（见健康教育）。

3．加强对局部暴发流行的控制

（1）通过措施 1-（1）提高及时发现小暴发点的能力。(见疫情监测一章)

（2）对发现的小暴发点及时采取紧急的传染源和媒介控制措施。

项目的实施和管理：

1．卫生部疾病控制司负责项目的督导和协调工作。

2．中国疾病预防控制中心寄生虫病预防控制所和云南省寄生虫病防治所和海南省热带病防治研究所负责项目的技术督导。

3. 两省卫生厅和疟疾防治机构负责项目的组织实施，蚊帐采购和对抗疟药供应和规范使用的监督和管理。

4．当地的疾病防治机构和预防医学会等共同负责对乡村医生、农场医生和个体医生进行疟疾诊治技术培训。

5．无国界卫生组织将参与对边远农村地区村医的技术培训并参与对当地村民的健康教育和提供医疗服务。

受益人群

项目覆盖地区 36 个县，包括云南省中老边境地区 2 个县 3 892 947 人，中缅边境地区 17 个县 1 572 087 人，中越边境地区 6 个县，和海南省山区 10 个县 3 500 000 人，共 9 000 000 人将成为项目的直接受益人群，云南和海南两省与项目覆盖地区相毗邻的 3200 万受威胁人群也将从中受益。

C.2 目标和指标(提供有关这一部分的目标信息。)

主要目标(说明结束时预计的情况)

项目地区的疟疾发病率下降 50%，限制云南省多重抗药性恶性疟的传播和扩散，阻断海南省多重抗药性恶性疟的传播。

具体目标:(与指标有关,包括基线数据,目前形势和全年指标)(指南第 34-37 段)

1. 通过加强项目地区乡村医院、诊所对疟疾的诊断条件和提高乡村医生、农场医生和个体医生对疟疾的治疗水平,以降低项目地区的疟疾发病率和死亡率。
2. 通过加强对抗疟药品销售和规范使用的管理和在多重抗药性恶性疟流行地区推广以青蒿素为主的联合用药,以减缓 恶性疟原虫抗药性的发展。
3. 通过健康教育提高乡村医生的职业道德,人群的自我保护意识和村民接受规范诊治的依从性和自觉性,并提供必要的帮助,以减少当地疟疾特别是多重抗药性恶性疟的传播和扩散。
4. 通过及时发现小暴发点并采取有效的控制措施,以减少当地的暴发流行。

指标	基线	目标				
	2001	2002	2003	2004	2005	2006
血检率(%)	60	65	70	75	85	90
正规治疗率(%)	35	50	60	65	70	80
蚊帐使用率(%)	40	45	55	65	70	80
浸帐率(%)	20	50	65	75	80	85

C.3 规划监测和评价计划:(继本部分之后的关于检查和评价程序概况)(指南第 34-37 段)

验证指标	验证方法	评价者
拥有镜检站的乡的比例(%)	检查工作记录	督导组
得到培训的乡村医生的比例(%)	检查培训报告	督导组
正规治疗病人比例(%)	检查工作记录	督导组
蚊帐保护率(人 / 帐)	现场调查	督导组
杀虫剂浸帐率(%)	现场调查	督导组
疟疾发病率(%)	疫情报告和现场调查	督导组
抗性恶性疟比例(%)	疫情报告	督导组
疟疾死亡病例数	疫情报告	督导组
中小学生的疟防知识知晓率(%)	同健康教育部分	同健康教育部分

C.4 时期：(估计期限)

开始和结束日期：

自：2002 年 3 月　　　　至：2006 年 12 月

这项资助要求所覆盖的时期：

自：2002 年　　　　至：2006 年

C.5 实施计划，包括向合作伙伴的资源分配(指南第 40 段)

(美元)

	预算类目 (请根据你的计划填写)							
实施合作伙伴	人力资源	后勤和供应	培训和指导	扩大的服务范围	商品或产品 *	数据和信息系统	其他 (解释)	总计
政府	0	1 360 80	680 40	362 88	1 678 32	453 60		453 600
民间社会 **	0	237 600	118 800	63 360	293 040	79 200		792 000
私立部门	0	118 800	59 900	61 680	146 520	39 600		396 000
援助方	0	172 800	86 400	46 080	213 120	56 000		574 400
其他	0	151 200	75 600	40 320	186 480	50 400		504 000
总计	0	680 400	340 700	211 440	839 160	225 200		2 720 000
* 包括药物								

** 包括防治机构，预防医学会和无国界卫生组织

1. 由卫生部疾病控制司和中国疾病预防控制中心共同负责制订适合不同抗性地区的抗疟药品使用原则和联合用药方案。

2. 由两省卫生厅和疟疾防治机构负责对抗疟药品的供应和规范使用进行监督和管理。

3．由当地卫生行政机构负责在项目实施地区的每个乡镇医院建立镜检站，由当地疟疾防治机构负责为乡村诊所提供必要的镜检设备或快速诊断试纸条以及向无

蚊帐者提供蚊帐并在项目地区推广杀虫剂浸泡蚊帐的使用。

4．由当地疟疾防治机构和预防医学会共同参与对乡村医生、农场医生和个体医生进行卫生法律，法规教育和疟疾诊治技能培训。无国界卫生组织参与对乡村医生的培训并指导对病人的合理、正规的治疗。

5．由当地疟疾防治机构，预防医学会和无国界卫生组织共同与参对当地居民疟疾防治知识的健康教育，由当地疟疾防治机构和教育部门共同参与对当地小学生进行疟疾防治知识的健康教育（见健康教育一章）。

6．由当地防治机构对发现的小暴发点及时采取控制措施进行流行病学调查，查清暴发流行范围、主要传播媒介、疟原虫种类；选择适合的抗疟药进行传染源控制并采用杀虫剂进行媒介控制。

C 部分：主要部分 C–3

（应为建议的每一主要部分准备另份 C 部分页篇，即如需要时提供更多的复制件。）

建议部分 –3— 健康教育与健康促进（以数码分别标识各部分：3 / 4）

C.1 说明:(描述建议的这一部分(例如针对疾病的干预措施),建议所要实现的目标,受益者,执行伙伴和实施战略)。

理由

云南边境地区和海南山区大多为少数民族聚居地，经济状况比较落后，居民的文化程度较低，健康保护意识较差。为最严重的疟疾流行区和多重抗性恶性疟传播和扩散地区。

有效的疟防措施较为欠缺，尤其是用于健康教育的投入极为有限，居民缺乏疟疾防护知识，乡村医生和个体医生缺乏疟疾防治技术，对疟疾的正确诊断和正规治疗水平有待提高。因此，疟防工作存在较大困难。

目的

1．通过加强健康教育提高边境居民的健康保护意识和服药的依从性。

2．通过加强不同层次的管理和技术人员的培训,提高各级疟防人员的疟疾诊断和治疗能力,尤其是乡村医生和个体医生。

3．通过健康教育提高中小学生对疟疾防治知识的知晓率。

受益者

本项目的覆盖范围包括云南省 26 个边境县和海南省 10 个有恶性疟流行的山区县，覆盖人口约分别为 5 800 000 和 3 500 000，因此总共约 9 300 000 居民将接受健康教育，约 3 600 名乡村医生和个体医生将接受疟疾防治知识的培训；项目区所有的中小学生将接受疟疾防治知识教育，其中海南有中小学校 1180 所，学生 60.22 万，云南有中小学校 1300 所，学生 73 万。

执行伙伴

为了达到预期目的，争取多方参与，以下几个部门各司其职，相互配合：

卫生部负责项目的管理和协调。

省的省级卫生部门组织各省的项目实施。

中国疾病预防控制中心寄生虫病预防控制所和有关健康教育机构负责技术指导、健康教育材料的设计、培训教材编写等。

非政府组织积极参与项目的实施，主要对乡村医生和个体医生的培训提供帮助及部分健康教育活动。

教育部门在中小学生健康教育课程中增加疟疾防治知识的内容，与卫生部门共同编写有关教材。

策略和措施

在项目区以多种形式对居民开展健康教育

内容：

疟疾的危害和预防

治疗的常识和非足量全程服药的危害

提供方便易懂易服包装的药物

方式：

医生与病人交流

当地卫生宣传员与居民交流

广播电视媒体

居民易懂的宣传画

在中小学校对学生开展健康教育

对乡村医生和个体医生进行培训，并开展卫生法律法规和职业道德教育。

C.2 目标和指标(提供有关这一部分的目标信息。)

主要目标(说明结束时预计的情况)

通过加强健康教育提高边境居民的自我保护意识和水平；重点加强乡村和个体医生的技术培训，职业道德和法律法规教育和中小学生的疟防知识教育，以降低疟疾的传播。

具体目标:(与指标有关,包括基线数据,目前形势和全年指标)(指南第 34-37 段)

1. 项目地区的乡村医生和个体医生将得到培训并通过考核，掌握疟疾诊断和治疗的基本知识，提高职业道德和法律法规意识；

2. 项目地区 90% 以上的成年居民将了解疟疾防治的基本知识；

3. 所有家庭将收到有关疟疾预防和诊治的小册子；

4. 项目地区的中小学生掌握基本的疟防知识。

指标	基线	目标				
	2001*	2002	2003	2004	2005	2006
接受培训的乡村医生的比例(%)		70	80	90	95	>95
乡村医生正确诊治疟疾病人的比例(%)	70	75	80	85	90	90
收到健康宣教材料的家庭的比例(%)		80	85	90	95	>95
居民疟防知识知晓比例(%)	20	50	70	90	>90	>90
中小学生疟防知识的知晓率		50	70	90	95	>95
蚊帐使用率(%)	40	50	60	65	75	80
医生正规处方率(%)	40	60	65	70	75	80

* 为估计数

C.3 规划监测和评价计划：(继本部分之后的关于检查和评价程序概况) (指南第 34-37 段)

1. 掌握基线：在项目的初始年(2002 年)，每个县选择 1 个村和 1 所学校进行自我保护意识和疟防知识水平的问卷调查。
2. 项目期间每年年底进行 1 次问卷调查以了解和评价项目实施的进展情况和健康教育和人员培训的效果。
3. 在项目的最后一年(2006 年)，根据目标和指标以及每年度的进展对整个健康教育和培训项目进行终末评价。
成立专门的督导小组，由卫生部门和卫生无国界组织成员组成，负责检查和考核乡村医生和个体医生接受培训的效果，通过问卷调查和考核等形式检查乡村医生和个体医生对疟疾诊断和治疗的正确率。
成立 1 个专门的考查小组，由卫生部门和卫生无国界组织成员组成，负责对居民和中小学生掌握疟疾知识和健康防护意识的评价。
每年度各校对中小学生疟疾防治知识的知晓率进行抽查，考核效果。

监督和评价活动	2002	2003	2004	2005	2006
基线调查	每个县选 1 个村和 1 所学校，共 36 个县				
年度评价	36 个项目县，每县选 1 个村对乡村医生和个体医生进行培训后问卷调查； 对当地居民和流动人口进行问卷调查； 对中小学生疟疾防治知识的知晓率进行考核。	同 2002 年	同 2002 年	同 2002 年	同 2002 年
终末评价					36 个县，每县选 1 个村对乡村医生和个体医生进行培训后问卷调查； 对当地居民和流动人口进行问卷调查； 汇总和分析年度评价的结果对中小学生疟疾防治知识的知晓率进行考核。

C.4 时期：(估计期限)

开始和结束日期：

自：　2002 年　　　　至：　2006 年

这项资助要求所覆盖的时期：
自：2002 年　　　　至：　2006 年

C.5 实施计划，包括向合作伙伴的资源分配（指南第 40 段）

（美元）

实施合作伙伴	人力资源	后勤和供应	培训和指导	扩大的服务范围	商品或产品 *	数据和信息系统	其他（解释）	总计
	预算类目（请根据你的计划填写）							
政府	30 000	30 000	250 000	50 000	40 000	100 000		500 000
民间社会 **	15 000	25 000	50 000	50 000	35 000	25 000		200 000
私立部门	10 000	15 000	75 000	40 000	30 000	30 000		200 000
援助方	5 000	5 000	15 000	15 000	5 000	5 000		50 000
其他	10 000	5 000	25 000	2 500	2 500	5 000		50 000
总计	70 000	80 000	415 000	157 500	112 500	165 000		1 000 000
* 包括药物								

** 包括防治机构、预防医学会、无国界卫生组织和红十字会

1. 健康教育

由健康教育和疟疾防治机构准备各种宣传材料，培训健康教育工作人员；

由政府部门指定或组织选拔并培训专职或兼职健康教育人员（省级：每省 4 名；县级：每县 5 名；乡级：每乡 10 名；村级：每村 1—2 名），负责当地居民的健康教育工作；

非政府组织，如卫生无国界组织、预防医学会和红十字会参与部分健康教育活动；

在项目区中小学每学年上 1—2 次疟疾防治疟疾健康教育活动，课时安排在流行高峰季节前的 4、5 月份，由教育部门安排执行；

充分利用各种宣传媒体和材料，对不同人群进行不同层次的健康教育，提高居民的疟防知识，增强他们的参与意识，改善其服药依从性。

2. 培训

疟疾防治部门负责对乡村医生和个体医生的培训，非政府组织，预防医学会、无国界卫生组织和红十字会培训部分乡村医生和个体医生并提供部分健康教育的宣传材料；

在项目地区将进行 4 个层次的培训，主要培训对象为：乡村医生、个体医生、专业人员、卫生管理人员等，重点为乡村医生和个体医生的培训。

省级专业培训：每省 5 名专业人员进行为期 2 个月的培训，学习疟疾控制和管理技术。10 名专业人员将参加卫生部英语培训中心的学习，为期 1 年。10 名专业人员参加为期 3 个月的电脑培训；

区与县级专业人员培训：共约 100 名专业人员接受为期 2 个月的专业培训，培训内容为：疟疾控制和管理、计算机应用技术、健康教育、显微镜诊断、Dipstick 快速诊断技术、浸泡蚊帐技术等。

乡级工作人员培训：共约 400 名乡级工作人员接受 1 个月的技术培训，内容为：疟疾防治的基本知识和技能、显微镜诊断技术、Dipstick 快速诊断技术、蚊帐浸泡技术、健康教育知识等；

乡村医生和个体医生培训：每年约 3600 名乡村医生和个体医生将接受疟防基本知识和健康教育知识的培训，培训期为 10 天，个体医生和乡村医生将了解和掌握疟疾报告、疟疾诊断技术、疟疾正规治疗方案以及抗疟药使用和配伍，同时进行职业道德、卫生法律、法规教育。

学校教师的培训：对项目地区中小学校医和讲授生理卫生的教师进行培训。

培训活动的安排如下：

1）2002—2003 年举办 2 期由 50 人参加的管理培训班；

2）2003—2006 年，每年每县举办 2 期 50 名学员的疟疾诊断和正规治疗学习班；

3）2003—2004 年，举办 1 期 30 名学员的网络技术培训班；

4）2002—2003 年，举办 1 期健康教育和卫生经济学习班。

C 部分：主要部分 C-4

（应为建议的每一主要部分准备另份 C 部分页篇，即如需要时提供更多的复制件。）

建议部分 4——建立南方边境区域哨点监测和疟疾联防信息网络（以数码分别标识各部分：4/4）

C.1 说明：(描述建议的这一部分(例如针对疾病的干预措施)，建议所要实现的目标，受益者，执行伙伴和实施战略)。

疫情漏报是目前中国疟疾流行区存在的一个严重问题。疫情漏报导致传染源的积累不仅是中国南方疟疾高传播地区出现疟疾暴发流行的最主要原因之一，也是多重抗药性恶性疟在当地迅速传播的重要因素。不适当用药和不全程用药也是当地多重抗药性恶性疟不断扩散的重要因素之一。根据 2000 年在云南和海南两省进行的疟疾疫情漏报调查，两省实际疟疾病例数应在 210 000 例以上，是疫情报告数的 18—25 倍。恶性疟的比例在 30%-90% 之间。已发现云南省 90% 以上的恶性疟对氯喹已有抗性，对哌喹的抗性已超过 60%，对其他抗疟药如法西达、氨酚喹等的抗性也在逐年升高。

因此，本项目通过建立哨点监测，改进疫情报告和建立疟疾疫情信息网，加强该地区的疟疾疫情和对恶性疟原虫抗药性的监测，以减少当地疟疾暴发流行，降低多重抗药性恶性疟的传播和扩散。

该项目的覆盖范围包括云南和海南两省 36 个县 930 万人口。项目覆盖范围内的 930 万人口将成为项目的直接受益者。

项目实施主要包括：

1．在项目覆盖各县建立监测点，在流行季节进行传染源的被动和主动侦查；

2．每个省在项目覆盖范围中选择 2-3 个点作为抗性监测点，进行疟原虫对抗疟药的抗性监测；

3．在项目覆盖县各乡镇卫生院，村医以及个体医生进行技术培训和法律教育，改进疫情报告的质量

4．在项目覆盖各县建立疫情信息站，每个省建立 1 个疫情信息中心，加强对疟疾疫情信息的收集及时处理；

项目实施职责和管理：

1．卫生部疾病控制司负责项目的督导和协调工作。

2．中国疾病预防控制中心寄生虫病预防控制所负责项目的技术督导。

3．云南省寄生虫病防治所和海南省热带病防治研究所负责项目 1、2、4 的实施。

4．当地的疾病防治机构和预防医学会等共同负责对乡镇卫生院、村医以及个体医生进行技术培训和法律教育。

5．由项目官员和专家组成的督导组，每季度对项目的执行情况进行检查和指导。

C.2 目标和指标(提供有关这一部分的目标信息。)

主要目标(说明结束时预计的情况)

加强项目地区疟疾疫情报告和疟原虫的抗性监测。

具体目标:(与指标有关,包括基线数据,目前形势和全年指标)(指南第 34—37 段)
建立疟疾疫情和疟原虫抗性的监测哨点,能了解疟疾疫情和疟原虫抗性的变化。
改善疫情报告系统,5 年内使项目县疫情漏报比 2000 年减少 90% 以上。
建立疟疾疫情信息网络,5 年内使项目覆盖地区能做到每月报告一次疫情,以减少当地疟疾暴发流行,降低多重抗药性恶性疟的传播和扩散。

指标	基线	目标				
	2001*	2002	2003	2004	2005	2006
监测哨点数		36	36	36	36	36
以县为单位信息网覆盖率(%)		100	100	100	100	100
漏报率(%)	>85	60	50	30	20	10
以乡为单位血检站覆盖率(%)		80	85	90	95	100
发热病人血检率(%)		60	70	80	90	90

* 为估计数

C.3 规划监测和评价计划:(继本部分之后的关于检查和评价程序概况)(指南第 34—37 段)

验证指标	验证方法	评价者
提供的仪器设备	工作记录	督导组
培训的防疫人员	工作记录	督导组
建立的血检站	工作记录	督导组
建立的监测哨点	工作记录	督导组
建立的药物抗性监测点	工作记录	督导组
发热病人血检情况	报告和督导	督导组
恶性疟对药物的敏感性	报告和督导	督导组
监测哨点资料收集	报告和督导	督导组
信息网络	报告和督导	督导组
病例报告	报告和督导	督导组

C.4 时期：(估计期限)
开始和结束日期：
自：　2002　　　　　　　　　至：2006
这项资助要求所覆盖的时期：
自：　2002　　　　　　　　　至：2006

C.5 实施计划，包括向合作伙伴的资源分配（指南第 40 段）

（美元）

预算类目（请根据你的计划填写）								
实施合作伙伴	人力资源	后勤和供应	培训和指导	扩大的服务范围	商品或产品 *	数据和信息系统	其他(解释)	总计
政府	4 250	4 582	9 166	41 660	3 500	9 166		34 832
民间社会 **	123 250	132 918	265 834	120 834	101 500	265 834		1 010 168
私立部门	8 850	9 500	0	8 650	7 250	2 400		72 550
援助方								
其他								
总计	136 350	147 000	275 000	133 650	112 250	277 400		1 117 550
* 包括药物								

** 包括防治机构、预防医学会和无国界卫生组织

在每个县随机抽取 1 个常年有疟疾流行的乡作为疟疾疫情监测哨点，由地、县专业人员收集和整理下列信息：

人口资料：包括人口数、流动人口及相关的资料。

疟疾影响因素资料：包括气温、湿度、雨量、暴露行为、主要农作物等。

疟疾流行情况：包括发热病人数、疟疾病人数和病程、主动侦察和被动侦察数等。

卫生服务资料：包括乡村医生和个体医生数，抗疟药的用量、处理的蚊帐数。

2．每个省选择 2—3 个点作为抗性监测点，采用 WHO 推荐的体外测试和体内 4 周测试法，由地、县专业人员每年监测 30—40 例病人对 6—8 种药物的敏感性，

持续5年。

3. 改善疟疾监测系统，由地、县专业人员进行培训：

（1）在每村，至少选择和培训1名乡村医生，由其负责采集和送检发热病人的血片。

（2）要求个体医生保留疟疾治疗 处方，及时报告疫情。

（3）各县疾控中心、各乡级卫生院及各个体行医诊所应填报疟疾疫情卡，县疾控中心/防疫站寄防科除督促这些部门填制疫情卡外，必须按月收集较完整的疫情数。

4. 由云南省寄生虫病防治所和海南省热带病防治研究所负责在项目各县建立疫情信息站，每个省建立1个疫情信息中心，加强对疟疾疫情信息的收集并及时进行分析处理。

附件1：辅助文件表

请注意：列入建议中的文件请标明文件号

总体文件：	附件编号
减贫战略文件（PRSP）	1
中国2001—2005年疟疾防治规划	2
疟疾具体文件：	附件编号
2000年中国疟疾形势分析	3
云南省疟疾防治“十五”规划（2001—2005）	4
海南省疟疾防治“十五‘规划（2001—2005）	5
云南省疟疾漏报调查	6
7. 海南省疟疾发病及疫情漏报情况调查	7
交叉文件/活动：	附件编号
8. 湄公河遏制疟疾项目：中国控制云南省疟疾2002—2003年实施计划	8
9. 湄公河疾病监测项目（M B D S）	9

第二节　项目标书英文版

THE GLOBAL FUND

To Fight Aids, Tuberculosis and Malaria Interim Secretariat

Geneva, 31 January 2002

GFATM/B1/6A

GUIDELINES FOR PROPOSALS

PROPOSAL FORM

Guidelines for Proposals set out detailed conditions of support and criteria for review of proposals. Reference is made in this form to relevant sections of the Guidelines.

For the use of the Global Fund Secretariat:
Date Received:
ID No:

This form is divided into 3 sections:

SECTION A seeks summary information on the overall proposal, total funding sought and information related to general eligibility criteria, including details of the Country Coordinating Mechanism;

SECTIOB B seeks further detail on the overall proposal, its objectives, how it will be monitored and demonstration of additionality;

SECTION C seeks detail, including budgetary information, separately on each component of the proposal.

For additional pages, please mark clearly whether SECTION A, B or C.

SECTION A: OVERVIEW INFORMATION

A.1. Country（or region）:

People's Republic of China

A.2. Proposal Title:

Malaria control in high transmission regions of China

A.3. **Spell out which of the three health problems or combination of them this proposal aims to address** (HIV/AIDS, TB and/or malaria) (*Guidelines para.4*):

Malaria

A.4 What are the additional outcomes expected from this proposal? (*Guidelines, para. 8 and Annex 1, II 3*).

1. Improved quality of life of local populations and the public health conditions in rural areas of the regions.

2. Improved tourism environment, enhanced economic development and reduction in poverty in rural areas in the southern part of China.

3. Enhanced infectious disease surveillance in rural areas of the border regions.

A.5. Total Amount Requested from the Global Fund:（in US$, by year）

Components (described in Section C)	Year 1	Year 2	Year 3	Year 4	Year 5	合计
	(bugdet)		(estimated)			
Component 1	470 732	392 277	313 822	235 366	156 911	1 569 108
Component 2	816 000	680 000	544 000	408 000	272 000	2 720 000
Component 3	300 000	250 000	200 000	150 000	100 000	1 000 000
Component 4	335 265	279 388	223 510	167 633	111 755	1 117 550
TOTAL (outlined in Section B)	1 921 997	1 601 665	1 281 332	960 999	640 666	6 406 658

A.6. Disease burden（Refer to official documentation or sources of epidemiological data on the prevalence and magnitude of HIV/AIDS, TB and/or malaria in the country/region/area）**or potential disease burden**（indicators such as incidence of new infections etc）（Guidelines para.6）

Although malaria has been basically controlled in most parts of China, the southern and central parts still face a serious malaria situation. Yunnan and Hainan Provinces are the two provinces with the highest malaria endemicity in China, with the sum of cases in these two provinces accounting for more than 70% of the total in the country. Based on the report of the malaria situation in China in 2000, the actual number of malaria cases in Yunnan Province and Hainan Province were estimated to be 140,000 and 70,000 cases, respectively. Of these cases, falciparum malaria accounted for 17% and 32.5%, respectively, in Yunnan and Province and Hainan Province were estimated to be 140,000 and 70,000 cases, respectively. Of these cases, falciparum malaria accounted for 17% and 32.5%, respectively, in Yunnan and Hainan. Malaria comprised 12.5% of all reported infectious disease cases（72,460）in

Yunnan Province in 2000（Roll Back Malaria Programme for Control of Malaria in Yunnan Province in China）. Most of the malaria cases occurred in the 26 counties bordering Laos, Myanmar and Vietnam, accounting for 66.8% of the cases in the whole province. In Hainan Province, the major problem is falciparum malaria in the population living in 10 mountainous counties, whose malaria cases account for 97% of the whole province. Malaria among children has been increasing as a public health problem. The serious malaria burden in the two provinces is attributed to the following:

1. **Special problems related to mobile populations:** Yunnan Province is located at the southern border of China with a total borderline of 4,061 kilometers. 26 counties in the southern and western part of the province border with Laos, Myanmar and Vietnam, where are all endemic for malaria. As a result of the greater opening up of the borders, and economic development in China, the annual mobile population reached 10 million in the border areas in recent years. Moreover, the malaria infections are not limited by the borders and are easily transmitted across the border, leading to increased transmission and prevalence of malaria on both sides of the borders. Meanwhile, because of the mobility and status of mobile populations in the borders areas, it is difficult to diagnose and treat infected people timely to control the spread of disease and to institute effective treatment measures.
   Hainan Province is one of the regions of China where the reform and opening to outside was started early and mobile populations from other part of China are estimated to be about 2 million. Besides the high prevalence level of malaria in the two provinces, they have also served as a source of spread of P. falciparum cases to other regions of China.
2. **Multi-drug resistance of P. falciparum:** Based on surveys of the sensitivity of *Plasmodium falciparum* to different anti-malarial drugs, resistance to not only chloroquine but also to piparaquine, fansidar and amodiaquine has been detected, while the sensitivity to artemisinin derivatives and pyronaridine has declined dramatically. Contributing to this is the quite widespread incorrect use and abuse of anti-malarial drugs in these provinces, which leads to drug resistance.
3. **Difficulties to control malaria vectors:** In Yunnan and Hainan provinces, the key malaria vectors are *An. minimus* and *An. dirus*, these two mosquitoes co-exist in most areas and lack of effective control strategies for these vectors in current.
4. **Poverty and malaria:** Most of the border regions of Yunnan Province and mountainous regions of Hainan Province are inhabited by minority nationalities. In these areas, the economic status is very backwards, the education background of residents is poor, and the consciousness of health protection in communities is low. This contributes to inadequate malaria control activities in these areas. Malaria not only results in disease-induced poverty, but also hinders economic development.
5. **Serious incompletness in report of malaria cases:** According to the survey on missing in report of malaria cases in Yunnan and Hainan provinces conducted in 2000, the rate of missing malaria reports was 88.8% and 94.6%, respectively. The actual malaria cases were estimated to be 18 to 25 times more than the reported number.

Potential disease burden

There are two potential dangerous malaria burdens in China owing to mobile population from Hainan and Yunnan provinces: 1) Falciparum malaria, which was once rampant in the central parts of China, has been eliminated in recent years, but potential transmission factors and malaria vectors still widely exist in these cleared areas. In recent years, all the falciparum malaria reported in other regions were the result of imported cases from these two provinces. This poses a continuing potential threat to the densely populated central part of China. 2) The importation of falciparum malaria to the central provinces can result in the spread of multi-drug resistant Plasmodium falciparum to densely populated part of China and to other countries.

A.7. Economic situation: (Refer to official indicators such as GNP per capita, HDI or other information on resource availability) (Guidelines para.6)

China is a developing country with approximately 1.3 billion population. Over 80% of the population lives in rural areas. The national level of GDP per capita was US$909 in 2000. The HDI is 0.718, ranked at 87th in the world in 2001. However, there are great economic variations in different parts of China. The economic development in the south-west and middle-west parts of the country is lower than other parts of China and the level of GDP per capita is also lower in the south-west and middle-west parts of China. Yunnan and Hainan are two of the provinces with lower economic development.

Yunnan province, with a population of 41 million, one-third of them minority nationalities, had a GDP per capita of US$488 in 2000. However, the income per capita of farmers was only US$153 (Yuan1387.25 RMB). The GDP per capita in rural areas in the border region is less than $100.(Annual report of Yunnan province in 2000).

Hainan, with a population of 7.8 millions in 2000 had a GDP per capita of US$808. The major *P. falciparum* endemic areas are in mountainous areas in middle part of Hainan province mainly among minority nationality villagers. The income per capita of the farmers in endemic areas was only US$100 (Yuan835RMB) in 2000. (Annual report of Hainan province in 2000).

A.8 Political commitment:(government contribution to the financing of the proposal <u>or</u> public spending on health <u>or</u> existence of supportive national policies or presence of a national counterpart in the proposal, or other indicator)(*Guidelines para. 6*).

1. The government of China will actively support and promote the cooperation for malaria control among target provinces and counties;
2. Once the financial support for the project is approved, the China government will offer corresponding support while all project funds will only be used for the project activities;
3. The project will be included under the China national malaria control program as an important component;
4. During the implementation of the project, the National Ministry of Health and Institute of Parasitic Diseases, Chinese Center for Disease Control and Prevention will perform the functions of organizing, coordinating, implementing, managing and supervising the project.

A.9 Links with existing activities: (What links are there between this proposal and other current activities supported, for example, through, national health strategies, Poverty Reduction Strategies and Sector-Wide Approaches? Provide copies of these as supporting documentation, noting them in Attachment 1)

1. WHO Roll Back Malaria Program

The proposed objectives of the project are consistent with the objectives of the WHO Roll Back Malaria Program, which will enhance and extend the malaria control project in southern part of China especially in Yunnan and Hainan province.

2. Mekong Basin Disease Surveillance (MBDS) Project

The malaria surveillance is one of four subprojects in Mekong Basin Disease Surveillance Project. The proposed objectives of the project will not only enhance malaria surveillance in Yunnan and Hainan province but also provide the favorable model for improving the surveillance of other infected diseases in these areas.

3. The "Tenth-five" National Program for Malaria Control in China and The "Tenth-five" Provincial Program for Diseases Control.

The two parts of malaria control and surveillance in Yunnan Province in the proposed project are considered as one of the parts of the "Tenth-five" National Program for Malaria Control in China as well as the important part of the provincial "Tenth-five" Program for Diseases Control in the two provinces.

4. Poverty Reduction Project in the west of China

Poverty Reduction Project in the west and middle of china and Development project of the west and middle of China are fulfilling currently. It provides opportunities for the west to reduce poverty of minorities with poor income caused by illness, to improve the environment of investment and promote development of local economy.

A.10 Profile of the Country Coordinating Mechanism（CCM）– If not submitted by a CCM, please move directly to A.14.（***Guidelines para. 9-14***）

Various agencies and partners (including NGOs and Research Institutions) that are supporting this proposal are co-ordinated and organised through a country coordinating mechanism which is referred to in this document as CCM.

7. Name of the CCM:

Country Coordinating Mechanism for Malaria Control

8. Date of constitution of the current CCM:

Feb. 2002

9. Organizational structure（e.g., secretariat, sub-committee, stand-alone）:

In order to meet the requirements of the Global Fund to Fight Against AIDS, TB and Malaria, the Country Coordinating Mechanism for Malaria Control was established in February 2002. Some of the international and national agencies are the members of CCM. It is responsible for coordinating the projects of the Global Fund to Fight Against Malaria nationwide. Two meetings have already been held by the CCM for discussing the proposal.

10. Frequency of meetings（e.g. monthly, quarterly）:

The CCM meetings will be held twice per year.

11. Major functions and responsibilities of the CCM:

1）To submit the proposals to the Global Fund once they are reviewed and approved by the CCM.

2）To coordinate the projects among the multi-sectors when implementing the proposal.

3）To monitor and evaluate the progress of the proposal.

6. Major strategies to enhance CCM's role and functions in the next 12 months:

1）To establish the secretariat of the CCM.

2）To strengthen the publicities of the Global Fund to increase public involvement of the Global Fund.

3）To organize CCM meetings to discuss the implementation plans.

4）To learn the internal or international best practice and solve existing problems of malaria control program.

5）To organize training programs at national and local level to improve the capabilities of the program managers and technical staff.

A.11 Please provide the total number and composition of members of CCM: Malaria

People living with HIV/TB/malaria	
NGOs/Community-based organisation	2
Private Sector	
Religious/Faith groups	
Academic/Educational Sector	
Govemment Sector	7
Other (International bilateral, multilateral agencies and NGOs)	10
TOTAL	19

A.12. Signatures:

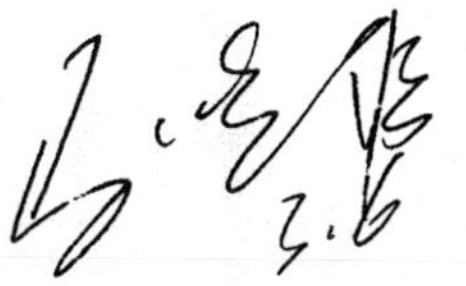

Chair of Country Coordination Mechanism: Dr. Ma Xiaowei,
Vice Minister
Ministry of Health, P. R., China
Chair Name and COntact Information: 1 Xizhimenwai South Rd
Beijing 100044, China

CCM Member Signature

Agency/Organization	Name/title	date	signature

See next page.

CCM 成员在下方签字认可这项申请，认可这项申请对伙伴机构或个人不产生任何财政（法律）承诺。

Members of CCM sign below to endorse this proposal. Endorsement of this proposal does not imply any financial (or legal) commitment on the part of partner agency or individual.

CCM Member Signature for Malaria

单位 organization	姓名 Name	职务 Title	签字 Signature	备注 Remarks
WHO	Janos Annus	Representative of WHO and Chairperson of UN Theme Group on Health	[signature]	representing **
Health Unlimited	Zhu Weixing	Regional manager for east Nsia		

**:LLO, UNAIDS, UNICEF, UNDP, UNESCO, UNFAP, WFP, World Bank, WHO

CCM 成员在下方签字认可这项申请，认可这项申请对伙伴机构或个人不产生任何财政（法律）承诺。

Member of CCM sign below to endorse this proposal. Endorsement of this proposal does not imply any financial (or legal) commitment on the part of partner agency or individul.

CCM Member Signature for Malaria 疟疾

单位 Organization	姓名 Name	职务 Title	签字 Signature
中国卫生部 Ministry of Health, P.R. China	刘培龙 Mr. Liu, Peilong	司长 Director General	[signature]

代表单位：

Representing:

外交部

Ministry of Foreign Affairs

国家计委

State Development Planning Commission

教育部

Ministry of Justice

财政部

Ministry of Finance

国家药品监督管理局

State Drug Administration

国家中医药管理局

State Administration of Chinese Traditional Medicine

共青团中央

Youth League of China

中国红十字总会

Red Cross Society of

A.13. In case the Global Fund Secretariat has queries on this submission,

please contact:

Name: Hao Yang

Title/Address: Director of Division of Endemic & Parasitic Disease Control
Department of Disease Control
MOH

Tel.No.: 86-10-68792376

Fax No.: 86-10-68792514

E-mail: haoyang@chsi3.moh.gov.cn

A.14. If submitting not under a CCM, but as an individual or a partnership of non-governmental organizations (NGOs) or from private sector, please explain clearly the circumstances, conditions and/or reasons why not applying under a CCM.

SECTION B: OVERALL PROPOSAL

B.1 Summary of overall proposal: (Synopsis of proposal, describing overall objectives, GFATM will be involved, the beneficiaries, listing the major health components and the synergies between the different components. [more detail on separate components is sought in section C]).

Although malaria has been basically controlled in most parts of China, the southern regions such as Yunnan and Hainan Provinces still face a serious malaria situation. Malaria cases in the two provinces account for more than 70% of the total in China (300,000 cases). With the changes in social and economic development, the mobile population is increasing significantly in these areas, with the potential to result in a significant increase of malaria transmission, especially the multi-drug resistant *P. falciparum,* particularly in the border region of Yunnan Province and in the mountainous areas of Hainan Province. This proposal seeks support for enhancing malaria control in high malaria transmission areas in southern parts of China, particularly in the border areas, focused on limiting the spread of multi-drug resistant malaria transmission.

In order to limit the spread of multi-drug resistant malaria transmission in the southern part of China and reduce the threat of multi-drug resistant malaria spread to the other parts of China where *P. falciparum* has been controlled, the Ministry of Health has recently adopted the "Tenth-five" year National Program for Malaria Control in China to enhance the malaria control in Yunnan and Hainan provinces. Yunnan and Hainan provincial governments also give priority to malaria control in the "Tenth-five" year Provincial Programmes for Disease Control. WHO Roll Back Malaria Program in Mekong Region has taken Yunnan and Hainan provinces as programme areas, providing limited funding. Although the national and provincial government have added the financial budget for malaria control program, it is urgently needed to get more funding to rapidly increase the malaria control program work in high transmission areas. Reduced *P. falciparum* malaria will also reduce the risk of spread of multi-drug falciparum malaria to neighboring countries, carried by mobile populations and the large numbers of tourists who visit Hainan and Yunnan provinces.

The main objectives of this proposal are: (1) malaria incidence in Yunnan Province will be decreased by 50% from year 2000 levels by the end of the project in 2006, (2) Falciparum malaria in Hainan Province will be eliminated, and (3) the spread of multi-drug resistant malaria transmission in target areas and beyond will be effectively limited through the implementation of the proposed project during 2002 to 2006.

The target areas include 26 border counties in Yunnan Province with a population of about 5.8 millions and 10 mountainous counties in Hainan Province with a population of about 3.5 millions, thus a total population 9.3 millions will directly benefit from the project. Considering the malaria transmission among 1.2 millions mobile population, about 50 millions people in the central parts of China will indirectly benefit from the project. In addition, about 20 millions people around the target areas will benefit from the project.

The proposed project includes four components:

1. Malaria management of mobile populations: Through enhancing health education for mobile populations and improving their access to diagnosis and treatment of malaria to decrease malaria incidence in mobile population; to reduce the epidemics in the border areas of Yunnan Province and

the mountainous areas of Hainan Province; especially limit the transmission and spread of multi-drug resistant falciparum malaria.

2. Strengthening malaria control in the endemic areas of southern China. To reduce malaria incidence and confine the spread of multi-drug resistant *P. falciparum* into other areas by improving the ability of rapid diagnosis and standard treatment in local village and township clinics, distributing legally and using standard treatment course, improving awareness of villager's self-protection, and strengthening case management, and controlling outbreaks.
3. Health education and health promotion: Through strengthening health education efforts for local residents and students in primary and middle schools to improve their awareness of health protection; through enhancing the training on village/private doctors to promote their capacity for correct malaria diagnosis and treatment.
4. Strengthen the malaria surveillance and information system: Improve surveillance of multi-drug resistance and establish a malaria information network and for joint malaria control in southern border regions in China to rapidly share information. To reduce the outbreaks of malaria and transmission and spread of multi-drug resistant *P. falciparum* in local areas by improving case reporting and establishing malaria information networks through establishment of malaria surveillance sentinel sites.

The proposed four components are closely related to each other to achieve the main objectives among the different target populations. In order to control malaria in target areas and to limit the spread of multi-drug resistant falciparum malaria in target areas and in the central part of China, malaria management of mobile population must be enhanced in the 26 border counties of Yunnan Province and the 10 high epidemic counties of Hainan Province. In addition, local malaria control and malaria surveillance are necessary to lessen malaria burden in local areas and to stabilize the malaria situation. Because the economic status of the target areas is low, and consciousness of protection in communities is poor, village/private doctors in these areas need training on correct diagnosis and treatment of malaria. Thus a component about health education and training is specially proposed to improve the awareness of self-protection of local residents as well as mobile population and to promote high quality malaria control of village/private doctors in target areas.

B.2 Programmatic monitoring and evaluation: *(Guidelines para. 34-37) (The proposal needs to include an outline of the monitoring and evaluation process that will be followed in relation to the overall proposal, including timelines, and baseline data, responsibility for collection, proposed/anticipated use of the information to be collected and involvement of target population with monitoring and evaluation. [Section C requests monitoring and evaluation information on major components])*

Routine supervision and evaluation of project

A Leading committee in national level will meet once a year at the beginning of the year to discuss the project progress, results, effectiveness and situation of finance, then plan the project direction, emphases and coordination with partners in all aspects.

The technical supervision committee at national level will conduct at least one supervision visit in every year. 2 or 3 member will go to field to supervise the activities implemented in the whole area.

The Project office in the local areas will have meetings once a year at the beginning of the year to discuss the project progress, result, effectiveness, problems and situation of finance in the past year, then recommend the possible solution and plan the project direction, emphases, coordination with partner in all aspect and arrange the activities of project in the year.

The Project office in the area will frame or revise the criteria for supervision and send out 2 or 3 staffs to fulfill twice a year for supervising activities implemented in the whole province and at least 2 of project counties.

The Project office will analyze the developments of the GFATM project in the project areas quarterly and submit progress reports twice a year.

SUPPORTIVE-SUPERVISION

Currently, supervision in China tends to be very authoritative, with a system of rewards and punishments. Under the project, it is intended to improve supervision activities to follow the modern method of supportive-supervision. The purpose of supportive-supervision is to ensure that the program activities are timely and appropriately carried out as planned. During the supportive-supervision process, staff will not simply criticize the implementing institutions, but work with them to solve problems. During the process, we should make our best effort to detect problems early, to look for their reasons, and to discuss them, and then help to solve the problems detected as much as possible.

The program implementation will be supervised at each level. MOH will supervise the Health Bureau of Yunnan Province (YNHB) and Hainan Province. These organizations will supervise local professional or technical institutions such as Yunnan Institute of Parasitic Diseases (YIPD). These institutions will in turn supervise county level Epidemic Prevention Stations (EPS). County levels should train and supervise township levels and village health workers (VHW). Township community hospitals are responsible for managing and supervising VHW.

1. **Supportive-supervision by GFATM** （The methods，time and places will be developed in a workplan after approval of the project by GFATM. ）

Supportive-supervision by MOH

Officials from MOH will visit the project area for supervision. Firstly, they will coordinate an Annual Working Conference on GFATM on malaria in Yunnan or Hainan Province. Then they will inspect the field to supervise the program progress.

Supportive-supervision by provinces

Yunnan Institute of Parasitic Diseases and Hainan Provincial Institute of Tropical Diseases will conduct regularly supervision twice a year to the project areas.

EVALUATION

Evaluation is the systemic collection and use of data to improve the health programmes and to guide the allocation of their resources, and to make sure the project is carried out in terms of the work plan.

1. Evaluation by GFATM (The methods, time and places will be developed in a work plan after approval by GFATM.)

2. Evaluation by MOH (The methods, time and places will be developed depending on MOH' s arrangements.)

3. Evaluation by Province or districts

Technical or professional institutions such as YIPD will send the above four supportive-supervision working groups to project counties to evaluate the program implementation, outcomes and impacts. The following framework will be used as reference in evaluation.

Reference working framework for support-supervision and evaluation

In order to improve the overall quality of programme implementation, supportive-supervision and evaluation are needed at all stages of implementation and should be planned from the outset. Therefore the following steps are used as the structure of evaluation for the programme.

In the supervision and evaluation frameworks, the column of means of verification indicates how to collect the data needed. How to do a special survey for some indicators should be designed according to epidemiology principle and methods. As for these indicators listed, they can be used selectively in different malaria areas according to different situation. Other suitable indicators will also be added when needed.

B.3. Financial management *(Guidelines para. 19-22, 38-40) (Describe arrangements in place for financial management, including suggested disbursement mechanisms and plans)*

Funding disbursement mechanisms:

In order to supervise work funded by the Global Fund to Fight Against AIDS, TB and Malaria, the National Project Coordinating Office for Malaria Control (Hereafter referred to "Project Office") will be established under the CCM. 2 financial officers will be appointed to work in the Project Office. The major tasks will be:

1. Coordination the process for developing and approving projects, including developing criteria and procedures for application and disbursement of funds to partners.
2. Technical management and supervision of project work funded.
3. financial management and supervision, including the production of financial reports, to be submitted to the Secretariat of the Global Fund through the CCM.
4. Arrangement for external audit of the project work, and of the fund disbursement process.

Funding disbursement plan and procedures:

1. The project office will develop annual workplans, which will be submitted to the CCM for approval.
2. On the basis of these annual plans, specific annual workplans will be requested from project partners. These workplans will set out measurable indicators of progress for use in monitoring. Partners' workplans will be submitted to the technical working group for review, amendment and approval.
3. Once the detailed plans of the implementing partners are approved, the project office will allocate

60% of the budget to the implementing partners. A following 30% will be provided on receipt of mid term reports. Once the projects are completed and on receipt of technical and financial reports the project office will allocate the remaining 10% of funds.

The project office will conduct the program monitoring and supervision in collaboration with the technical working group. This will include financial supervision as well as technical assistance.

5.The project office will request external auditors to conduct independent audits of project partners.

Audit:

Audit of both the project office and project partners will be conducted by the State Audit Bureau.

B.4 Statement of Budget Requirements, Financial Commitments and Unmet Needs

2002 (Guidelines para. 8, Annex1, III.2) (Demonstrate the additionality of the proposal)

(US$)

	Budget Categorires (please fill in according to plan)							
	Human Resources	Logistics & supplies	Training & Super-vision	Outreach Services	Commod-ities or products*	Data & infor-mation systems	Other (explain)	TOTAL
BUDGET QUIREMENTS	2 067 930	1 043 407	912 424	424 278	1 161 494	477 603		6 087 134
Financial commit-ments, by source								
Govern-ment	1 137 697	334 963	307 937	125 822	373 982	166 307		2 446 707
Civil Society	699 531	66 346	48 844	35 026	73 785	26 546		950 077
Private sector	105 103	74 338	63 293	36 260	75 377	30 052		384 421
Donors	64 100	36 560	30 906	15 216	44 624	13 661		205 067
Other	61 500	32 240	25 120	9 064	38 296	12 645		178 865
TOTAL OMMIT-MENTS	2 067 930	544 447	476 100	221 387	606 064	249 211		4 165 137
UNMET NEEDS	0	498 960	436 324	202 891	555 430	228 392		1 921 997

*including drugs

B.5　Duration (provide an estimate):

Beginning and end dates:

From:　2002　To:　2006

Period to be covered by this request for financing:

From:　2002　To:　2006

SECTION C--1: MAJOR COMPONENTS

(separate Section C pages should be prepared for each major component of the proposal i.e. make more copies if needed.)

PROPOSAL COMPONENT 1. Malaria control in mobile population---- (Number separate components 1 to 4)

C.1 Description: (Describe this component of the proposal (e.g. disease-specific intervention), what it seeks to accomplish, who are the beneficiaries, who will be the implementing partners and strategies for implementation).

Rationale

Yunnan and Hainan are the two most malaria endemic provinces in China. The international borderline in Yunnan province is 4100 km long, with 62 official border crossing points but people usually do not cross at the official border points, cross small streams, or cross roads to visit China and return home. Both sides of the border are high malaria endemic areas and are the top multi-drug resistant malaria region in South-east Asia and in the world. There are an estimated 10 million international trips each year in Yunnan. Yunnan and Hainan are the only current falciparum malaria endemic provinces in China. The Mobile population also is moving to Hainan Province because of the availability of jobs with economic development, putting them at high risk for malaria infection. These mobile populations may not have been previously exposed to malaria so they not only have higher rates of malaria, but also serve as a transmission source to spread malaria, especially multi-drug resistant malaria, to other provinces. The rate of multi-drug resistance is worsening due to the increasing mobile population and difficulties of implementing malaria control among this population group. Key issues related to this population are the high infection rate, lack of access to examination facilities and poor knowledge of malaria and malaria protection among the mobile populations.

The project in this component will focus on decreasing malaria incidence in mobile population and reducing their role as a malaria transmission source for exporting malaria to other areas.

Beneficiaries population

10 millions mobile population along the border areas;

9.3 millions local villagers in target areas;

20 millions residents living in the areas near the target areas;

50 millions residents living in the middle part of China where P. falciparum transmission has been controlled.

Strategies and Activities

The professional institutions will set up microscope examination stations (MES) supplied with necessary facilities and qualified professional staff in the hospitals and clinics near frontier station and the following work will be carried out:

Mobile population with fever will be got early diagnosis and immediate treatment at the clinics;To deliver health education materials to mobile population when cross the international line and to carry out health education for mobile population.

The professional institutions at different levels will supply early diagnosis by microscopy or rapid diagnosis test, fever cases in mobile population in local areas in the programmed regions will be examined and the positive will be given standard treatment to prevent exporting malaria patients and carriers, especially multi-drug resistance malaria.

Professional institutions will set up mobile clinics with microscope to follow up temporal residences where there is dense mobile population.

Chinese Association of Preventive Medicine, Red Cross and Health Unlimited will help train the doctors and microscope examination staffs who work at the hospitals and clinics near frontier station.

C.2 Objectives and indicators (Provide information on objectives for this component.)

Main objective (Describe the expected end situation)

To decrease malaria incidence in mobile population and reduce malaria endemic in target areas especially to limit multi-drug resistant P falciparum spread to other areas.

Specific objectives: (Related to indicators, including baseline data, current situation and annual targets) (Guidelines para. 34-37)

1. To improve the accessibility of diagnosis and prompt treatment of malaria in mobile population;
2. To raise the self-protection and increase the awareness of malaria in mobile population.

Indicator	Baseline	Targets				
	2001*	2002	2003	2004	2005	2006
% of frontiers with MES		50	100	100	100	100
Blood examination rate of fever cases among mobile population (%)		50	60	60	70	80
Percentage of mobile population receiving health education (%)		50	60	70	80	90
Percentage of prompt regular treatment of malaria cases among mobile population (%)	30	40	45	55	65	80

* Baseline data are estimated

C 3. Programmatic monitoring and evaluation plans: (An outline of the monitoring and evaluation process that will be followed for this component.)

A supervision group consisting of members of health sector Red Cross and Health Unlimited will supervise the implementation and evaluate the progress every year.

Monitoring and evaluation indicator	Means of verification	Evaluators
Distribution of RDT assays or microscopy in public and private health facilities	Work records	Supervisor
Distribution of IEC materials	Work records	Supervisor
The percentage of malaria cases early diagnosed and prompt treated	Work records	Supervisor
Training course holding for village doctor and private sector	Report	Supervisor
Awareness of malaria increased in mobile population	Special investigation	Professionals

C 4. Duration: (provide an estimate)

Beginning and end dates:

From:……………2002…………….To:………2006………

Period to be covered by this request for financing:

From:……………2002…………….To:………2006………

C. 5 Implementation plans including resource allocations to partners (Guidelines para. 40)

(US$)

	Budget Categories (please fill in according to plan)							
Implementation	Human Resources	logistics and supplies	Training & Supervision	Outreach Services	Commodities or Products*	Data & information systems	Other (explain)	TOTAL
Government	329 513	215 752	275 378	109 838	54 919	28 244	0	1 013 644
Civil Society**	23 537	58 842	33 893	15 691	7 846	4 707	0	144 515
Private sector	117 683	117 683	63 549	31 382	15 691	9 415	0	355 403
Donors	0	0	50 839	0	0	941	0	51 781
Other	0	0	0	0	0	3 766	0	3 766
TOTAL	470 732	392 277	423 659	156 911	78 455	47 073	0	1 569 108
*Including drugs								

**including professional institutions, Chinese Association of Preventive Medicine, Red Cross and Health Unlimited

At the beginning, a baseline survey will be carried out to get baseline information on awareness of malaria and consciousness of self-protection and positive rate of malaria in mobile population by local professional institutions.

Technical institutions are in charge of training qualified professional staff for MES, Chinese Association of Preventive Medicine, Red Cross and Health Unlimited will join the training. Totally 130 persons will be trained.

MES will be set up around each frontier stations and supply with necessary facilities and qualified professional staff by professional institutions gradually, in first year at least 31 will be set up. All fever cases in mobile population will be examined for malaria and the positive will be treated and the manual of malaria will be delivered at nearest clinics.

Red Cross and Health Unlimited will take part in part of health education works to mobile populations.

The mobile MES will follow up temporal residences with dense mobile population and examine the febrile monthly.

SECTION C-2: MAJOR COMPONENTS

(separate Section C pages should be prepared for each major component of the proposal i.e. make more copies if needed.)

PROPOSAL COMPONENT 2—Strengthening malaria control in endemic areas of southern China

C.1 **Description:** (Describe this component of the proposal (e.g. disease-specific intervention), what it seeks to accomplish, who are the beneficiaries, who will be the implementing partners and strategies for implementation).

Rationales

Yunnan and Hianan provinces are the top two provinces with serious malaria endemicity in China. Since the difficulty of controlling *An.dirus* faced in the control of malaria, early diagnosis, prompt treatment of malaria patients and strengthening self-protection in the population are the most cost effective way to control malaria in local area. They are the important ways to reduce transmission of multi-drug resistant *P. falciparum* imported by mobile population in local areas and confine the spread of multi-drug resistant *P. falciparum* into other areas by mobile population. Yunnan and Hainan province are mountainous and border areas with less developed economy and poor transportation. The populations are minority nationalities with low education, lack of microscopy and experienced professionals and poor awareness of self-protection. Therefore, the key point of this project is to reduce malaria incidence and confine the spread of multi-drug resistant *P. falciparum* into other areas by distributing legally and using standard treatment course, improving awareness of villager's self-protection, and strengthening case management, and controlling outbreaks.

Control strategies

1. Control of infectious resources

1) To improve the capacity of rapid diagnosis in township hospital and village doctor in project areas.

2) To improve prompt treatment of malaria cases provided by doctors from village, plantation and private section.

2. Prevention and control of drug-resistant falciparum malaria

1) To strengthen surveillance of *Plasmodium falciparum* sensitivity and to stop using drugs with obvious resistance.

To formulate anti-malarial policy and standard regiments, to treat malaria patients by using the standards.

To strengthen anti-malarial supply and management to make sure the standard use.

To recommend the combinations of anti-malarial drugs, especially including artemisinin derivatives.

To promote knowledge and skills of health workers and doctors in villages, state farms and private sectors in malaria diagnosis, treatment, medical ethics and attitudes to patients by intensive training.

To promote the compliance of patients to the standard regiments by health education.

3. Strengthen self-protection of population.
1) To popularized bednet treated by insecticides and provide bednet to the poor without it.
2) To provide health education for local residents and students (detailed in Health education section).
4.Strengthen controlling outbreak
1) To improve the ability of detection of outbreak spot by strengthening the capacity of rapid diagnosis.
2) To response quickly and control any malaria outbreak spots.

Implementation partners

Division of Endemic and Parasitic Diseases, Department of Diseases control, MOH will be responsible for supervision and coordination;

Institute of Parasitic Diseases, Chinese Center for Disease Prevention and Control, Yunnan Institute of Parasitic Diseases and Hainan Provincial Institute of Tropical Diseases will be responsible for supervision in techniques.

Health Bureaus of the two provinces and anti-malarial institutions will be responsible for the program organization and implementation, bednet order and distribution, anti-malarial supply, use, management and supervision.

Local anti-malarial agencies will be responsible for training village health workers, doctors in plantations and private sectors in malaria diagnosis and treatment.

Health unlimited will be in charge of professional training rural village doctors and providing health education to villagers in remote areas.

Population covered by project

The target population will be over 9,000,000 in high endemic areas in Yunnan and Hainan provinces including 2 Sino-Laos counties, with the population of 3,892,947; 17 Sino-Maynmer border counties with the population of 1,572,087; 6 Sino-Vietnam border counties in Yunnan and 10 counties with 3.5 million in mountain areas in Hainan. 32 millions living adjacent will benefit from the project too.

C.2 Objectives and indicators (Provide information on objectives for this component.)

Main objective (Describe the expected end situation)

To reduce malaria incidence in the target population by 50%, confine transmission and spread of multi-drug resistant falciparum malaria and stop transmission of of multi-drug resistant *P. falciparum* in Hainan.

Specific objectives: (Related to indicators, including baseline data, current situation and annual targets) (Guidelines para. 34-37)

To reduce malaria morbidity and mortality in project areas by improving rapid and correct diagnosis of patients and prompt treatment.

To delay the resistance development of Plasmodium falciparum by strengthening anti-malarial drugs supply and use management, and recommending the combinations of mainly including artemisinin derivatives in multi-resistant falciparum malaria endemics.

3 To reduce the spread of multi-drug resistant falciparum malaria by increasing awareness of villager' s self-protection and patients' compliance to the standard regiments by health education together with necessary help.

4 To reduce outbreaks of malaria by conducting activities to detect outbreak spot in small scope.

INDICATOR	Baseline	Targets				
	2001	2002	2003	2004	2005	2006
Blood examination rate (BER) (%)	60	65	70	75	85	90
% of standard treatment	35	50	60	65	70	80
Rate of bednet usage (%)	40	45	55	65	70	80
Ratio of ITNs (%)	20	50	65	75	80	85

C.3 Programmatic monitoring and evaluation plans: (An outline of the monitoring and evaluation process that will be followed for this component.) (Guidelines para. 34-37)

Verifiable indicators	Means of verification	Evaluators
% of township with BES	Work records	Supervising groups
% of village doctors trained	Work records	Supervising groups
% of patients treated regularly	Work records	Supervising groups
No of persons per bednet	Survey	Supervising groups
% of ITNs	Survey	Supervising groups
Malaria morbidity	Survey	Supervising groups
% of resistant falciparum malaria to drugs	Report and survey	Supervising groups
No. of death due to malaria	Report	Supervising groups
% of students with malaria knowledge in primary and middle school	Same as education section	Same as education section

C.4 Duration: (provide an estimate)

Beginning and end dates:

From: June, 2002 To: December,

2006

Period to be covered by this request for financing:

From:June, 2002 To: December, 2006

C.5 Implementation Plans including resource allocations to partners (*Guidelines para. 40*)
* including drugs

	Budget Categories (please fill in according to your plan) (US$)							
Implementing Partner	Human Resources	Logistics and supplies	Training & Supervision	Outreach Services	Commodities or Products*	Data & information systems	Other (explain)	TOTAL
Government	0	1 360 80	680 40	362 88	1 678 32	453 60		453 600
Civil Society**	0	237 600	118 800	63 360	293 040	79 200		792 000
Private sector	0	118 800	59 900	61 680	146 520	39 600		396 000
Donors	0	172 800	86 400	46 080	213 120	56 000		574 400
Other	0	151 200	75 600	40 320	186 480	50 400		504 000
TOTAL	0	680 400	340 700	211 440	839 160	225 200		2 720 000

**including professional institutions, Chinese Association of Preventive Medicine and NGO.

1. Department of Diseases control, MOH and Institute of Parasitic Diseases, Chinese Center for Disease Prevention and Control will work together to formulate anti-malarial policy and combined regiments for different endemic areas with drug-resistant levels.

2. Health Bureaus of the two provinces and anti-malarial institutions will be responsible for anti-malarial drugs supply, use management and supervision.

3. Local health administrative departments will be responsible for establishing microscopy examination stations in each township of target regions. Local anti-malarial agencies will be responsible for supplying microscopes or rapid diagnosis test (RDT), and bednets to the poor populations to popularize ITNs in target areas.

4. Local anti-malaria agencies and associations of preventive medicine will work together to train village health workers, doctors in state farms and private sectors in health regulation, technology of malaria diagnosis and treatment. Health unlimited will also be in charge of these professional training activities.

5. Local anti-malaria agencies, associations of preventive medicine and health unlimited will work together to do health education to local communities. Meanwhile health education will be carried out in primary and secondary schools by cooperation with education departments.

6. Local anti-malaria agencies will provide bed nets to the poor without it and popularize the net treated by insecticides by local professional institutes.

7. Local anti-malaria institutions are responsible for epidemiological surveys and control of outbreaks in time; detecting the scope of outbreak, major vectors and parasite species; treating and managing malaria cases and controlling the vectors with insecticides.

SECTION C-3: MAJOR COMPONENTS

(separate Section C pages should be prepared for each major component of the proposal i.e. make more copies if needed.)

PROPOSAL COMPONENT 3--- Health education and health promotion (training)

(Number separate components 3 /4)

C.1 Description: *(Describe this component of the proposal (e.g. disease-specific intervention), what it seeks to accomplish, who are the beneficiaries, who will be the implementing partners and strategies for implementation).*

Rationale

Most of the border regions of Yunnan Province and mountainous regions of Hainan Province are inhabited by minority nationalities. In these regions, economic conditions are poor, education background of residents is weak, and people's consciousness of protection is poor. They are the top malaria endemic areas and most serious regions of falciparum malaria with multi-drug resistance in China.

Effective control measures have not been fully successful, due to a lack of resources, particularly for health education. Residents are not aware of the knowledge of malaria prevention and self protection, township and village doctors do not understand basic techniques for malaria control. All of the above constraints hinder the control work. In addition, village/private doctors in these areas need to be trained on correct diagnosis and treatment of malaria.

Objectives:

1. To improve the awareness of residents' self-protection and patients' compliance with drug regiments by health education;
2. To train management and technical staff at different levels to improve their capacities on malaria diagnosis and treatment, and especially to train village/private doctors.
3. To raise the comprehension rate of students in primary and middle school on malaria, especially prevention and self-protection.

Target Population:

About 5.8 millions people in 26 border counties in Yunnan Province and about 3.5 millions people in 10 mountainous counties in Hainan Province, about 9.3 millions people will receive health education. About 3,600 village/private doctors will be trained by technique and knowledge of malarial control. All students in primary and middle schools of the programmed regions will have health education courses or activities on malaria, including 602,200 students from 1,180 schools in Hainan Province and 730,000 students from 1,300 schools in Yunnan Province.

Partners

Several partners will participate and cooperate in this project, they are:

1. Ministry of Health will be responsible for the management and coordination of the project;
2. The Health Bureaus in the two provinces will organize implementation of the project.
3. The Institutes of Parasitic Diseases, Chinese CDC and health education agencies will be responsible for guiding the training, and preparing training and health education materials;
4. NGOs will actively participate in the implementation of the project, mainly to participate in raining village/private doctors.
5. The Education sector will insert content of malaria control into the textbook on health education,

working together with health agencies to prepare the book.

Strategies and activities

1. In program regions, different kinds of health education activities will be carried out for residents;

Content:

Harm and prevention of malaria

Common sense of malaria treatment and the harm of uncompleted course of treatment

Supply of pre-packed drugs to increase compliance with drug regiments

Method:

Communication between doctors and patients

B. Communication between local health educators and residents

C. Malaria health education by broadcast network and television program

D. Delivering posters and leaflets with pictures.

2.Health education courses on malaria will be taught in primary and middle school;

3.Village and private doctors will receive training on malaria diagnosis and control techniques, and education on professional ethics, health law and regulations.

C.2 Objectives and indicators (Provide information on objectives for this component.)

Main objective (Describe the expected end situation)

To improve the awareness of self-protection and compliance with drug regiments of local residents by health education.

To train management staff and professional staff at different levels to improve their capacities on malaria, and especially to train village/private doctors.

To raise the comprehension rate of students in primary and middle school on malaria.

Specific objectives: (Related to indicators, including baseline data, current situation and annual targets) (Guidelines para. 34-37)

1. Medical workers and village/private doctors in target areas will be trained to master the diagnosis and standard treatment of malaria, professional ethics, health laws and regulations;
2. More than 90% adults should understand the basic knowledge of malaria control;
3. All families in focal villages should have books about malaria;
4. Students of primary and middle schools in the target areas will master basic malaria knowledge.

INDICATOR	Baseline	Targets				
	2001*	2002	2003	2004	2005	2006
Rate of bednet usage	40	50	60	65	75	80
Ratio of standard regiments and dosages prescribed by doctors (%)	40	60	65	70	75	80

* Baseline data are estimated.

C.3 Programmatic monitoring and evaluation plans: (An outline of the monitoring and evaluation process that will be followed for this component.) (Guidelines para. 34-37)

1) Collection of baseline data: in the beginning year of the project, select a village and 1 school in each border counties to conduct questionnaire survey for understanding the awareness of self-protection and the knowledge of malaria;
2) The evaluation of health education and training will be carried out to understand the implemental progress of project activities by questionnaire surveys in the end of each year;
3) The final evaluation of project activities will be carried out to inspect the accomplishment of various objectives and indices in terms of the each year's results of questionnaire survey in the end year of the project;
4) A monitoring and supervision group consisting of members of health sector, Red Cross and Health Unlimiteds, will be responsible of the evaluation on the improvement in diagnosis and treatment of malaria by village doctors and private doctors by questionnaire and examination;
5) An investigation group consisting of members of health sector, Red Cross and Health Unlimited, will be responsible of the questionnaire surveys to evaluate the improvement of health education in residents and students and their awareness of protection and the knowledge of malaria.

Monitoring and evaluation activities	2002	2003	2004	2005	2006
Baseline survey	1 village and 1school in each county, total 36 counties				
Annual evaluation	1 questionnaire survey to village/ private doctors in 36 counties selecting 1 village in each county; 1 questionnaire survey to residents including mobile population; To examine comprehension rate of students on malaria.	Same as the year 2002	Same as the year 2002	Same as the year 2002	Same as the year 2002.
Final evaluation					1 questionnaire survey to village/ private doctors in 36 counties selecting 1 village in each county; 1 questionnaire survey to residents including mobile population; Sum up and analysis of annual results; To examine comprehension rate of students on malaria.

C.4 Duration: (provide an estimate)

Beginning and end dates:

From: 2002 To: 2006

Period to be covered by this request for financing:

From: 2002 To: 2006

C.5 Implementation Plans including resource allocations to partners (Guidelines para. 40)

(US$)

	Budget Categories (please fill in according to your plan)							
Implementing Partner	Human Resources	Logistics and supplies	Training & Supervision	Outreach Services	Commodities or Products*	Data & information systems	Other (explain)	TOTAL
Government	30 000	30 000	250 000	50 000	40 000	100 000		500 000
Civil Society	15 000	25 000	50 000	50 000	35 000	25 000		200 000
Private sector	10 000	15 000	75 000	40 000	30 000	30 000		200 000
Donors	5 000	5 000	15 000	15 000	5 000	5 000		50 000
Other	10 000	5 000	25 000	2 500	2 500	5 000		50 000
TOTAL	70 000	80 000	415 000	157 500	112 500	165 000		1 000 000
*Including drugs								

**including professional institutions, Chinese Association of Preventive Medicine, Red Cross and Health Unlimited.

1. Health education:

Malaria control agencies will prepare for various propaganda materials and train health educators;

Chinese Association of Preventive Medicine, Red Cross and Health Unlimited will take part in part of health education;

1-2 health education courses or activities on malaria will be carried out yearly before peak endemic season in April to May in all schools in programmed regions. It will be arranged by education sector.

Full-time and/or part-time health educators (4 from each province, 5 each county, 10 each township and 1-2 each village) will be selected and receive training, they will take responsibility of health education in the area;

Fully utilize various mass media to carry out different types of health education to various population, raise the residents' knowledge level of malaria control, and enhance their consciousness of participation in malaria control measures, and improve the compliance of patients with drug administration;

2. Training:

Four-level (Provincial, District, County, Township) trainings will be carried out in the following subject: village doctors, private doctors, professionals, management staff, etc. with an emphasis in village doctors and private doctors.

Malaria control agencies will be in charge of training village and private doctors; Chinese Association of Preventive Medicine, Red Cross and Health Unlimited will train part of these doctors.

Professionals at provincial level: A total of 5 professionals each province will be trained for 2 months to learn the technology of malaria control and management. 10 professionals will be trained in the English Language Training Center of MOH for 1 year each. 10 professionals will be trained on computer science for 3 months each.

Professionals at district and county level: A total of 100 professionals will be trained for 2 months on the technology of malarial control and management, computer application, health education, microscopy diagnosis, dipstick technique, bed net emerged with insecticides.

Staff at township level: A total of 400 staff will be trained for 1 month on the following knowledge: basic knowledge and techniques on malaria control, diagnosis by microscopy or dipstick, bed net emerged with insecticides, identification of common mosquito species, and health education.

Village doctors and private doctors at township or village level: A total of 3600 doctors will be trained for 10 days each year to learn the preparation of the report on transmission situation, diagnosis techniques for malaria and standard treatment scheme as well as the basic principles of usage of anti-malaria medicine, combination and protection, and at same time, they will receive education on professional ethics, health related laws and regulations;

Training for teachers: School doctors in programmed regions will be trained, and teachers for Physical Health course trained by school doctors will be in charge of teaching students on malaria.

The schedule for training should be as follows:

1) One training course for management staff will be held during 2002-2003 with a total of 50 participants；

2) During 2003 to 2006, training courses for village and private doctors will hold annually on diagnosis techniques and routine treatment schemes, two courses will hold per year with a total of 50 participants for each, every doctors will be trained in turn；

3) During 2003 to 2004, one training course for network staff will be held with a total of 30 participants；

4) During 2002 to 2003, one training course for health education and health economics will be held.

SECTION C-4: MAJOR COMPONENTS

(separate Section C pages should be prepared for each major component of the proposal i.e. make more copies if needed.)

PROPOSAL COMPONENT 4 ---- Establishment of malaria sentinel surveillance stations and information network in southern part of China (Number separate components 4/4)

C.1 Description: (*Describe this component of the proposal (e.g. disease-specific intervention), what it seeks to accomplish, who are the beneficiaries, who will be the implementing partners and strategies for implementation*).

Incomplete reporting is a serious problem in the area of malaria surveillance in China. Accumulation of infections resulted from missing reports is not only one of the reasons for causing extended outbreaks in the areas with malaria transmission in southern China, but also an important factor for rapid spread of multi-drug resistant *P. falciparum* in this area. Inappropriate and incomplete dosages of treatment is one of the main reasons for the spread of multi-drug resistant P. falciparum. According to investigation of missing reports in Yunnan and Hainan provinces in 2000, the real number of malaria cases in the two provinces could be 210,000. It is 18-25 times the number reported. The percentage of falciparum malaria varied from 30% to 90%. It is found that 90% of cases with P. falciparum in Yunnan are resistant to chloroquine and 60% of them are resistant to piperaquine in 2000. The resistance to fansidar and amodiaquine is also rising.

Therefore, this project aims to reduce the number and intensity of outbreaks of malaria, malaria transmission and spread of multi-drug resistant P. falciparum in local areas by improving case reporting and establishing a network of malaria information from malaria surveillance sentinel sites.

9.3 million population in Yunnan and Hainan will be covered and benefit from the project.

Strategy

This component includes the following items:

To establish malaria surveillance sentinel sites to better understand the malaria situation by conducting active cases detection (ACD) and passive cases detection (PCD).

To establish sentinel sites for resistance sueveillance in the areas covered by the project (3 in Yunnan and 2 in Hainan).

To improve the quality of cases reported by providing training on cases reporting and promulgate the requirement for cases reporting according to laws in the township level and private sector.

To improve information collection, timely analysis by establishing a malaria information station in each project county and an information center in each project province.

The following agencies will be involved in the project:

Division of Endemic and Parasitic Diseases, Department of Diseases control, MOH will be responsible for supervision and coordination;

Institute of Parasitic Diseases, Chinese Center for Disease Prevention and Control will be responsible for technical supervision;

Yunnan Institute of Parasitic Diseases and Hainan Provincial Institute of Tropical Diseases will be in charge of implementation of activities items 1,2,4.

Anti-malaria professional agencies at prefecture and county levels and the Chinese Association of Preventive Medicine will be responsible for training township doctors (doctors in township hospital), village doctors and private doctors in Yunnan and Hainan province.

5) Project officers and experts from the Supervision Committee will inspect and supervise project progress quarterly.

C.2 Objectives and indicators (Provide information on objectives for this component.)

Main objective (Describe the expected end situation)

To strengthen malaria reporting information and surveillance of resistant to drugs in the project regions

Specific objectives: (Related to indicators, including baseline data, current situation and annual targets) (*Guidelines para.* 34-37)

To establish malaria surveillance sentinel sites in high epidemic areas to know malaria information and changes of resistance to drugs.

To improve malaria reporting system and reduce 90% of cases missing reported of 2000 during the following 5 years.

To reduce outbreak of malaria and transmission and spread of multi-drug resistant P. falciparum in the areas covered by project by establishing malaria information network and malaria cases reported monthly.

INDICATOR	Baseline	Targets				
	2001	2002	2003	2004	2005	2006
No. sentinel sites		36	36	36	36	36
Coverage rate of counties by network (%)		100	100	100	100	100
Missing report rate (%)	>85	60	50	30	20	10
Coverage rate of blood examination station in township (%)		80	85	90	95	100
BER (%)		60	70	80	90	90

C.3 Programmatic monitoring and evaluation plans: (An outline of the monitoring and evaluation process that will be followed for this component.) (Guidelines para. 34-37)

Verifiable indicators	Means of verification	Evaluators
Equipment supplied	Work records	Supervising and guiding groups
Trained health workers	Work records	Supervising and guiding groups
Establishment of blood examination station	Work records	Supervising and guiding groups
Establishment of sentinel sites	Work records	Supervising and guiding groups
Establishment of monitoring spots for drug resistance	Work records	Supervising and guiding groups
Examination of Blood slides of febrile	Reports and supervision	Supervising and guiding groups
Drug sensitivity to P.f.	Reports and supervision	Supervising and guiding groups
Data collection from sentinel sites	Reports and supervision	Supervising and guiding groups
Information network	Reports and supervision	Supervising and guiding groups
Case report	Reports and supervision	Supervising and guiding groups

C.4 Duration: (provide an estimate)

Beginning and end dates:

From: 2002 To: 2006

Period to be covered by this request for financing:

From: 2002 To: 2006

C.5 Implementation Plans including resource allocations to partners (*Guidelines para. 40*)

(US$)

	Budget Categories (please fill in according to your plan)							
Imple-menting Partner	Human Resources	Logistics and supplies	Training & Super-vision	Outreach Services	Commodi-ties or Products*	Data & infor-mation systems	Other (explain)	TOTAL
Government	4 250	4 582	9 166	4 166	3 500	9 166	0	34 832
Civil Society**	123 250	132 918	265 834	120 834	101 500	265 834	0	1 010 168
Private sector	8 850	9 500	0	8 650	7 250	2 400	0	72 550
Donors								
Other								
TOTAL	136 350	147 000	275 000	133 650	112 250	277 400	0	1 117 550
*Including drugs								

**including professional institutions, Chinese Association of Preventive Medicine ,Red Cross and Health Unlimited.

In each county supported by the project, 1 township will be randomly selected as surveillance sentinel from endemic townships with malaria annually reported. Staffs from prefecture and county will collect following information.

Demographic data, including population, mobile population and related information.

Effecting factors: including average temperature, humidity, rainfalls, exposure behavior, and main agricultural .

Malaria status, including number of febrile cases, number of cases and duration of illness, number of ACD and PCD.

Health service, such as number of village doctors, number of private clinics, amount of medicine used for treatment of malaria, number of treated mosquito nets.

Surveillance for resistance of antimalarials to P.falciparum. WHO-recommended *in vitro* micro test and in vivo 4-week method will be used for determining the sensitivity of 30-40 cases of falciparum malaria to 6-8 antimalarials in 2-3 monitoring spot of each province every year by staffs from prefecture and county levels. The surveillance will be continued for 5 years.

To improve malaria surveillance system and provide training on it by professionals in prefecture and county level.

In each village, at least 1 village doctor will be selected and trained to be in charge of collecting and sending blood slides of febrile cases.

Private doctors will be asked to keep the record of malaria cases and report malaria information to county CDC.

Case reporting records of malaria will be filled out by county CDC, township hospital, private section. County CDC will monitor and collect it monthly.

To set up information station in each project county and two provincial information center charged by Yunnan Institute of Parasitic Diseases and Hainan Provincial Institute of Tropic Diseases to strengthen data collection and timely analysis of malaria

Attachment: List of Supporting Documents

Please note which documents are being included with your proposal by indicating a document number

General documentation:	**Attachment #**
White Paper on Rural Poverty-relief Issued	1
National Program for Malaria Control 2001-2005	2
Malaria specific documentation:	**Attachment #**
The malaria situation in China in 2000	3
"Tenth-five" Provincial Program for Malaria Control in Yunnan Province (2001-2005)	4
" Tenth-five" Provincial Program for Malaria Control in Hainan Province (2001-2005)	5
6. Malaria Missing Report Survey in Yunnan Province in 2001	6
7. Malaria Missing Report Survey in Hainan Province in 2001	7
Crosscutting documents/activities	**Attachment #**
Roll Back Malaria Programme in Mekong River Countries	8
9. Mekong basin Disease Surveillance Project (MBDS)	9

附录

附录 1：终期总结报告附表

表 1 发热病人血检活动统计

SRs/SSRs		合计		2003		2004		2005		2006		2007		2008（5A）	
		计划开展	实际完成	计划开展	实际完成	计划开展	实际完成	计划开展	实际完成	计划开展	实际完成	计划开展	实际完成	计划开展	实际完成
云南	麻栗坡	25 260	49 858	1 500	2 997	10 000	15 174	5 420	12 869	4 360	12 965	3 700	5 237	280	616
	马关	25 480	59 245	1 500	1 373	10 000	14 317	5 420	14 829	4 360	13 105	3 700	13 464	500	2 157
	富宁	25 270	37 474	1 500	2 838	10 000	12 106	5 420	9 108	4 360	6 010	3 700	6 945	290	467
	绿春	24 040	24 264	1 500	1 194	6 000	4 683	6 450	5 528	5 650	6 560	4 200	5 155	240	1 144
	金平	27 600	88 298	1 500	3 161	10 000	22 836	6 450	20 426	5 150	21 286	3 700	20 031	800	558
	河口	31 285	38 632	1 500	2 413	7 000	5 004	8 140	14 861	7 570	7 222	6 675	7 757	400	1 375
	江城	24 040	27 566	1 500	2 784	7 000	5 782	6 450	6 324	5 150	6 058	3 700	6 218	240	400
	孟连	40 205	49 896	1 500	8 500	8 000	7 832	10 420	9 031	9 910	10 901	9 825	11 257	550	2 375
	澜沧	32 700	94 931	1 500	5 353	12 000	22 119	5 420	20 375	5 560	21 309	7 300	22 460	920	3 315
	西盟	47 465	58 546	1 500	2 367	12 500	12 742	12 410	15 985	10 380	14 205	10 025	12 576	650	671
	勐腊	45 725	59 600	1 500	3 657	11 500	10 845	11 120	10 494	10 460	14 449	10 225	17 988	920	2 167
	景洪	44 505	78 052	1 500	3 756	12 200	20 460	10 420	14 339	9 910	26 526	9 725	11 477	750	1 494
	勐海	21 660	23 748	1 500	1 341	6 000	5 782	5 420	5 680	4 760	6 952	3 800	3 813	180	180
	沧源	30 155	36 763	1 500	1 847	6 000	4 683	8 140	13 099	7 570	8 485	6 675	7 809	270	840
	福贡	20 120	18 991	1 500	4 385	5 000	1 060	5 420	2 619	4 360	6 437	3 600	4 040	240	450
	耿马	29 185	28 644	1 500	2 123	5 000	4 839	8 140	7 001	7 570	7 479	6 675	6 901	300	301
	贡山	20 370	15 780	1 500	2 810	4 000	1 270	5 800	4 796	5 050	4 090	3 900	2 646	120	168
	龙陵	29 260	62 538	1 500	7 391	10 000	13 406	6 450	17 467	5 300	15 839	5 560	7 930	450	505
	陇川	38 485	42 852	1 500	5 391	8 000	7 992	10 420	10 066	9 660	10 170	8 505	8 300	400	933
	泸水	20 310	17 178	1 500	1 584	5 000	2 447	5 420	2 620	4 360	4 871	3 600	5 298	430	358
	潞西	36 185	89 671	1 500	1 232	12 000	18 401	8 140	23 553	7 170	22 700	6 675	22 064	700	1 721
	瑞丽	45 165	62 652	1 500	9 576	10 000	9 356	12 410	14 838	10 580	12 600	10 225	13 870	450	2 412
	腾冲	47 455	58 914	1 500	3 535	11 000	10 716	12 530	14 079	10 490	19 092	11 075	8 941	860	2 551
	盈江	49 265	74 455	1 500	4 511	14 000	17 076	11 720	18 021	10 460	15 050	10 825	17 190	760	2 607
	镇康	27 510	20 119	1 500	2 191	9 000	6 600	6 450	2 252	5 850	5 093	4 410	3 573	300	410
	小计	808 700	1 218 667	37 500	88 310	221 200	257 528	200 000	290 260	176 000	299 454	162 000	252 940	12 000	30 175
海南	万宁	55 500	56 948	2 000	1 875	11 200	12 139	12 500	12 947	14 100	14 183	14 400	14 502	1 300	1 302
	陵水	46 600	46 480	2 000	2 256	10 000	10 338	11 400	10 503	11 200	11 276	11 200	11 336	800	771

续表

SRs/SSRs		合计		2003		2004		2005		2006		2007		2008（5A）	
		计划开展	实际完成	计划开展	实际完成	计划开展	实际完成	计划开展	实际完成	计划开展	实际完成	计划开展	实际完成	计划开展	实际完成
	三亚	54 400	62 775	2 000	3 811	12 500	13 512	11 900	16 129	13 500	15 105	13 100	12 743	1 400	1 475
	保亭	67 800	77 269	2 000	4 213	14 400	19 360	16 800	18 511	16 500	16 920	16 500	16 433	1 600	1 832
	乐东	87 200	94 172	2 000	4 728	14 800	22 127	21 500	17 950	23 200	23 073	23 400	23 930	2 300	2 364
	五指山	51 000	51 066	2 000	2 697	12 300	13 123	11 500	9 634	12 100	12 473	11 900	11 788	1 200	1 351
	琼中	89 200	80 942	2 000	2 868	16 200	13 853	21 900	15 378	23 300	22 837	23 500	23 692	2 300	2 314
	东方	53 700	55 040	2 000	2 153	11 200	12 442	12 400	12 414	13 500	13 506	13 400	13 351	1 200	1 174
	昌江	48 900	49 042	2 000	1 521	11 000	11 589	11 500	11 832	11 800	11 582	11 800	11 743	800	775
	白沙	79 700	81 441	2 000	3 453	15 400	17 489	18 600	17 447	20 800	21 137	20 800	19 633	2 100	2 282
	小计	634 000	655 175	20 000	29 575	129 000	145 972	150 000	142 745	160 000	162 092	160 000	159 151	15 000	15 640
河南	淮滨	50 000	58 315	10 000	12 620	10 000	13 705	10 000	10 864	10 000	10 651	10 000	10 475	0	0
	商城	0	0	0	0	0	0	0	0	0	0	0	0	0	0
	小计	50 000	58 315	10 000	12 620	10 000	13 705	10 000	10 864	10 000	10 651	10 000	10 475	0	0
湖北	枣阳	30 500	43 923	4 500	4 541	2 000	2 196	8 000	10 260	8 000	16 317	8 000	10 609	0	0
	曾都区	22 000	25 984	5 000	4 850	5 000	5 150	4 000	4 819	4 000	6 441	4 000	4 724	0	0
	小计	52 500	69 907	9 500	9 391	7 000	7 346	12 000	15 079	12 000	22 758	12 000	15 333	0	0
安徽	怀远	60 000	146 954	12 000	26 381	12 000	31 727	12 000	33 727	12 000	27 097	12 000	28 022	0	0
江苏	泗洪	37 600	42 279	4 000	4 157	6 000	6 302	9 200	9 525	9 200	9 782	9 200	12 513	0	0
	盱眙	10 400	11 211	1 000	763	1 000	852	2 800	2 702	2 800	4 240	2 800	2 654	0	0
	小计	48 000	53 490	5 000	4 920	7 000	7 154	12 000	12 227	12 000	14 022	12 000	15 167	0	0
广东	惠州市	43 000	55 675	8 000	8 760	11 000	11 650	8 000	18 984	8 000	8 514	8 000	7 767	0	0
	惠阳区	8 400	25 218	0	0	0	0	2 800	9 701	2 800	8 238	2 800	7 279	0	0
	徐闻	65 600	67 716	13 000	13 469	13 000	14 118	13 200	13 082	13 200	13 585	13 200	13 462	0	0
	小计	117 000	148 609	21 000	22 229	24 000	25 768	24 000	41 767	24 000	30 337	24 000	28 508	0	0
广西	百色	60 000	82 178	12 000	11 653	12 000	13 510	12 000	14 298	12 000	20 616	12 000	22 101	0	0
四川	筠连	40 000	33 177	0	0	4 000	2 090	12 000	6 681	12 000	12 030	12 000	12 376	0	0
贵州	榕江	59 000	63 773	11 000	2 868	12 000	18 373	12 000	12 917	12 000	17 521	12 000	12 094	0	0
总计		1 929 200	2 530 245	138 000	207 947	438 200	523 173	456 000	580 565	442 000	616 578	428 000	556 167	27 000	45 815

表 2 疟疾病人治疗活动统计

SRs/SSRs		合计		2003		2004		2005		2006		2007		2008（5A）	
		计划开展	实际完成	计划开展	实际完成	计划开展	实际完成	计划开展	实际完成	计划开展	实际完成	计划开展	实际完成	计划开展	实际完成
云南	麻栗坡	9 264	7 402	100	77	2 000	1 305	2 829	2 123	2 500	2 010	1 780	1 832	55	55
	马关	9 399	8 812	100	118	2 000	1 985	2 829	1 499	2 500	2 768	1 880	2 183	90	259
	富宁	9 259	8 076	50	48	2 000	1 330	2 829	2 086	2 500	2 501	1 780	1 947	100	164
	绿春	10 586	9 367	50	54	2 000	1 027	3 386	3 247	3 300	3 175	1 780	1 711	70	153
	金平	12 666	11 994	300	273	4 000	4 757	3 386	2 620	3 050	2 378	1 880	1 913	50	53
	河口	14 040	13 171	150	146	2 000	1 525	4 350	4 350	4 420	3 772	3 010	2 941	110	437
	江城	9 876	7 557	100	65	1 500	960	3 386	2 183	3 050	2 755	1 780	1 503	60	91
	孟连	18 859	16 527	800	1 028	2 000	825	5 589	5 069	5 820	4 534	4 480	4 670	170	401
	澜沧	11 999	11 887	150	132	2 000	1 209	2 829	3 290	3 150	3 149	3 700	3 896	170	211
	西盟	20 200	19 644	500	552	2 500	2 432	6 450	5 630	6 110	6 076	4 480	4 793	160	161
	勐腊	18 955	16 478	100	0	2 000	2 188	5 935	3 927	5 820	6 057	4 580	3 989	520	317
	景洪	17 839	16 045	100	0	2 000	1 946	5 599	3 700	5 420	5 018	4 480	4 774	240	607
	勐海	9 044	6 766	100	0	1 500	820	2 829	2 147	2 750	1 964	1 820	1 780	45	55
	沧源	13 740	20 025	50	0	2 000	936	4 350	12 942	4 220	3 347	3 010	2 563	110	237
	福贡	9 189	6 804	50	31	2 000	831	2 829	2 885	2 500	1 984	1 780	1 036	30	37
	耿马	14 590	13 974	400	434	2 500	2 010	4 350	4 465	4 220	3 977	3 010	2 977	110	111
	贡山	9 280	6 498	160	189	1 200	195	3 080	2 501	2 930	3 337	1 890	264	20	12
	龙陵	12 606	11 358	700	717	2 500	1 902	3 386	2 930	3 100	2 720	2 800	2 951	120	138
	陇川	18 559	16 487	750	777	2 500	1 657	5 569	4 642	5 620	5 609	3 960	3 642	160	160
	泸水	9 469	6 668	300	0	2 000	1 036	2 829	2 857	2 500	1 934	1 780	827	60	14
	潞西	15 520	18 635	850	5 343	3 000	2 689	4 350	4 037	4 170	3 897	3 010	2 442	140	227
	瑞丽	21 100	14 938	800	1 129	3 000	1 042	6 570	4 070	6 110	5 385	4 480	3 111	140	201
	腾冲	21 325	14 393	300	0	3 000	1 686	6 725	4 141	6 010	4 286	5 050	4 024	240	256
	盈江	21 380	20 686	850	2 435	3 500	2 315	6 230	2 470	5 870	8 576	4 710	4 670	220	220
	镇康	34 446	10 113	450	490	25 000	1 292	3 386	2 457	3 360	2 836	2 090	2 478	160	560
	小计	373 190	314 305	8 260	14 038	79 700	39 900	105 880	92 268	101 000	94 045	75 000	68 917	3 350	5 137
海南	万宁	7 300	6 865	200	152	3 800	3 264	1 020	1 140	1 490	1 481	710	747	80	81
	陵水	5 700	5 996	100	111	3 100	3 162	740	918	1 190	1 198	520	555	50	52
	三亚	9 210	7 984	1 000	267	4 400	3 859	1 330	1 369	1 640	1 613	750	777	90	99
	保亭	12 900	12 199	1 300	128	6 700	6 938	1 670	1 839	2 110	2 153	990	1 014	130	127

续表

SRs/SSRs		合计		2003		2004		2005		2006		2007		2008（5A）	
		计划开展	实际完成	计划开展	实际完成	计划开展	实际完成	计划开展	实际完成	计划开展	实际完成	计划开展	实际完成	计划开展	实际完成
	乐东	14 770	18 406	1 500	266	7 200	11 816	2 010	2 261	2 630	2 519	1 270	1 371	160	173
	五指山	7 340	7 377	800	194	3 800	3 782	830	1 368	1 280	1 325	580	654	50	54
	琼中	15 640	13 050	1 500	192	7 900	6 333	2 140	2 235	2 660	2 829	1 280	1 292	160	169
	东方	7 640	7 199	800	279	3 900	3 950	1 010	1 089	1 240	1 158	590	630	100	93
	昌江	6 390	6 653	500	273	3 300	3 490	830	1 145	1 190	1 116	520	569	50	60
	白沙	14 590	15 056	1 300	768	7 400	7 329	2 000	2 788	2 570	2 779	1 190	1 255	130	137
	小计	101 480	100 785	9 000	2 630	51 500	53 923	13 580	16 152	18 000	18 171	8 400	8 864	1 000	1 045
河南	淮滨	2 850	2 966	0	0	0	0	950	1 050	950	1 016	950	900	0	0
	商城	300	504	0	107	0	89	100	103	100	100	100	105	0	0
	小计	3 150	3 470	0	107	0	89	1 050	1 153	1 050	1 116	1 050	1 005	0	0
湖北	枣阳	13 900	20 729	2 500	2 569	6 000	5 939	1 800	3 704	1 800	5 118	1 800	3 399	0	0
	曾都区	1 600	1 678	300	368	700	710	200	200	200	200	200	200	0	0
	小计	15 500	22 407	2 800	2 937	6 700	6 649	2 000	3 904	2 000	5 318	2 000	3 599	0	0
安徽	怀远	5 000	39 358	1 000	3 344	1 000	21 465	1 000	8 820	1 000	1 709	1 000	4 020	0	0
江苏	泗洪	8 600	13 591	1 000	4 346	1 600	3 081	2 000	2 295	2 000	2 472	2 000	1 397	0	0
	盱眙	800	1 037	300	396	200	248	100	167	100	125	100	101	0	0
	小计	9 400	14 628	1 300	4 742	1 800	3 329	2 100	2 462	2 100	2 597	2 100	1 498	0	0
广东	惠州市	1 800	1 800	0	0	0	0	600	600	600	600	600	600	0	0
	惠阳区	2 400	2 415	0	0	0	0	800	810	800	805	800	800	0	0
	徐闻	3 200	3 400	500	542	500	565	500	552	900	912	800	829	0	0
	小计	7 400	7 615	500	542	500	565	1 900	1 962	2 300	2 317	2 200	2 229	0	0
广西	百色	6 000	2 208	0	0	0	578	2 000	1 630	2 000	0	2 000	0	0	0
四川	筠连	6 000	7 020	0	0	0	0	2 000	2 845	2 000	2 025	2 000	2 150	0	0
贵州	榕江	6 000	5 424	0	0	0	0	2 000	1 395	2 000	1 910	2 000	2 119	0	0
总计		533 120	517 220	22 860	28 340	141 200	126 498	133 510	132 591	133 450	129 208	97 750	94 401	4 350	6 182

表 3 杀虫剂浸泡蚊帐活动统计

SRs/SSRs		合计		2003		2004		2005		2006		2007		2008（5A）	
		计划开展	实际完成	计划开展	实际完成	计划开展	实际完成	计划开展	实际完成	计划开展	实际完成	计划开展	实际完成	计划开展	实际完成
云南	麻栗坡	8 660	7 250	1 800	0	4 900	0	860	2 892	1 100	4 358	0	0	0	0
	马关	7 160	5 559	1 800	0	3 400	0	860	413	1 100	5 146	0	0	0	0
	富宁	9 060	9 182	1 800	0	5 300	2 817	860	2 017	1 100	4 348	0	0	0	0
	绿春	9 030	10 225	1 800	0	4 900	3 554	1 030	1 263	1 300	5 408	0	0	0	0
	金平	7 530	6 966	1 800	0	3 400	0	1 030	800	1 300	6 166	0	0	0	0
	河口	9 730	6 857	1 800	0	4 900	197	1 330	0	1 700	6 560	0	0	0	0
	江城	7 530	9 384	1 800	0	3 400	300	1 030	815	1 300	8 269	0	0	0	0
	孟连	8 800	14 210	1 800	0	3 000	500	1 800	600	2 200	13 110	0	0	0	0
	澜沧	8 860	9 250	1 800	0	4 900	0	860	0	1 300	9 250	0	0	0	0
	西盟	9 400	10 305	1 800	0	3 400	200	2 000	1 000	2 200	9 105	0	0	0	0
	勐腊	11 300	10 306	1 800	0	5 400	130	1 900	1 120	2 200	9 056	0	0	0	0
	景洪	9 100	13 686	1 800	0	3 400	750	1 800	6 479	2 100	6 457	0	0	0	0
	勐海	9 260	5 739	1 800	0	5 400	0	860	0	1 200	5 739	0	0	0	0
	沧源	8 230	6 603	1 800	0	3 400	0	1 330	1 330	1 700	5 273	0	0	0	0
	福贡	7 960	5 753	1 800	0	4 200	0	860	343	1 100	5 410	0	0	0	0
	耿马	9 730	9 888	1 800	0	4 900	2 000	1 330	1 074	1 700	6 814	0	0	0	0
	贡山	7 410	3 790	1 800	0	3 400	198	910	910	1 300	2 682	0	0	0	0
	龙陵	7 580	13 290	1 800	0	3 400	0	1 080	2 489	1 300	10 801	0	0	0	0
	陇川	11 300	12 281	1 800	0	5 600	863	1 700	1 537	2 200	9 881	0	0	0	0
	泸水	9 160	5 955	1 800	0	5 400	0	860	200	1 100	5 755	0	0	0	0
	潞西	8 130	19 803	1 800	0	3 400	4 952	1 330	6 893	1 600	7 958	0	0	0	0
	瑞丽	11 400	18 586	1 800	0	5 400	5 258	2 000	5 566	2 200	7 762	0	0	0	0
	腾冲	9 650	11 594	1 800	0	3 400	0	2 250	2 315	2 200	9 279	0	0	0	0
	盈江	11 500	13 923	1 800	0	5 400	908	2 100	3 789	2 200	9 226	0	0	0	0
	镇康	7 530	10 685	1 800	0	3 400	0	1 030	0	1 300	10 685	0	0	0	0
	小计	225 000	251 070	45 000	0	107 000	22 627	33 000	43 845	40 000	184 598	0	0	0	0
海南	万宁	9 150	12 746	2 100	1 152	4 500	4 449	850	2 794	850	3 391	850	960	0	0
	陵水	8 750	7 105	2 100	425	4 000	4 000	600	627	1 450	1 432	600	621	0	0
	三亚	9 150	9 560	2 100	1 864	4 500	5 106	850	869	850	859	850	862	0	0
	保亭	10 950	11 117	2 100	1 000	6 000	6 049	1 000	1 070	950	2 101	900	897	0	0

续表

SRs/SSRs		合计		2003		2004		2005		2006		2007		2008（5A）	
		计划开展	实际完成	计划开展	实际完成	计划开展	实际完成	计划开展	实际完成	计划开展	实际完成	计划开展	实际完成	计划开展	实际完成
	保亭	10 950	11 117	2 100	1 000	6 000	6 049	1 000	1 070	950	2 101	900	897	0	0
	乐东	14 700	14 766	2 100	579	6 900	7 020	1 600	3 248	2 500	2 312	1 600	1 607	0	0
	五指山	11 050	2 877	2 100	410	6 850	0	650	746	700	759	750	962	0	0
	琼中	13 900	17 170	2 100	2 728	6 500	6 509	1 600	2 384	2 100	3 895	1 600	1 654	0	0
	东方	8 200	7 736	2 100	284	4 000	3 560	700	700	700	2 482	700	710	0	0
	昌江	8 050	9 930	2 100	1 013	4 000	4 005	650	3 549	650	705	650	658	0	0
	白沙	14 100	20 962	2 100	7 735	6 500	6 530	1 500	2 544	2 500	2 698	1 500	1 455	0	0
	小计	108 000	113 969	21 000	17 190	53 750	47 228	10 000	18 531	13 250	20 634	10 000	10 386	0	0
河南	淮滨	0	0	0	0	0	0	0	0	0	0	0	0	0	0
	商城	0	0	0	0	0	0	0	0	0	0	0	0	0	0
	小计	0	0	0	0	0	0	0	0	0	0	0	0	0	0
湖北	枣阳	0	0	0	0	0	0	0	0	0	0	0	0	0	0
	曾都区	0	0	0	0	0	0	0	0	0	0	0	0	0	0
	小计	0	0	0	0	0	0	0	0	0	0	0	0	0	0
安徽	怀远	0	0	0	0	0	0	0	0	0	0	0	0	0	0
江苏	泗洪	0	0	0	0	0	0	0	0	0	0	0	0	0	0
	盱眙	0	0	0	0	0	0	0	0	0	0	0	0	0	0
	小计	0	0	0	0	0	0	0	0	0	0	0	0	0	0
广东	惠州市	0	0	0	0	0	0	0	0	0	0	0	0	0	0
	惠阳区	0	0	0	0	0	0	0	0	0	0	0	0	0	0
	徐闻	0	0	0	0	0	0	0	0	0	0	0	0	0	0
	小计	0	0	0	0	0	0	0	0	0	0	0	0	0	0
广西	百色	0	0	0	0	0	0	0	0	0	0	0	0	0	0
四川	筠连	0	0	0	0	0	0	0	0	0	0	0	0	0	0
贵州	榕江	0	0	0	0	0	0	0	0	0	0	0	0	0	0
总计		333 000	365 039	66 000	17 190	160 750	69 855	43 000	62 376	53 250	205 232	10 000	10 386	0	0

表 4 乡村 / 个体医生和镜检员培训活动统计

SRs/SSRs		合计		2003		2004		2005		2006		2007		2008（5A）	
		计划开展	实际完成	计划开展	实际完成	计划开展	实际完成	计划开展	实际完成	计划开展	实际完成	计划开展	实际完成	计划开展	实际完成
云南	麻栗坡	292	375	110	136	40	84	40	41	62	74	40	40	0	0
	马关	532	622	160	212	240	267	40	42	52	57	40	44		
	富宁	307	372	30	75	140	147	45	45	52	55	40	50	0	0
	绿春	437	768	120	158	180	213	45	186	52	171	40	40	0	0
	金平	302	376	110	135	45	90	45	45	62	66	40	40	0	0
	河口	302	331	120	149	45	48	45	42	52	52	40	40	0	0
	江城	302	354	110	135	45	51	45	50	62	78	40	40	0	0
	孟连	243	439	60	128	40	68	40	62	63	91	40	90	0	0
	澜沧	314	487	140	225	40	50	40	60	54	95	40	57	0	0
	西盟	373	469	150	191	40	65	40	78	103	94	40	41	0	0
	勐腊	222	317	40	90	40	81	40	46	62	60	40	40	0	0
	景洪	322	398	140	157	40	49	40	40	62	62	40	90	0	0
	勐海	282	330	100	135	40	42	40	40	62	73	40	40	0	0
	沧源	532	596	110	142	290	312	40	42	52	60	40	40	0	0
	福贡	272	414	100	195	40	49	40	48	52	82	40	40	0	0
	耿马	420	497	100	140	140	145	40	59	100	113	40	40	0	0
	贡山	190	294	40	80	30	44	30	22	50	69	40	79	0	0
	龙陵	325	493	140	224	40	52	40	43	65	94	40	80	0	0
	陇川	390	457	130	190	70	74	50	51	100	102	40	40	0	0
	泸水	230	421	30	185	60	64	40	45	60	87	40	40	0	0
	潞西	252	507	60	194	45	55	45	131	62	89	40	38	0	0
	瑞丽	433	624	50	141	190	192	50	133	103	114	40	44	0	0
	腾冲	402	599	50	155	160	160	50	102	102	102	40	80	0	0
	盈江	442	852	50	359	200	257	50	71	102	116	40	49	0	0
	镇康	242	358	60	165	40	40	40	40	62	71	40	42	0	0
	小计	8 360	11 750	2 310	4 096	2 280	2 699	1 060	1 564	1 710	2 127	1 000	1 264	0	0
海南	省本级	330	427	150	188	60	65	60	111	60	63	0	0	0	0
	万宁	200	280	80	155	80	83	40	42	0	0	0	0	0	0
	陵水	200	186	80	73	80	77	40	36	0	0	0	0	0	0
	三亚	280	281	80	82	80	76	40	35	40	45	40	43	0	0

续表

SRs/SSRs		合计		2003		2004		2005		2006		2007		2008（5A）	
		计划开展	实际完成	计划开展	实际完成	计划开展	实际完成	计划开展	实际完成	计划开展	实际完成	计划开展	实际完成	计划开展	实际完成
	保亭	240	257	40	41	80	108	40	42	40	30	40	36	0	0
	乐东	200	207	40	42	40	42	40	41	40	40	40	42	0	0
	五指山	240	498	120	378	40	40	40	40	40	40	0	0	0	0
	琼中	160	160	0	0	80	80	40	40	40	40	0	0	0	0
	东方	180	197	0	0	80	100	40	40	60	57	0	0	0	0
	昌江	150	169	30	31	80	97	40	41	0	0	0	0	0	0
	白沙	320	333	120	122	80	80	40	41	40	48	40	42	0	0
	小计	2 500	2 995	740	1 112	780	848	460	509	360	363	160	163	0	0
河南	淮滨	0	0	0	0	0	0	0	0	0	0	0	0	0	0
	商城	0	0	0	0	0	0	0	0	0	0	0	0	0	0
	小计	0	0	0	0	0	0	0	0	0	0	0	0	0	0
湖北	枣阳	0	0	0	0	0	0	0	0	0	0	0	0	0	0
	曾都区	0	0	0	0	0	0	0	0	0	0	0	0	0	0
	小计	0	0	0	0	0	0	0	0	0	0	0	0	0	0
安徽	怀远	0	0	0	0	0	0	0	0	0	0	0	0	0	0
江苏	泗洪	0	0	0	0	0	0	0	0	0	0	0	0	0	0
	盱眙	0	0	0	0	0	0	0	0	0	0	0	0	0	0
	小计	0	0	0	0	0	0	0	0	0	0	0	0	0	0
广东	惠州市	0	0	0	0	0	0	0	0	0	0	0	0	0	0
	惠阳区	0	0	0	0	0	0	0	0	0	0	0	0	0	0
	徐闻	0	0	0	0	0	0	0	0	0	0	0	0	0	0
	小计	0	0	0	0	0	0	0	0	0	0	0	0	0	0
广西	百色	0	0	0	0	0	0	0	0	0	0	0	0	0	0
四川	筠连	0	0	0	0	0	0	0	0	0	0	0	0	0	0
贵州	榕江	0	0	0	0	0	0	0	0	0	0	0	0	0	0
总计		10 860	14 745	3 050	5 208	3 060	3 547	1 520	2 073	2 070	2 490	1 160	1 427	0	0

表 5 中小学生疟疾知识培训活动统计

SRs/SSRs		合计		2003		2004		2005		2006		2007		2008（5A）	
		计划开展	实际完成	计划开展	实际完成	计划开展	实际完成	计划开展	实际完成	计划开展	实际完成	计划开展	实际完成	计划开展	实际完成
云南	麻栗坡	230	287			100	140	40	55	65	67	25	25	0	0
	马关	245	407			100	140	40	40	80	81	25	146		
	富宁	230	300			100	140	40	70	65	65	25	25	0	0
	绿春	235	311			100	140	40	76	70	70	25	25	0	0
	金平	280	336			100	140	80	88	75	83	25	25	0	0
	河口	280	401			100	140	40	53	100	159	40	49	0	0
	江城	240	298			100	140	40	48	75	86	25	24	0	0
	孟连	355	610			100	140	60	66	140	156	55	248	0	0
	澜沧	270	389			100	140	40	75	80	124	50	50	0	0
	西盟	400	461			100	140	90	90	150	160	60	71	0	0
	勐腊	400	397			100	140	100	55	140	142	60	60	0	0
	景洪	385	500			100	140	80	20	140	248	65	92	0	0
	勐海	230	272			100	140	40	42	65	65	25	25	0	0
	沧源	270	327			100	140	40	47	90	100	40	40	0	0
	福贡	230	334			100	140	40	86	65	83	25	25	0	0
	耿马	300	417			100	140	60	74	100	163	40	40	0	0
	贡山	240	371			100	140	40	96	75	110	25	25	0	0
	龙陵	295	357			100	140	80	99	80	82	35	36	0	0
	陇川	360	423			100	140	80	82	130	141	50	60	0	0
	泸水	230	270			100	140	40	45	65	75	25	10	0	0
	潞西	300	677			100	140	60	65	100	266	40	206	0	0
	瑞丽	410	463			100	140	100	113	150	150	60	60	0	0
	腾冲	430	511			100	140	100	138	170	170	60	63	0	0
	盈江	400	517			100	140	90	102	150	204	60	71	0	0
	镇康	255	329			100	157	40	42	80	93	35	37	0	0
	小计	7 500	9 965	0	0	2 500	3 517	1 500	1 767	2 500	3 143	1 000	1 538	0	0
海南	万宁	200	235	0	0	100	100	100	135	0	0	0	0	0	0
	陵水	200	215	0	0	100	100	100	115	0	0	0	0	0	0
	三亚	200	259	0	0	100	100	100	159	0	0	0	0	0	0
	保亭	200	310	0	0	100	101	100	209	0	0	0	0	0	0

续表

SRs/SSRs		合计		2003		2004		2005		2006		2007		2008（5A）	
		计划开展	实际完成	计划开展	实际完成	计划开展	实际完成	计划开展	实际完成	计划开展	实际完成	计划开展	实际完成	计划开展	实际完成
	乐东	200	314	0	0	100	100	100	214	0	0	0	0	0	0
	五指山	200	225	0	0	100	100	100	125	0	0	0	0	0	0
	琼中	200	311	0	0	100	100	100	211	0	0	0	0	0	0
	东方	200	241	0	0	100	100	100	141	0	0	0	0	0	0
	昌江	200	242	0	0	100	100	100	142	0	0	0	0	0	0
	白沙	200	327	0	0	100	100	100	227	0	0	0	0	0	0
	小计	2 000	2 679	0	0	1 000	1 001	1 000	1 678	0	0	0	0	0	0
河南	淮滨	0	0	0	0	0	0	0	0	0	0	0	0	0	0
	商城	0	0	0	0	0	0	0	0	0	0	0	0	0	0
	小计	0	0	0	0	0	0	0	0	0	0	0	0	0	0
湖北	枣阳	0	0	0	0	0	0	0	0	0	0	0	0	0	0
	曾都区	0	0	0	0	0	0	0	0	0	0	0	0	0	0
	小计	0	0	0	0	0	0	0	0	0	0	0	0	0	0
安徽	怀远	0	0	0	0	0	0	0	0	0	0	0	0	0	0
江苏	泗洪	0	0	0	0	0	0	0	0	0	0	0	0	0	0
	盱眙	0	0	0	0	0	0	0	0	0	0	0	0	0	0
	小计	0	0	0	0	0	0	0	0	0	0	0	0	0	0
广东	惠州市	0	0	0	0	0	0	0	0	0	0	0	0	0	0
	惠阳区	0	0	0	0	0	0	0	0	0	0	0	0	0	0
	徐闻	0	0	0	0	0	0	0	0	0	0	0	0	0	0
	小计	0	0	0	0	0	0	0	0	0	0	0	0	0	0
广西	百色	0	0	0	0	0	0	0	0	0	0	0	0	0	0
四川	筠连	0	0	0	0	0	0	0	0	0	0	0	0	0	0
贵州	榕江	0	0	0	0	0	0	0	0	0	0	0	0	0	0
总计		9 500	12 644	0	0	3 500	4 518	2 500	3 445	2 500	3 143	1 000	1 538	0	0

表 6 张贴疟疾宣传海报活动统计

SRs/SSRs		合计		2003		2004		2005		2006		2007		2008（5A）	
		计划开展	实际完成	计划开展	实际完成	计划开展	实际完成	计划开展	实际完成	计划开展	实际完成	计划开展	实际完成	计划开展	实际完成
云南	麻栗坡	5 100	3 959			1 800	2 300	1 300	0	1 000	1 042	1 000	617	0	0
	马关	5 300	5 821			1 800	2 300	1 300	1 300	1 000	1 000	1 200	1 221		
	富宁	5 100	5 359			1 800	2 300	1 300	1 300	1 000	1 157	1 000	602	0	0
	绿春	5 300	4 780			1 800	2 300	1 300	0	1 100	1 880	1 100	600	0	0
	金平	5 300	3 500			1 800	2 300	1 300	0	1 100	1 000	1 100	200	0	0
	河口	6 800	7 380			2 400	2 900	1 600	1 700	1 400	1 514	1 400	1 266	0	0
	江城	5 500	5 770			2 000	2 500	1 300	1 320	1 100	1 140	1 100	810	0	0
	孟连	9 300	18 703			3 400	3 900	2 100	2 035	2 000	10 570	1 800	2 198	0	0
	澜沧	5 500	6 461			1 800	2 300	1 300	1 300	1 200	1 061	1 200	1 800	0	0
	西盟	10 300	9 870			4 200	4 700	2 500	1 500	1 800	1 800	1 800	1 870	0	0
	勐腊	10 700	4 936			4 200	4 700	2 500	0	2 000	120	2 000	116	0	0
	景洪	9 500	8 508			3 400	3 400	2 100	491	2 000	2 212	2 000	2 405	0	0
	勐海	5 100	5 079			1 800	2 300	1 300	1 150	1 000	1 079	1 000	550	0	0
	沧源	5 700	6 980			1 800	2 300	1 100	1 650	1 400	1 830	1 400	1 200	0	0
	福贡	5 000	6 010			1 800	2 300	1 200	1 200	1 000	1 910	1 000	600	0	0
	耿马	6 800	7 100			2 400	2 900	1 600	1 600	1 400	1 400	1 400	1 200	0	0
	贡山	5 000	5 316			1 800	2 300	1 200	1 000	1 000	1 416	1 000	600	0	0
	龙陵	5 300	4 888			1 800	2 300	1 300	0	1 100	1 300	1 100	1 288	0	0
	陇川	8 500	9 100			2 400	2 900	2 100	2 012	2 000	2 388	2 000	1 800	0	0
	泸水	5 100	5 200			1 800	2 300	1 300	1 300	1 000	1 000	1 000	600	0	0
	潞西	6 600	7 261			2 400	2 900	1 600	1 523	1 300	1 600	1 300	1 228	0	10
	瑞丽	9 500	9 800			3 400	3 900	2 100	2 100	2 000	2 000	2 000	1 800	0	0
	腾冲	10 700	8 846			4 200	4 700	2 500	346	2 000	2 000	2 000	1 800	0	0
	盈江	10 700	10 073			4 200	4 700	2 500	1 055	2 000	2 518	2 000	1 800	0	0
	镇康	5 300	6 102			1 800	2 200	1 300	200	1 100	2 502	1 100	1 200	0	0
	小计	173 000	176 802	0	0	62 000	73 900	41 000	26 082	35 000	47 439	35 000	29 371	0	10
海南	万宁	6 400	8 510	1 000	1 850	3 000	4 850	800	0	800	1 000	800	810	0	0
	陵水	5 100	6 736	0	0	3 000	5 030	700	0	700	1 010	700	696	0	0
	三亚	5 600	7 716	0	0	3 000	6 030	900	0	900	900	800	786	0	0
	保亭	13 400	14 440	3 000	3 140	7 000	9 000	1 100	0	1 100	1 100	1 200	1 200	0	0

续表

SRs/SSRs		合计		2003		2004		2005		2006		2007		2008（5A）	
		计划开展	实际完成	计划开展	实际完成	计划开展	实际完成	计划开展	实际完成	计划开展	实际完成	计划开展	实际完成	计划开展	实际完成
	乐东	7 200	7 810	0	0	3 000	5 000	1 400	0	1 400	1 400	1 400	1 410	0	0
	五指山	5 400	7 350	0	0	3 000	5 450	800	0	800	1 100	800	800	0	0
	琼中	7 500	8 700	0	0	3 000	5 200	1 500	0	1 500	2 000	1 500	1 500	0	0
	东方	5 100	6 895	0	0	3 000	5 200	700	0	700	1 000	700	695	0	0
	昌江	5 100	6 900	0	0	3 000	5 200	700	0	700	1 000	700	700	0	0
	白沙	7 200	7 781	0	0	3 000	5 000	1 400	0	1 400	1 400	1 400	1 381	0	0
	小计	68 000	82 838	4 000	4 990	34 000	55 960	10 000	0	10 000	11 910	10 000	9 978	0	0
河南	淮滨	0	0	0	0	0	0	0	0	0	0	0	0	0	0
	商城	0	0	0	0	0	0	0	0	0	0	0	0	0	0
	小计	0	0	0	0	0	0	0	0	0	0	0	0	0	0
湖北	枣阳	0	0	0	0	0	0	0	0	0	0	0	0	0	0
	曾都区	0	0	0	0	0	0	0	0	0	0	0	0	0	0
	小计	0	0	0	0	0	0	0	0	0	0	0	0	0	0
安徽	怀远	0	0	0	0	0	0	0	0	0	0	0	0	0	0
江苏	泗洪	0	0	0	0	0	0	0	0	0	0	0	0	0	0
	盱眙	0	0	0	0	0	0	0	0	0	0	0	0	0	0
	小计	0	0	0	0	0	0	0	0	0	0	0	0	0	0
广东	惠州市	0	0	0	0	0	0	0	0	0	0	0	0	0	0
	惠阳区	0	0	0	0	0	0	0	0	0	0	0	0	0	0
	徐闻	0	0	0	0	0	0	0	0	0	0	0	0	0	0
	小计	0	0	0	0	0	0	0	0	0	0	0	0	0	0
广西	百色	0	0	0	0	0	0	0	0	0	0	0	0	0	0
四川	筠连	0	0	0	0	0	0	0	0	0	0	0	0	0	0
贵州	榕江	0	0	0	0	0	0	0	0	0	0	0	0	0	0
总计		241 000	259 640	4 000	4 990	96 000	129 860	51 000	26 082	45 000	59 349	45 000	39 349	0	10

表 7 疟防广播电视宣传活动统计

SRs/SSRs		合计		2003		2004		2005		2006		2007		2008（5A）	
		计划开展	实际完成	计划开展	实际完成	计划开展	实际完成	计划开展	实际完成	计划开展	实际完成	计划开展	实际完成	计划开展	实际完成
云南	麻栗坡	7	11			2	6	2	2	3	3				
	马关	7	10			2	5	2	2	3	3				
	富宁	7	10			2	5	2	2	3	3				
	绿春	7	11			2	6	2	2	3	3				
	金平	7	10			2	5	2	2	3	3				
	河口	7	26			2	5	2	18	3	3				
	江城	7	20			2	6	2	11	3	3				
	孟连	7	32			2	5	2	16	3	11				
	澜沧	7	23			2	6	2	12	3	5				
	西盟	7	17			2	5	2	6	3	6				
	勐腊	7	9			2	5	2	3	3	1				
	景洪	7	27			2	5	2	9	3	13				
	勐海	7	13			2	6	2	2	3	5				
	沧源	7	20			2	5	2	6	3	9				
	福贡	7	13			2	6	2	4	3	3				
	耿马	7	11			2	6	2	2	3	3				
	贡山	7	11			2	6	2	2	3	3				
	龙陵	7	10			2	5	2	2	3	3				
	陇川	7	46			2	6	2	17	3	23				
	泸水	7	25			2	5	2	16	3	4				
	潞西	7	25			2	6	2	16	3	3				
	瑞丽	7	10			2	5	2	2	3	3				
	腾冲	7	10			2	5	2	2	3	3				
	盈江	7	12			2	6	2	3	3	3				
	镇康	7	44			2	5	2	36	3	3				
	小计	175	456	0	0	50	136	50	195	75	125	0	0	0	0
海南	万宁	6	6	0	0	2	2	1	1	1	1	2	2	0	0
	陵水	6	6	0	0	2	2	1	1	1	1	2	2	0	0
	三亚	6	6	0	0	2	2	1	1	1	1	2	2	0	0
	保亭	6	6	0	0	2	2	1	1	1	1	2	2	0	0

续表

SRs/SSRs		合计		2003		2004		2005		2006		2007		2008（5A）	
		计划开展	实际完成	计划开展	实际完成	计划开展	实际完成	计划开展	实际完成	计划开展	实际完成	计划开展	实际完成	计划开展	实际完成
	乐东	6	6	0	0	2	2	1	1	1	1	2	2	0	0
	五指山	6	6	0	0	2	2	1	1	1	1	2	2	0	0
	琼中	6	6	0	0	2	2	1	1	1	1	2	2	0	0
	东方	6	6	0	0	2	2	1	1	1	1	2	2	0	0
	昌江	6	6	0	0	2	2	1	1	1	1	2	2	0	0
	白沙	6	6	0	0	2	2	1	1	1	1	2	2	0	0
	小计	60	60	0	0	20	20	10	10	10	10	20	20	0	0
河南	淮滨	2	2	0	0	2	2	0	0	0	0	0	0	0	0
	商城	0	0	0	0	0	0	0	0	0	0	0	0	0	0
	小计	2	2	0	0	2	2	0	0	0	0	0	0	0	0
湖北	枣阳	2	2	0	0	2	2	0	0	0	0	0	0	0	0
	曾都区	0	0	0	0	0	0	0	0	0	0	0	0	0	0
	小计	2	2	0	0	2	2	0	0	0	0	0	0	0	0
安徽	怀远	2	2	0	0	2	2	0	0	0	0	0	0	0	0
江苏	泗洪	2	2	0	0	2	2	0	0	0	0	0	0	0	0
	盱眙	0	0	0	0	0	0	0	0	0	0	0	0	0	0
	小计	2	2	0	0	2	2	0	0	0	0	0	0	0	0
广东	惠州市	2	2	0	0	2	2	0	0	0	0	0	0	0	0
	惠阳区	0	0	0	0	0	0	0	0	0	0	0	0	0	0
	徐闻	0	0	0	0	0	0	0	0	0	0	0	0	0	0
	小计	2	2	0	0	2	2	0	0	0	0	0	0	0	0
广西	百色	2	2	0	0	2	2	0	0	0	0	0	0	0	0
四川	筠连	2	2	0	0	2	2	0	0	0	0	0	0	0	0
贵州	榕江	2	2	0	0	2	2	0	0	0	0	0	0	0	0
总计		251	532	0	0	86	172	60	205	85	135	20	20	0	0

表 8 M&E 指标完成情况统计

SRs/SSRs		疟疾调查推断发病率 (1/10 000)			海南 10 个项目县的恶性疟调查推断发病率 (1/10 000)			目标地区中小学生能够正确回答至少 3 个与疟疾相关问题的比例 (%)			发热病人在症状出现 2 天内求诊的比例 (%)			拥有杀虫剂浸泡蚊帐的家庭比例 (%)			网络直报疟疾病人比例 (%)		
		基线调查值	项目目标	终期调查值	基线调查值	项目目标	终期调查值	基线调查值	项目目标	终期调查值	基线调查值	项目目标	终期调查值	基线调查值	项目目标	终期调查值	基线调查值	项目目标	终期调查值
NPO 统计		云南 : 197 海南 : 385	云南 : 97 海南 : 192	云南 : 65.88 海南 : 31.13	9.06	<1	0.40	60.00	85.00	93.18	44.12	90.00	89.95	13.98	30.00	37.60	7.12	40.00	38.92
云南	全省	197.00	97.00	65.88	/	/	/	58.20	85.00	94.83	37.95	90.00	92.36	4.30	30.00	32.36	8.80	40.00	45.30
	麻栗坡	5.18	2.59	17.00	/	/	/	0.00	85.00	87.36	38.75	90.00	90.63	0.00	30.00	31.80	0.00	40.00	46.67
	马关	35.38	17.69	17.57	/	/	/	0.00	85.00	92.11	32.94	90.00	92.81	0.00	30.00	34.46	0.00	40.00	37.50
	富宁	1.26	0.63	4.16	/	/	/	0.00	85.00	85.98	48.18	90.00	89.94	0.00	30.00	31.42	0.00	40.00	40.74
	绿春	8.54	4.27	17.18	/	/	/	0.00	85.00	88.78	29.67	90.00	92.90	0.00	30.00	30.12	0.00	40.00	42.86
	金平	32.53	16.27	79.87	/	/	/	0.00	85.00	88.08	16.82	90.00	91.20	0.00	30.00	34.56	0.00	40.00	42.31
	河口	28.85	14.43	87.73	/	/	/	0.00	85.00	96.10	49.54	90.00	93.62	0.00	30.00	32.27	0.00	40.00	46.67
	江城	34.42	17.21	22.54	/	/	/	0.00	85.00	99.74	59.38	90.00	94.65	0.00	30.00	32.65	0.00	40.00	50.00
	孟连	1 089.12	544.56	185.87	/	/	/	0.00	85.00	99.05	50.27	90.00	99.07	0.00	30.00	31.37	0.00	40.00	42.42
	澜沧	84.59	42.30	30.33	/	/	/	0.00	85.00	99.48	37.86	90.00	93.60	0.00	30.00	33.38	0.00	40.00	40.98
	西盟	4 270.90	2 135.45	340.54	/	/	/	0.00	85.00	95.78	35.22	90.00	93.64	0.00	30.00	30.25	0.00	40.00	45.24
	勐腊	445.36	222.68	131.58	/	/	/	0.00	85.00	93.11	37.36	90.00	52.48	0.00	30.00	24.12	0.00	40.00	40.54
	景洪	399.90	199.95	4.45	/	/	/	0.00	85.00	85.46	77.21	90.00	93.37	0.00	30.00	38.34	0.00	40.00	47.62
	勐海	296.30	148.15	36.18	/	/	/	0.00	85.00	96.20	14.29	90.00	97.20	0.00	30.00	35.45	0.00	40.00	46.67
	沧源	34.54	17.27	61.78	/	/	/	0.00	85.00	97.26	52.99	90.00	45.24	0.00	30.00	32.41	0.00	40.00	60.00
	福贡	5.02	2.51	25.57	/	/	/	0.00	85.00	91.76	16.33	90.00	97.95	0.00	30.00	32.29	0.00	40.00	27.27
	耿马	22.51	11.26	45.39	/	/	/	0.00	85.00	97.29	23.01	90.00	93.95	0.00	30.00	36.98	0.00	40.00	33.33
	贡山	27.58	13.79	142.10	/	/	/	0.00	85.00	99.44	61.78	90.00	93.41	0.00	30.00	31.31	0.00	40.00	35.00
	龙陵	20.99	10.50	40.82	/	/	/	0.00	85.00	99.49	25.00	90.00	99.66	0.00	30.00	30.11	0.00	40.00	58.33
	陇川	296.12	148.06	70.24	/	/	/	0.00	85.00	89.22	32.11	90.00	90.39	0.00	30.00	39.66	0.00	40.00	44.44
	泸水	1.13	0.57	9.83	/	/	/	0.00	85.00	99.79	38.14	90.00	96.02	0.00	30.00	30.28	0.00	40.00	50.00
	潞西	12.94	6.47	153.77	/	/	/	0.00	85.00	95.82	19.07	90.00	97.47	0.00	30.00	32.76	0.00	40.00	46.88
	瑞丽	273.67	136.84	380.43	/	/	/	0.00	85.00	96.78	40.40	90.00	95.92	0.00	30.00	31.60	0.00	40.00	48.39
	腾冲	187.19	93.60	36.43	/	/	/	0.00	85.00	100.00	48.80	90.00	90.82	0.00	30.00	31.42	0.00	40.00	56.76
	盈江	188.10	94.05	218.72	/	/	/	0.00	85.00	99.25	38.43	90.00	100.00	0.00	30.00	30.84	0.00	40.00	51.43
	镇康	26.18	13.09	44.14	/	/	/	0.00	85.00	95.63	16.92	90.00	93.02	0.00	30.00	30.10	0.00	40.00	47.62
海南	全省	385.00	192.00	31.13	9.06/10000	<1	0.40	62.57	85.00	89.39	54.61	90.00	85.27	38.91	30.00	52.38	5.02	40.00	33.38
	万宁	385.00	192.00	21.46	9.06	<1	0.02	62.57	85.00	90.14	54.61	90.00	88.81	38.91	30.00	51.60	5.02	40.00	44.94
	陵水	385.00	192.00	42.40	9.06	<1	0.12	62.57	85.00	89.78	54.61	90.00	88.33	38.91	30.00	51.28	5.02	40.00	25.16
	三亚	385.00	192.00	5.21	9.06	<1	0.79	62.57	85.00	90.83	54.61	90.00	85.07	38.91	30.00	54.66	5.02	40.00	44.23
	保亭	385.00	192.00	81.76	9.06	<1	0.06	62.57	85.00	89.95	54.61	90.00	84.02	38.91	30.00	60.82	5.02	40.00	33.62
	乐东	385.00	192.00	39.97	9.06	<1	0.57	62.57	85.00	88.60	54.61	90.00	84.13	38.91	30.00	51.02	5.02	40.00	16.18
	五指山	385.00	192.00	18.97	9.06	<1	0.09	62.57	85.00	89.23	54.61	90.00	85.78	38.91	30.00	50.34	5.02	40.00	45.45
	琼中	385.00	192.00	61.89	9.06	<1	0.10	62.57	85.00	88.32	54.61	90.00	85.76	38.91	30.00	48.98	5.02	40.00	24.44
	东方	385.00	192.00	26.94	9.06	<1	0.72	62.57	85.00	88.71	54.61	90.00	88.53	38.91	30.00	51.98	5.02	40.00	41.43
	昌江	385.00	192.00	14.00	9.06	<1	0.30	62.57	85.00	87.23	54.61	90.00	86.14	38.91	30.00	51.28	5.02	40.00	46.15
	白沙	385.00	192.00	64.75	9.06	<1	0.54	62.57	85.00	90.62	54.61	90.00	82.95	38.91	30.00	51.14	5.02	40.00	44.07

表 9 预算执行情况统计

单位：元　　　　　　　　　　　　　　　　　　　　　　　　　　　　预算数折算汇率 1:8

PR/SRs/SSRs	合计				2003－2004				2005				2006				2007				2008（5A）			
	预算数	到款数	支出数	执行率(%)	预算数	到款数	支出数	执行率(%)	预算数	到款数	支出数	执行率(%)	预算数	到款数	支出数	执行率(%)	预算数	到款数	支出数	执行率(%)	预算数	到款数	支出数	执行率(%)
中央	9 000 232.00	8 010 529.64	7 720 347.62	85.78	3 449 192.00	3 152 233.06	1 974 291.83	62.63	2 196 016.00	1 311 433.82	1 566 525.82	71.33	1 545 392.00	2 639 288.71	1 255 254.10	81.23	1 142 328.00	907 574.05	1 803 275.59	157.86	667 304.00	0.00	1 121 000.28	167.99
采购	14 602 360.00	15 013 798.77	14 662 815.46	100.41	10 110 920.00	10 583 488.58	8 239 153.19	77.85	2 749 440.00	2 833 263.63	2 183 874.33	79.43	1 366 600.00	1 349 560.76	2 868 311.63	209.89	375 400.00	369 626.36	1 371 476.32	365.34	0.00	(122 140.55)	0.00	0.00
云南 省本级	2 814 616.00	3 235 613.13	3 238 582.26	115.06	1 540 000.00	1 539 981.83	1 198 388.46	77.82	432 000.00	225 216.68	432 068.26	191.85	394 000.00	794 083.96	802 762.47	203.75	272 000.00	627 243.09	139 424.51	51.26	176 616.00	49 087.57	665 938.56	377.05
麻栗坡	419 760.00	344 867.23	344 867.23	82.16	205 696.00	139 150.00	139 150.00	100.00	64 900.00	42 984.97	42 984.97	100.00	65 136.00	87 433.90	87 069.66	133.67	51 760.00	75 298.36	52 354.21	101.15	32 268.00	0.00	23 308.39	72.23
马关	352 236.00	351 785.90	351 785.90	99.87	144 000.00	144 000.00	144 075.63	100.05	64 900.00	42 984.98	43 408.89	100.99	65 136.00	87 311.02	85 945.32	131.95	53 440.00	77 489.90	55 737.04	104.30	24 760.00	0.00	22 619.02	91.35
富宁	351 340.00	344 703.60	344 703.60	98.11	145 200.00	139 150.00	139 238.97	100.06	64 820.00	42 823.66	42 872.62	100.11	65 136.00	87 247.83	87 200.20	133.87	51 720.00	75 482.11	52 512.82	101.53	24 464.00	0.00	22 878.99	93.52
绿春	364 064.00	372 582.14	372 582.14	102.34	144 680.00	144 680.00	136 841.59	94.58	70 200.00	48 238.49	56 285.03	116.68	72 040.00	103 319.05	102 597.67	142.42	52 880.00	76 344.60	54 422.51	102.92	24 264.00	0.00	22 435.34	92.46
金平	388 000.00	369 472.01	369 472.01	95.22	162 000.00	150 780.00	150 392.35	99.74	70 200.00	48 238.49	47 312.87	98.08	70 240.00	92 539.21	93 973.83	133.79	52 480.00	77 914.31	54 182.00	103.24	33 080.00	0.00	23 610.96	71.38
河口	598 420.00	420 644.03	420 644.03	70.29	340 600.00	170 190.00	157 556.16	92.58	79 560.00	58 548.20	70 889.27	121.08	83 952.00	104 891.77	105 178.06	125.28	64 080.00	87 014.06	61 481.29	95.94	30 228.00	0.00	25 539.25	84.49
江城	359 384.00	356 607.60	356 607.60	99.23	142 680.00	142 680.00	127 345.22	89.25	70 200.00	48 238.49	62 135.23	128.81	70 240.00	92 520.64	88 416.08	125.88	52 040.00	73 168.47	49 223.75	94.59	24 224.00	0.00	29 487.32	121.73
孟连	499 196.00	491 737.53	491 737.53	98.51	185 112.00	186 440.00	175 668.24	94.22	92 708.00	74 645.59	84 918.98	113.76	110 616.00	128 702.58	126 504.90	114.36	77 600.00	101 949.36	82 188.20	105.91	33 160.00	0.00	22 457.21	67.72
澜沧	362 988.00	370 594.99	370 594.99	102.10	132 520.00	140 500.00	123 879.54	88.17	64 900.00	42 984.97	58 218.10	135.44	71 656.00	93 880.33	91 339.20	127.47	68 160.00	93 229.69	72 688.50	106.64	25 752.00	0.00	24 469.65	95.02
西盟	533 860.00	517 032.19	517 032.19	96.85	226 960.00	199 980.00	198 484.79	99.25	101 656.00	83 176.35	84 259.50	101.30	102 328.00	130 412.21	131 071.00	128.09	79 040.00	103 463.63	79 899.15	101.09	23 876.00	0.00	23 317.75	97.66
勐腊	541 820.00	500 050.29	500 050.29	92.29	227 040.00	193 726.07	200 163.38	103.32	96 252.00	75 403.79	66 269.10	87.89	113 456.00	128 104.30	129 989.52	114.57	79 360.00	102 816.13	73 493.63	92.61	25 712.00	0.00	30 134.66	117.20
景洪	500 984.00	492 038.39	492 038.39	98.21	186 740.00	186 740.00	184 373.92	98.73	92 748.00	74 645.59	74 968.35	100.43	110 296.00	128 297.48	128 074.20	116.12	77 440.00	102 355.32	56 231.71	72.61	33 760.00	0.00	48 390.21	143.34
勐海	381 824.00	345 995.11	345 995.11	90.62	165 480.00	142 650.00	141 443.31	99.15	64 900.00	42 984.98	42 340.81	98.50	67 096.00	85 343.56	86 283.07	128.60	52 240.00	75 016.57	53 880.77	103.14	32 108.00	0.00	22 047.15	68.67
沧源	418 004.00	414 350.77	414 350.77	99.13	166 740.00	166 740.00	148 152.91	88.85	79 560.00	58 548.20	77 348.78	132.11	83 152.00	104 425.78	104 489.60	125.66	64 080.00	84 636.79	60 831.42	94.93	24 472.00	0.00	23 528.06	96.14
福贡	344 740.00	343 806.23	343 806.23	99.73	139 200.00	139 113.93	138 168.32	99.32	64 900.00	42 976.87	44 020.41	102.43	65 136.00	86 900.41	86 974.70	133.53	51 400.00	74 815.02	47 618.12	92.64	24 104.00	0.00	27 024.68	112.12
耿马	438 372.00	429 643.81	429 643.81	98.01	166 900.00	166 740.00	166 705.20	99.98	79 560.00	58 548.20	58 564.54	100.03	95 152.00	116 395.35	116 668.33	122.61	64 240.00	87 960.26	64 698.28	100.71	32 520.00	0.00	23 007.46	70.75
贡山	399 424.00	387 176.39	387 176.39	96.93	178 400.00	178 240.00	147 101.72	82.53	67 112.00	62 806.03	88 991.82	141.69	69 560.00	72 844.97	77 311.09	111.14	52 480.00	73 285.39	45 807.50	87.29	31 872.00	0.00	27 954.26	87.74
龙陵	392 876.00	384 821.35	384 821.35	97.95	146 780.00	146 780.00	143 465.81	97.74	70 360.00	48 238.49	51 533.00	106.83	83 280.00	105 285.89	104 182.18	125.10	60 416.00	84 516.97	62 193.22	102.94	32 040.00	0.00	23 447.14	73.18
陇川	480 332.00	478 196.20	478 196.20	99.56	192 600.00	192 590.00	190 570.30	98.95	92 308.00	74 439.00	76 483.39	102.75	97 416.00	112 838.37	113 110.23	116.11	73 128.00	98 328.83	74 195.77	101.46	24 880.00	0.00	23 836.51	95.81
泸水	356 284.00	340 871.50	340 871.50	95.67	142 320.00	142 150.00	135 513.25	95.22	64 900.00	42 984.98	32 819.11	76.35	65 136.00	81 150.16	98 089.80	150.59	51 400.00	74 586.36	42 802.09	83.27	32 528.00	0.00	31 647.25	97.29
潞西	416 904.00	416 793.80	416 793.80	99.97	166 072.00	166 740.00	162 584.91	97.90	79 560.00	58 548.20	61 740.98	105.45	81 912.00	102 997.63	103 745.33	126.65	64 080.00	88 507.97	62 282.04	97.19	25 280.00	0.00	26 440.54	104.59
瑞丽	530 284.00	507 818.91	507 818.91	95.76	208 860.00	198 780.00	174 023.38	83.32	101 816.00	83 589.58	107 979.80	129.18	115 208.00	121 904.21	122 561.70	106.38	79 520.00	103 545.12	78 578.00	98.82	24 880.00	0.00	24 676.03	99.18
腾冲	504 108.00	510 791.10	510 791.10	101.33	175 000.00	174 640.00	174 847.23	99.91	103 748.00	69 317.38	69 362.63	100.07	116 464.00	158 862.69	158 178.39	135.82	82 960.00	107 971.03	82 851.91	99.87	25 936.00	0.00	25 550.94	98.52
盈江	516 724.00	508 286.49	508 286.49	98.37	186 740.00	186 740.00	173 497.08	92.91	100 112.00	77 602.42	91 078.55	117.37	114 656.00	137 644.18	136 534.94	119.08	81 520.00	106 299.89	83 409.95	102.32	33 696.00	0.00	23 765.97	70.53
镇康	381 856.00	374 331.48	374 331.48	98.03	150 000.00	149 830.00	142 429.72	94.95	70 200.00	48 238.49	55 770.64	115.61	73 200.00	95 507.69	95 601.42	130.60	55 736.00	80 755.30	56 335.90	101.08	32 720.00	0.00	24 193.80	73.94
小计	13 648 400.00	13 610 612.17	13 613 581.30	99.74	5 968 320.00	5 629 731.83	5 114 061.39	85.69	2 404 080.00	1 676 953.07	2 024 625.63	120.73	2 521 600.00	3 440 845.17	3 463 852.89	137.37	1 865 200.00	2 813 994.53	1 699 324.29	91.11	889 200.00	49 087.57	1 311 717.10	147.52
海南 省本级	1 361 299.00	1 050 408.34	743 311.67	54.60	734 506.00	414 619.52	401 192.90	54.62	90 196.00	165 226.13	130 947.90	79.25	211 807.00	216 077.78	62 120.40	29.33	104 790.00	233 484.91	21 734.00	20.74	220 000.00	21 000.00	127 316.47	57.87
万宁	478 136.00	463 888.00	486 244.14	101.70	264 991.00	243 991.00	243 233.80	91.79	80 527.00	100 527.00	108 692.14	108.12	50 838.00	51 838.00	43 719.60	86.00	67 530.00	67 532.00	68 137.60	100.90	14 250.00	0.00	22 461.00	157.62
陵水	370 870.00	348 528.00	378 554.30	102.07	205 370.00	184 148.00	184 046.10	89.62	69 600.00	79 275.00	87 120.00	109.90	43 700.00	44 619.00	45 620.00	104.39	40 540.00	40 486.00	40 239.20	99.26	11 660.00	0.00	21 529.00	184.64
三亚	490 140.00	473 352.00	498 524.22	101.71	274 050.00	252 557.00	251 833.20	91.89	74 560.00	93 960.00	91 611.05	97.50	68 319.00	69 773.00	73 236.97	107.20	58 051.00	57 062.00	57 394.00	98.87	15 160.00	0.00	24 449.00	161.27
保亭	545 673.00	559 780.00	602 357.23	110.39	286 440.00	267 459.00	267 958.86	93.55	85 337.00	126 354.00	141 572.14	112.04	91 923.00	97 431.00	87 048.56	94.70	67 103.00	68 536.00	81 340.68	121.22	14 870.00	0.00	24 436.99	164.34
乐东	553 787.00	523 506.00	544 259.90	98.28	277 600.00	236 446.00	236 161.90	85.07	92 397.00	122 443.00	99 138.00	80.97	81 440.00	82 477.00	82 814.50	101.69	86 090.00	82 140.00	101 850.50	118.31	16 260.00	0.00	24 295.00	149.42
五指山	387 480.00	373 383.00	395 527.56	102.08	217 210.00	196 202.00	194 171.40	89.39	64 250.00	84 202.00	71 007.45	84.33	48 240.00	49 186.00	51 068.50	105.86	43 790.00	43 793.00	57 098.21	130.39	13 990.00	0.00	22 182.00	158.56
琼中	648 341.00	643 509.00	690 323.15	106.48	362 873.00	340 161.00	339 166.10	93.47	91 580.00	132 154.00	115 055.70	87.06	84 431.00	82 798.00	120 904.36	143.20	94 067.00	88 396.00	85 423.67	90.81	15 390.00	0.00	29 773.32	193.46
东方	511 470.00	496 080.00	545 695.30	106.69	264 000.00	245 206.00	244 990.30	92.80	99 370.00	117 908.00	124 381.00	105.49	66 650.00	66 371.00	66 292.00	99.46	67 200.00	66 595.00	85 858.50	127.77	14 250.00	0.00	24 173.50	169.64
昌江	391 489.00	399 489.00	422 866.70	108.01	223 260.00	210 576.00	210 575.70	94.32	61 978.00	81 232.00	81 222.50	99.99	49 042.00	46 879.00	38 210.60	77.91	43 839.00	60 802.00	69 165.40	157.77	13 370.00	0.00	23 592.50	177.21

续表

PR/SRs/SSRs	合计				2003 - 2004				2005				2006				2007				2008（5A）			
	预算数	到款数	支出数	执行率(%)	预算数	到款数	支出数	执行率(%)	预算数	到款数	支出数	执行率(%)	预算数	到款数	支出数	执行率(%)	预算数	到款数	支出数	执行率(%)	预算数	到款数	支出数	执行率(%)
白沙	553 635.00	571 574.00	608 349.72	109.88	254 100.00	242 136.00	238 429.72	93.83	91 725.00	137 137.00	103 069.20	75.16	90 410.00	90 410.00	138 952.80	153.69	101 800.00	101 891.00	102 311.00	100.50	15 600.00	0.00	25 587.00	164.02
小计	6 292 320.00	5 903 497.34	5 916 013.89	94.02	3 364 400.00	2 833 501.52	2 811 759.98	83.57	901 520.00	1 240 418.13	1 153 817.08	93.02	886 800.00	897 859.78	809 988.29	91.34	774 800.00	910 717.91	770 552.76	99.45	364 800.00	21 000.00	369 895.78	101.40
河南 省本级	386 397.50	358 180.41	334 947.86	86.68	218 700.00	195 380.21	192 115.05	87.84	79 785.00	51 378.78	45 817.96	89.18	46 652.00	77 082.40	53 391.20	114.45	25 260.50	30 532.42	27 576.00	109.17	16 000.00	3 806.60	16 047.65	100.30
淮滨	439 379.00	457 622.77	473 870.85	107.85	114 150.00	114 150.00	113 510.25	99.44	132 975.00	88 222.47	88 907.10	100.78	95 134.00	158 326.30	158 366.00	166.47	79 770.00	96 924.00	96 886.50	121.46	17 350.00	0.00	16 201.00	93.38
商城	163 423.50	167 386.91	175 636.91	107.47	32 900.00	32 900.00	32 900.00	100.00	53 190.00	34 174.61	34 174.61	100.00	41 164.00	66 748.30	66 748.30	162.15	27 919.50	33 564.00	33 564.00	120.22	8 250.00	0.00	8 250.00	100.00
小计	989 200.00	983 190.09	984 455.62	99.52	365 750.00	342 430.21	338 525.30	92.56	265 950.00	173 775.86	168 899.67	97.19	182 950.00	302 157.00	278 505.50	152.23	132 950.00	161 020.42	158 026.50	118.86	41 600.00	3 806.60	40 498.65	97.35
湖北 省本级	504 798.88	528 769.33	529 550.64	104.90	211 466.97	205 630.21	129 823.70	61.39	136 268.01	31 523.58	38 266.60	121.39	91 760.76	225 429.84	131 623.50	143.44	46 703.15	61 985.70	215 198.70	460.78	18 600.00	4 200.00	14 638.14	78.70
枣阳	319 351.27	335 780.00	335 780.00	105.14	87 412.70	85 000.00	160 472.40	183.58	103 745.59	24 000.00	54 094.80	225.40	65 421.56	160 722.00	130 857.00	200.02	49 771.42	66 058.00	(31 552.00)	(63.39)	13 000.00	0.00	21 907.80	168.52
曾都区	151 449.84	169 515.00	169 545.00	111.95	53 270.33	51 800.00	51 800.00	97.24	25 936.40	6 000.00	6 000.00	100.00	25 767.68	63 303.80	63 303.80	245.67	36 475.43	48 411.20	48 441.20	132.81	10 000.00	0.00	0.00	0.00
小计	975 600.00	1 034 064.33	1 034 875.64	106.08	352 150.00	342 430.21	342 096.10	97.14	265 950.00	61 523.58	98 361.40	159.88	182 950.00	449 455.64	325 784.30	178.07	132 950.00	176 454.90	232 087.90	174.57	41 600.00	4 200.00	36 545.94	87.85
安徽 省本级	672 968.58	310 038.43	310 401.22	46.12	344 390.00	212 430.21	135 997.46	39.49	225 214.12	6 743.76	79 758.00	1 182.69	69 802.43	69 802.43	39 607.50	56.74	11 962.03	11 962.03	1 561.00	13.05	21 600.00	9 100.00	53 477.26	247.58
怀远	424 871.42	677 204.70	677 204.70	159.39	130 000.00	130 000.00	130 000.00	100.00	40 735.88	40 735.88	40 735.88	100.00	113 147.57	338 804.58	338 804.58	299.44	120 987.97	167 664.24	87 579.57	72.39	20 000.00	0.00	80 084.67	400.42
小计	1 097 840.00	987 243.13	987 605.92	89.96	474 390.00	342 430.21	265 997.46	56.07	265 950.00	47 479.64	120 493.88	253.78	182 950.00	408 607.01	378 412.08	206.84	132 950.00	179 626.27	89 140.57	67.05	41 600.00	9 100.00	133 561.93	321.06
江苏 省本级	717 144.00	592 283.45	594 379.91	82.88	361 150.00	230 430.21	130 110.52	36.03	173 998.00	93 642.90	188 126.50	200.90	104 598.00	215 045.77	174 071.17	166.42	54 598.00	39 164.57	42 664.10	78.14	22 800.00	14 000.00	59 407.62	260.56
泗洪	133 496.00	167 154.00	167 274.58	125.30	44 000.00	44 000.00	44 094.70	100.22	33 624.00	40 000.00	39 932.22	99.83	28 024.00	35 000.00	35 092.94	125.22	17 784.00	48 154.00	38 629.00	217.21	10 064.00	0.00	9 525.72	94.65
盱眙	245 960.00	232 359.50	232 359.50	94.47	68 000.00	68 000.00	68 000.00	100.00	58 328.00	38 860.00	38 860.00	100.00	50 328.00	28 000.00	28 000.00	55.64	60 568.00	97 499.50	59 593.60	98.39	8 736.00	0.00	37 905.90	433.90
小计	1 096 600.00	991 796.95	994 013.99	90.65	473 150.00	342 430.21	242 205.22	51.19	265 950.00	172 502.90	266 918.72	154.73	182 950.00	278 045.77	237 164.11	129.63	132 950.00	184 818.07	140 886.70	105.97	41 600.00	14 000.00	106 839.24	256.83
广东 省本级	192 900.00	183 027.73	183 820.40	95.29	70 000.00	61 779.21	61 779.21	88.26	53 950.00	35 481.16	31 860.73	89.80	38 950.00	59 781.89	42 218.20	108.39	20 000.00	18 103.47	29 368.50	146.84	10 000.00	7 882.00	18 593.76	185.94
惠州市	233 550.00	213 800.00	213 800.00	91.54	80 000.00	45 000.00	45 000.00	56.25	60 000.00	28 800.00	28 800.00	100.00	45 000.00	93 000.00	93 000.00	206.67	36 950.00	47 000.00	40 000.00	108.25	11 600.00	0.00	7 000.00	60.34
惠阳区	204 000.00	187 800.00	187 800.00	92.06	86 000.00	65 000.00	65 000.00	75.58	60 000.00	25 800.00	25 800.00	100.00	30 000.00	65 000.00	65 000.00	216.67	20 000.00	32 000.00	27 000.00	135.00	8 000.00	0.00	5 000.00	62.50
徐闻	235 850.00	221 800.00	221 800.00	94.04	86 850.00	70 000.00	70 000.00	80.60	60 000.00	27 800.00	27 858.40	100.21	45 000.00	82 000.00	81 933.60	182.07	32 000.00	42 000.00	32 028.00	100.09	12 000.00	0.00	9 980.00	83.17
小计	866 300.00	806 427.73	807 220.40	93.18	322 850.00	241 779.21	241 779.21	74.89	233 950.00	117 881.16	114 319.13	96.98	158 950.00	299 781.89	282 151.80	177.51	108 950.00	139 103.47	128 396.50	117.85	41 600.00	7 882.00	40 573.76	97.53
广西 百色	929 100.00	784 045.00	784 045.00	84.39	385 650.00	241 779.21	235 450.20	61.05	233 950.00	182 769.27	163 483.05	89.45	158 950.00	199 810.90	75 605.00	47.57	108 950.00	156 185.62	270 836.85	248.59	41 600.00	3 500.00	38 669.90	92.96
小计	929 100.00	784 045.00	784 045.00	84.39	385 650.00	241 779.21	235 450.20	61.05	233 950.00	182 769.27	163 483.05	89.45	158 950.00	199 810.90	75 605.00	47.57	108 950.00	156 185.62	270 836.85	248.59	41 600.00	3 500.00	38 669.90	92.96
四川 省本级	475 162.00	449 333.43	451 131.51	94.94	230 000.00	181 979.21	178 352.21	77.54	96 640.00	37 985.69	41 663.22	109.68	71 219.00	150 955.13	78 784.00	110.62	45 003.00	73 399.02	95 981.30	213.28	32 300.00	5 014.38	56 350.78	174.46
筠连	381 058.00	354 087.67	354 087.67	92.92	82 770.00	59 800.00	63 427.00	76.63	137 310.00	84 846.80	81 219.80	95.73	87 731.00	141 651.87	94 108.80	107.27	63 947.00	67 789.00	91 162.10	142.56	9 300.00	0.00	24 169.97	259.89
小计	856 220.00	803 421.10	805 219.18	94.04	312 770.00	241 779.21	241 779.21	77.30	233 950.00	122 832.49	122 883.02	100.04	158 950.00	292 607.00	172 892.80	108.77	108 950.00	141 188.02	187 143.40	171.77	41 600.00	5 014.38	80 520.75	193.56
贵州 省本级	740 450.00	645 975.09	646 771.44	87.35	330 650.00	216 779.21	214 541.96	64.88	206 950.00	109 388.73	32 399.19	29.62	118 300.00	198 022.13	156 072.06	131.93	62 950.00	117 235.02	115 004.20	182.69	21 600.00	4 550.00	128 754.03	596.08
榕江	158 650.00	138 650.00	138 650.00	87.39	25 000.00	25 000.00	22 780.00	91.12	27 000.00	27 000.00	29 214.80	108.20	40 650.00	40 650.00	16 164.44	39.76	46 000.00	46 000.00	43 045.03	93.58	20 000.00	0.00	27 445.73	137.23
小计	899 100.00	784 625.09	785 421.44	87.36	355 650.00	241 779.21	237 321.96	66.73	233 950.00	136 388.73	61 613.99	45.18	158 950.00	238 672.13	172 236.50	108.36	108 950.00	163 235.02	158 049.23	145.07	41 600.00	4 550.00	156 199.76	375.48
总计	51 253 272.00	49 713 251.36	49 095 615.46	95.79	25 935 192.00	24 535 792.67	20 284 421.04	78.21	10 250 656.00	8 077 222.28	8 045 815.72	99.61	7 687 992.00	10 796 691.76	10 320 159.00	134.24	5 125 328.00	6 303 544.64	7 009 196.61	136.76	2 254 104.00	(0.00)	3 436 023.09	152.43

表 10 物资情况统计

品目	分配时间（年）	单价（人民币元）	金额（人民币元）	单位	数量											合计
					云南	海南	广东	广西	四川	贵州	河南	湖北	安徽	江苏	中央	
磷酸氯 / 伯喹片剂	2004	2.65	397 500.00	人份	50 000	50 000	6 250	6 250	6 250	6 250	6 250	6 250	6 250	6 250	0	150 000
双氢青蒿素片剂	2004	16.50	495 000.00	人份	10 000	20 000	0	0	0	0	0	0	0	0	0	30 000
蒿甲醚针剂	2004	33.00	396 000.00	人份	5 000	5 000	0	0	0	0	0	0	0	0	2 000	12 000
氟氯氰菊酯	2004	153.00	45 900.00	升	100	100	13	13	13	13	13	13	13	13	0	300
一次性注射器	2004	0.45	4 590.00	支	5 100	5 100	0	0	0	0	0	0	0	0	0	10 200
三目多功能显微镜	2004	46 597.65	465 976.50	台	1	1	1	1	1	1	1	1	1	1	0	10
双目生物显微镜	2004	3 973.47	794 694.00	台	100	60	5	5	5	5	5	5	5	5	0	200
台式电脑	2004	9 712.00	563 300.00	台	27	12	2	2	2	2	2	2	2	2	3	58
笔记本电脑	2004	16 180.00	647 200.00	台	5	4	2	2	2	2	2	2	2	2	15	40
服务器	2004	39 410.00	39 410.00	台	0	0	0	0	0	0	0	0	0	0	1	1
激光彩色打印机	2004	19 990.00	19 990.00	台	0	0	0	0	0	0	0	0	0	0	1	1
激光打印机	2004	1 780.00	1 780.00	台	0	0	0	0	0	0	0	0	0	0	1	1
数码相机	2004	7 840.00	39 200.00	台	1	1	0	0	0	0	0	0	0	0	3	5
蚊帐	2004	20.00	60 000.00	顶	2 000	1 000	0	0	0	0	0	0	0	0	0	3 000
磷酸氯 / 伯喹片剂	2005	2.65	605 525.00	人份	150 000	14 000	0	0	0	0	750	13 750	43 750	6 250	0	228 500
青蒿琥酯片剂	2005	10.80	216 000.00	人份	20 000	0	0	0	0	0	0	0	0	0	0	20 000
蒿甲醚针剂	2005	33.00	198 000.00	人份	5 000	1 000	0	0	0	0	0	0	0	0	0	6 000
溴氰菊酯	2005	105.00	682 500.00	公斤	4 000	2 000	0	0	0	0	0	500	0	0	0	6 500
一次性注射器	2005	0.34	2 050.00	支	5 000	1 000	0	0	0	0	0	0	0	0	0	6 000
双目生物显微镜	2005	3 999.84	607 975.68	台	100	40	3	0	3	0	0	3	3	0	0	152
台式电脑	2005	10 729.00	472 056.00	台	12	0	3	0	3	3	0	3	3	2	15	44
笔记本电脑	2005	13 900.00	250 200.00	台	0	0	0	0	1	0	1	1	1	0	14	18
激光打印机	2005	2 300.00	64 400.00	台	1	12	2	0	0	0	1	1	0	0	11	28
数码相机	2005	5 100.00	66 300.00	台	1	0	2	0	0	1	1	0	1	0	7	13
蚊帐	2005	17.50	385 000.00	顶	13 000	9 000	0	0	0	0	0	0	0	0	0	22 000
蚊帐	2005	24.18	531 960.00	顶	13 000	9 000	0	0	0	0	0	0	0	0	0	22 000
解剖镜	2005	1 800.00	7 200.00	台	0	0	0	0	0	0	0	0	0	0	4	4
喷墨彩色打印机	2005	19 990.00	19 990.00	台	0	0	0	0	0	1	0	0	0	0	0	1
多媒体投影仪	2005	17 850.00	53 550.00	台	1	1	0	0	0	0	0	0	0	0	1	3
传真机	2005	2 710.00	8 130.00	台	1	0	0	0	0	1	0	0	0	0	1	3
复印机	2005	18 029.99	18 029.99	台	1	0	0	0	0	0	0	0	0	0	0	1
便携式复印打印连体机	2005	2 450.00	2 450.00	台	0	0	0	0	0	0	0	0	0	0	1	1
专业摄像机	2005	27 500.00	27 500.00	台	0	0	0	0	0	0	0	0	0	0	1	1
面包车	2005	215 775.53	215 775.53	辆	0	1	0	0	0	0	0	0	0	0	0	1
越野车	2005	183 500.00	917 500.00	辆	5	0	0	0	0	0	0	0	0	0	0	5
丰田 4800 越野车	2005	299 146.93	604 813.86	辆	2	0	0	0	0	0	0	0	0	0	0	2
125cc 摩托车	2005	3 658.79	157 327.97	辆	33	10	0	0	0	0	0	0	0	0	0	43
面包车	2005	283 365.54	283 365.54	辆	0	0	0	0	0	0	0	0	0	0	1	1
皮卡车	2005	82 800.00	165 600.00	辆	0	2	0	0	0	0	0	0	0	0	0	2
台式电脑	2006	7 300.00	29 200.00	台	0	0	0	0	0	0	0	0	0	0	4	4
笔记本电脑	2006	17 300.00	69 200.00	台	0	0	0	0	0	0	0	0	0	0	4	4
皮卡车	2006	88 800.00	355 200.00	辆	0	4	0	0	0	0	0	0	0	0	0	4
蒿甲醚针剂	2006	36.60	43 920.00	支	1 000	200	0	0	0	0	0	0	0	0	0	1 200
溴氢菊酯	2006	90.00	180 000.00	公斤	2 000	0	0	0	0	0	0	0	0	0	0	2 000
青蒿琥酯片剂	2006	14.52	50 820.00	瓶	3 500	0	0	0	0	0	0	0	0	0	0	3 500
蒿甲醚针剂	2006	36.60	128 100.00	支	2 000	1 500	0	0	0	0	0	0	0	0	0	3 500
摩托车	2006	3 800.00	539 600.00	辆	0	142	0	0	0	0	0	0	0	0	0	142
越野车	2006	183 600.00	1 101 600.00	辆	6	0	0	0	0	0	0	0	0	0	0	6
数码相机 IXUS750	2006	3 440.00	37 840.00	台	0	0	0	0	0	0	0	1	0	0	10	11
显微镜	2007	3 756.85	578 554.90	台	50	72	4	4	4	4	4	4	4	4	0	154
越野车 途胜	2007	128 000.00	128 000.00	辆	0	1	0	0	0	0	0	0	0	0	0	1
复方磷酸哌喹	2007	0.34	68 000.00	片	150 000	50 000	0	0	0	0	0	0	0	0	0	200 000
蒿甲醚针剂	2007	36.60	54 900.00	盒	0	1 500	0	0	0	0	0	0	0	0	0	1 500
青蒿琥酯片剂	2007	12.80	38 400.00	盒	3 000	0	0	0	0	0	0	0	0	0	0	3 000
磷酸伯 / 氨喹	2007	4.10	426 400.00	人份	63 000	0	4 000	4 000	4 000	4 000	4 000	4 000	13 000	4 000	0	104 000
注射器（5ml）	2007	0.38	2 850.00	支	0	7 500	0	0	0	0	0	0	0	0	0	7 500
长效蚊帐	2007	37.43	262 010.00	顶	5 000	2 000	0	0	0	0	0	0	0	0	0	7 000
合计			14 628 334.97													

表 11 固定资产分配表

品目	分配时间（年）	采购时间（年.月.日）	型号	单价（人民币元）	金额（人民币元）	单位	数量											合计
							云南	海南	广东	广西	四川	贵州	河南	湖北	安徽	江苏	中央	
三目多功能显微镜	2004	2004.03.22	OLYMPUS SZX9	46 597.65	465 976.50	台	1	1	1	1	1	1	1	1	1	1	0	10
双目生物显微镜	2004	2004.03.22	OLYMPUS CX21	3 973.47	794 694.00	台	100	60	5	5	5	5	5	5	5	5	0	200
台式电脑	2004	2004.01.05	DELL GX270SMT	9 712.00	563 300.00	台	27	12	2	2	2	2	2	2	2	2	3	58
笔记本电脑	2004	2004.01.05	东芝 PORTEGE A100	16 180.00	647 200.00	台	5	4	2	2	2	2	2	2	2	2	15	40
服务器	2004	2004.3	DELL 4600	39 410.00	39 410.00	台	0	0	0	0	0	0	0	0	0	0	1	1
激光彩色打印机	2004	2004.3	Hp 4600	19 990.00	19 990.00	台	0	0	0	0	0	0	0	0	0	0	1	1
激光打印机	2004	2004.3	Hp1010	1 780.00	1 780.00	台	0	0	0	0	0	0	0	0	0	0	1	1
数码相机	2004	2004.3	SONY V1	7 840.00	39 200.00	台	1	1	0	0	0	0	0	0	0	0	3	5
双目生物显微镜	2005	2004.12	OLYMPUS CX21	3 999.84	607 975.68	台	100	40	3	0	3	0	0	3	3	0	0	152
台式电脑	2005	2004.11.03	DELL 280SMT	10 729.00	472 056.00	台	12	0	3	0	3	3	0	3	3	2	15	44
笔记本电脑	2005	2004.11.03	东芝 PORTEGE A100	13 900.00	250 200.00	台	0	0	0	0	1	0	1	1	1	0	14	18
激光打印机	2005	2004.11.03	HP 1015	2 300.00	64 400.00	台	1	12	2	0	0	0	1	1	0	0	11	28
数码相机	2005	2004.11.03	SONY 717	5 100.00	66 300.00	台	1	0	2	0	0	1	1	0	1	0	7	13
解剖镜	2005	2004.12	Pxs-V1	1 800.00	7 200.00	台	0	0	0	0	0	0	0	0	0	0	4	4
喷墨彩色打印机	2005	2004.12	HP4600	19 990.00	19 990.00	台	0	0	0	0	0	1	0	0	0	0	0	1
多媒体投影仪	2005	2004.12	LG RD-JT30	17 850.00	53 550.00	台	1	1	0	0	0	0	0	0	0	0	1	3
传真机	2005	2004.12	KX-FL 553	2 710.00	8 130.00	台	1	0	0	0	0	1	0	0	0	0	1	3
复印机	2005	2004.12	V330	18 029.99	18 029.99	台	0	0	0	0	0	0	0	0	0	0	1	1
便携式复印打印连体机	2005	2004.12	FC 298	2 450.00	2 450.00	台	0	0	0	0	0	0	0	0	0	0	1	1

续表

品目	分配时间（年）	采购时间（年.月.日）	型号	单价（人民币元）	金额（人民币元）	单位	数量											合计
							云南	海南	广东	广西	四川	贵州	河南	湖北	安徽	江苏	中央	
专业摄像机	2005	2004.12	SONY PD190	27 500.00	27 500.00	台	0	0	0	0	0	0	0	0	0	0	1	1
面包车	2005	2005.07.08	丰田海狮 TRH213L-JDMNK	215 775.53	215 775.53	辆	0	1	0	0	0	0	0	0	0	0	0	1
越野车	2005	2005.03.30	ZN6452WAG 帕拉丁越野车	183 500.00	917 500.00	辆	5	0	0	0	0	0	0	0	0	0	0	5
丰田 4800 越野车	2005	2005.07.08	丰田霸道 GRJ120L-GKAGKV	299 146.93	604 813.86	辆	2	0	0	0	0	0	0	0	0	0	0	2
125cc 摩托车	2005	2004.12.08	隆鑫 LX125-A	3 658.79	157 327.97	辆	33	10	0	0	0	0	0	0	0	0	0	43
面包车	2005	2005.11.23	丰田 普瑞维亚	283 365.54	283 365.54	辆	0	0	0	0	0	0	0	0	0	0	1	1
皮卡车	2005	2004.12.05	长城赛铃 CC1027S	82 800.00	165 600.00	辆	0	2	0	0	0	0	0	0	0	0	0	2
台式电脑	2006	2006.05.17	DELL GX520	7 300.00	29 200.00	台	0	0	0	0	0	0	0	0	0	0	4	4
笔记本电脑	2006	2006.05.17	IBM T43-26680RC	17 300.00	69 200.00	台	0	0	0	0	0	0	0	0	0	0	4	4
皮卡车	2006	2006.09.12	NISSAN ZN1021U2S	88 800.00	355 200.00	辆	0	4	0	0	0	0	0	0	0	0	0	4
摩托车	2006	2006.10.31	隆鑫 125CC	3 800.00	539 600.00	辆	0	142	0	0	0	0	0	0	0	0	0	142
越野车	2006	2006.11.30	ZN6452WAG 帕拉丁越野车	183 600.00	1 101 600.00	辆	6	0	0	0	0	0	0	0	0	0	0	6
数码相机 IXUS750	2006	2006.05.21	佳能 IXUS 750	3 440.00	37 840.00	台	0	0	0	0	0	0	0	1	0	0	10	11
显微镜	2007	2006.09.12	OLYMPLUS CX21	3 756.85	578 554.90	台	50	72	4	4	4	4	4	4	4	4	0	154
越野车 途胜	2007	2006.12.01	现代途胜 4X4	128 000.00	128 000.00	辆	0	1	0	0	0	0	0	0	0	0	0	1
固定资产合计					9 352 909.97													

表 12 卫生产品分配表

品目	分配时间	单价	金额(元)	单位	数量											合计
					云南	海南	广东	广西	四川	贵州	河南	湖北	安徽	江苏	中央	
蒿甲醚针剂	2004	2.65	397 500.00	人份	50 000	50 000	6 250	6 250	6 250	6 250	6 250	6 250	6 250	6 250	0	150 000
双氢青蒿素片剂	2004	16.50	495 000.00	人份	10 000	20 000	0	0	0	0	0	0	0	0	0	30 000
蒿甲醚针剂	2004	33.00	396 000.00	人份	5 000	5 000	0	0	0	0	0	0	0	0	2 000	12 000
氟氯氰菊酯	2004	153.00	45 900.00	升	100	100	13	13	13	13	13	13	13	13	0	300
一次性注射器	2004	0.45	4 590.00	支	5 100	5 100	0	0	0	0	0	0	0	0	0	10 200
蚊帐	2004	20.00	60 000.00	顶	2 000	1 000	0	0	0	0	0	0	0	0	0	3 000
蒿甲醚针剂	2005	2.65	605 525.00	人份	150 000	14 000	0	0	0	0	750	13 750	43 750	6 250	0	228 500
青蒿琥酯片剂	2005	10.80	216 000.00	人份	20 000	0	0	0	0	0	0	0	0	0	0	20 000
蒿甲醚针剂	2005	33.00	198 000.00	人份	5 000	1 000	0	0	0	0	0	0	0	0	0	6 000
溴氰菊酯	2005	105.00	682 500.00	公斤	4 000	2 000	0	0	0	0	0	500	0	0	0	6 500
一次性注射器	2005	0.34	2 050.00	支	5 000	1 000	0	0	0	0	0	0	0	0	0	6 000
蚊帐	2005	17.50	385 000.00	顶	13 000	9 000	0	0	0	0	0	0	0	0	0	22 000
蚊帐 2	2005	24.18	531 960.00	顶	13 000	9 000	0	0	0	0	0	0	0	0	0	22 000
蒿甲醚针剂	2006	36.60	43 920.00	支	1 000	200	0	0	0	0	0	0	0	0	0	1 200
溴氢菊酯	2006	90.00	180 000.00	公斤	2 000	0	0	0	0	0	0	0	0	0	0	2 000
青蒿琥酯片	2006	14.52	50 820.00	瓶	3 500	0	0	0	0	0	0	0	0	0	0	3 500
蒿甲醚针剂	2006	36.60	128 100.00	支	2 000	1 500	0	0	0	0	0	0	0	0	0	3 500
复方磷酸哌喹	2007	0.34	68 000.00	片	150 000	50 000	0	0	0	0	0	0	0	0	0	200 000
蒿甲醚针剂	2007	36.60	54 900.00	盒	0	1 500	0	0	0	0	0	0	0	0	0	1 500
青蒿琥酯片剂	2007	12.80	38 400.00	盒	3 000	0	0	0	0	0	0	0	0	0	0	3 000
磷酸伯 / 氨喹	2007	4.10	426 400.00	人份	63 000	0	4 000	4 000	4 000	4 000	4 000	4 000	13 000	4 000	0	104 000
注射器(5ml)	2007	0.38	2 850.00	支	0	7 500	0	0	0	0	0	0	0	0	0	7 500
长效蚊帐	2007	37.43	262 010.00	顶	5 000	2 000	0	0	0	0	0	0	0	0	0	7 000
卫生产品合计			5 275 425.00													

附录 2：终期评估报告附表

表 1 全球基金疟疾项目单位基本情况表

<table>
<tr><td colspan="2">评估时间</td><td colspan="2">评估组长</td><td colspan="2">评估组组长</td><td></td></tr>
<tr><td colspan="2">被评估单位全称</td><td colspan="5"></td></tr>
<tr><td colspan="2">单位主管部门</td><td colspan="5"></td></tr>
<tr><td colspan="2" rowspan="2">开户银行情况</td><td colspan="2">开户银行名称</td><td colspan="3"></td></tr>
<tr><td colspan="2">开户账号</td><td colspan="3"></td></tr>
<tr><td colspan="2">单位地址</td><td colspan="3"></td><td>邮编</td><td></td></tr>
<tr><td colspan="2">单位负责人</td><td></td><td>职务</td><td></td><td>电话</td><td></td></tr>
<tr><td colspan="2">项目负责人</td><td></td><td>职务</td><td></td><td>电话</td><td></td></tr>
<tr><td colspan="2">财务负责人</td><td></td><td>职务</td><td></td><td>电话</td><td></td></tr>
<tr><td colspan="2">单位性质</td><td colspan="3"></td><td>单位人数</td><td></td></tr>
<tr><td rowspan="11">项目办人员情况</td><td>姓名</td><td>职称（岗位）</td><td>学历</td><td>联系电话</td><td colspan="2">E-mail</td></tr>
<tr><td></td><td></td><td></td><td></td><td></td><td></td></tr>
<tr><td></td><td></td><td></td><td></td><td></td><td></td></tr>
<tr><td></td><td></td><td></td><td></td><td></td><td></td></tr>
<tr><td></td><td></td><td></td><td></td><td></td><td></td></tr>
<tr><td></td><td></td><td></td><td></td><td></td><td></td></tr>
<tr><td></td><td></td><td></td><td></td><td></td><td></td></tr>
<tr><td></td><td></td><td></td><td></td><td></td><td></td></tr>
<tr><td></td><td></td><td></td><td></td><td></td><td></td></tr>
<tr><td></td><td></td><td></td><td></td><td></td><td></td></tr>
<tr><td></td><td></td><td></td><td></td><td></td><td></td></tr>
</table>

表 2 工作计划完成情况调查评估表

填表单位：　　　　　　　　　　　　　　　　　　　　　　　　填表日期：　年　月　日

评估项目	评估指标	年度	计划目标（A）	实际完成（A）	完成率 (%)（A）	评分 (B)*	预算 (A)	实际支出 (A)	执行率 (%)(A)	备注
目标 1：使云南省边境地区流动人口更好地获得疟疾诊断和合理治疗（10 分）	边境流动人口发热病人血检（5 分）	2003								
		2004								
		2005								
		2006								
		2007								
		合计								
	边境流动人口疟疾病人规范治疗（5 分）	2003								
		2004								
		2005								
		2006								
		2007								
		合计								
目标 2：使目标地区当地居民得到更好的早期诊断和个人防护（35 分）	项目地区居民发热病人血检（5 分）	2003								
		2004								
		2005								
		2006								
		2007								
		合计								

续表

填表单位：　　　　　　　　　　　　　　　　　　　　填表日期：　年　月　日

评估项目	评估指标	年度	计划目标（A）	实际完成（A）	完成率(%)（A）	评分(B)*	预算(A)	实际支出(A)	执行率(%)(A)	备注
	项目地区居民疟疾病人规范治疗（5分）	2003								
		2004								
		2005								
		2006								
		2007								
		合计								
	乡、村医生/个体医生培训（5分）	2003								
		2004								
		2005								
		2006								
		2007								
		合计								
	镜检员培训（5分）	2003								
		2004								
		2005								
		2006								
		2007								
		合计								
	药浸蚊帐（5分）	2003								
		2004								
		2005								
		2006								
		2007								
		合计								

续表

填表单位：　　　　　　　　　　　　　　　　　　　　　　　　填表日期：　年　月　日

评估项目	评估指标	年度	计划目标(A)	实际完成(A)	完成率(%)(A)	评分(B)*	预算(A)	实际支出(A)	执行率(%)(A)	备注
	高危人群预防服药(5分)	2003								
		2004								
		2005								
		2006								
		2007								
		合计								
	疟疾暴发流行控制(5分)	2003								
		2004								
		2005								
		2006								
		2007								
		合计								
目标3：使云南省和海南省流行区居民更有效地采取疟疾预防措施，及时治疗(20分)	健康教育材料印制(4分)	2003								
		2004								
		2005								
		2006								
		2007								
		合计								
	健康教育人员培训(4分)	2003								
		2004								
		2005								
		2006								
		2007								
		合计								

续表

填表单位：　　　　　　　　　　　　　　　　　　　　填表日期：　年　月　日

评估项目	评估指标	年度	计划目标(A)	实际完成(A)	完成率(%)(A)	评分(B)*	预算(A)	实际支出(A)	执行率(%)(A)	备注
	云南和海南项目县用广播进行疟疾知识宣传(4分)	2003								
		2004								
		2005								
		2006								
		2007								
		合计								
	云南和海南项目县中小学生疟防知识课(4分)	2003								
		2004								
		2005								
		2006								
		2007								
		合计								
	云南和海南项目县在公共场所张贴疟疾知识宣传画(4分)	2003								
		2004								
		2005								
		2006								
		2007								
		合计								
目标4：优化云南、海南及其他八个项目省的疟疾控制项目管理(35分)	项目地区哨点病例主动监测(5分)	2003								
		2004								
		2005								
		2006								
		2007								
		合计								

续表

填表单位：　　　　　　　　　　　　　　　　　　填表日期：　年　月　日

评估项目	评估指标	年度	计划目标（A）	实际完成（A）	完成率(%)（A）	评分(B)*	预算(A)	实际支出(A)	执行率(%)(A)	备注
	项目地区药物抗性监测（5分）	2003								
		2004								
		2005								
		2006								
		2007								
		合计								
	项目地区媒介监测（5分）	2003								
		2004								
		2005								
		2006								
		2007								
		合计								
	项目地区专项调查（5分）	2003								
		2004								
		2005								
		2006								
		2007								
		合计								
	疫情报告网络运行维护	2003	/	/	/	/				
		2004	/	/	/	/				
		2005	/	/	/	/				
		2006	/	/	/	/				
		2007	/	/	/	/				
		合计	/	/	/	/				
	项目办日常管理	2003	/	/	/	/				
		2004	/	/	/	/				
		2005	/	/	/	/				
		2006	/	/	/	/				
		2007	/	/	/	/				
		合计	/	/	/	/				

续表

填表单位：　　　　　　　　　　　　　　　　填表日期：　年　月　日

评估项目	评估指标	年度	计划目标(A)	实际完成(A)	完成率(%)(A)	评分(B)*	预算(A)	实际支出(A)	执行率(%)(A)	备注
	项目会议(5分)	2003								
		2004								
		2005								
		2006								
		2007								
		合计								
	项目督导(10分)	2003								
		2004								
		2005								
		2006								
		2007								
		合计								
		总计								

表 3　考核指标达标情况调查评估表

填表单位：　　　　　　　　　　　　　　　　　　　　填表日期：　年　月　日

评估项目	评估指标	基线 (A)		终期目标 (A)	终期调查 (A)		指标达标率 (%) (A)	评分 (B)	评分说明	备注
		值	年月	值	值	年月				
疟疾调查推断发病率(40 分)	疟疾调查推断发病率 (40 分)								根据指标达标率评分 指标达标率≥ 90% 评分 40 :80%—90% 评分 30 :60%—80% 评分 20 :50%—60% 评分 10 < 50% 评分 0	
居民疟防知识与行为改变(40 分)	目标地区中小学生能够正确回答至少 3 个与疟疾相关问题的比例(10 分)								根据指标达标率评分 指标达标率≥ 90% 评分 10 :80%—90% 评分 7 :60%—80% 评分 5 :50%—60% 评分 3 < 50% 评分 0	
	发热病人在症状出现 2 天内求诊的比例(15 分)								根据指标达标率评分 指标达标率≥ 90% 评分 15 指标达标率：80%—90% 评分 12 指标达标率：60%—80% 评分 10 指标达标率：50%—60% 评分 5 指标达标率< 50% 评分 0	
	拥有杀虫剂浸泡蚊帐的家庭比例(15 分)								根据指标达标率评分 指标达标率≥ 90% 评分 15 :80%—90% 评分 12 :60%—80% 评分 10 :50%—60% 评分 5 < 50% 评分 0	
网络直报疟疾病人比例(20 分)	网络直报疟疾病人比例(20分)								根据指标达标率评分 指标达标率≥ 90% 评分 20 :80%—90% 评分 15 :60%—80% 评分 10 :50%—60% 评分 5 < 50% 评分 0	
得分总计										

注：本表请根据终期评估传面调查结果填写。

表 4　项目管理能力评估表

填表单位：　　　　　　　　　　　　　　　　　　　　　　填表日期：　年　月　日

评估项目	评估指标	评估方式	评分	评分说明	备注
项目办公室建设和运转情况(30 分)	项目办机构健全、规章制度完善(20 分)	查阅文件，实地调查		项目办工作正常运行　5 分 项目办人员职责清晰　5 分 项目办工作规章制度齐全　10 分	
	各项目省、县按计划召开或参加项目年会、例会(10 分)	查阅文件		按照工作计划召开或参加会议　5 分 会议记录齐全　5 分	
项目工作计划和总结(30 分)	制定项目年度和季度工作计划(6 分)	查阅文件		制定了项目年度工作计划　3 分 制定了项目季度工作计划　3 分	
	制定各项具体活动的实施方案(4 分)	查阅文件		各项项目活动都有实施方案　4 分	
	项目工作记录规范(10 分)	查阅文件		项目工作有记录　7 分 项目工作记录细致清楚　3 分	
	项目活动有总结(4 分)	查阅文件		项目活动结束后都有总结　4 分	
	按规定及时上报项目报表和报告(6 分)	查阅文件，实地调查		及时上报项目报表和报告　3 分 报表填写规范　3 分	
项目培训(40 分)	按计划组织开展项目培训活动(15)	查阅文件，实地调查		按工作计划开展或参加培训　5 分 培训内容针对当前项目需要　5 分 培训的记录、资料齐全　5 分	
	项目管理和执行人员按要求参加有关的项目培训(25)	查阅文件，实地调查		根据项目执行人员培训覆盖率评分 覆盖率≥ 90% 评分 25 :80%—90% 评分 20 :60%—80% 评分 15 :50%—60% 评分 5 < 50% 评分 0	
得分总计					

表 5　M&E 管理能力评估表

填表单位：　　　　　　　　　　　　　　　　　填表日期：　年　月　日

评估指标	评估方式	评分	评分说明	备注
有专人负责项目数据、报表的收集、审核、汇总和上报工作（20 分）	查阅文件，实地调查		专人负责报表的收集、汇总和上报　10 分 专人负责报表的审核　10 分	
项目季度报表上报及时、填写规范、数据准确（20 分）	查阅文件		报表上报及时　5 分 报表填写规范　5 分 报表数据准确　10 分	
项目办有制定或使用指导 M&E 工作的指南和模板（15 分）	查阅文件		有 M&E 工作的指南和模板　15 分	
组织开展或参加相关培训（15 分）	查阅文件，实地调查		组织开展或参加相关培训　5 分 培训记录、资料齐全，内容有针对性　10 分	
项目督导规范、有成效（30 分）	查阅文件，实地调查		按照工作计划开展督导　5 分 有督导通知、督导报告　5 分 督导过程有记录　10 分 督导后跟踪整改情况　10 分	
得分总计				

表 6 项目资金收支情况表

填表单位： 填表日期： 年 月 日

周期序号	年度	科目	目标 1		目标 2		目标 3		目标 4		合计	
			人民币	百分比	人民币	百分比	人民币	百分比	人民币	百分比	人民币	百分比
项目一期	2003—2004	预算										
		到款										
		支出										
项目二期	2005	预算										
		到款										
		支出										
	2006	预算										
		到款										
		支出										
	2007	预算										
		到款										
		支出										
	2008	预算										
		到款										
		支出										
累计		预算										
		到款										
		支出										
		结余										

注：①预算数根据工作计划填写（折算汇率 1：8），到款数为实际收到拨款数，支出数为实际支出数，结余数为截止 07 年 12 月 31 日项目资金结余数。

②预算拨付率＝到款数 / 预算数；预算执行率＝支出数 / 预算数；资金结余率＝结余数 / 到款数。

表 7　财务人员情况调查表

填表单位：　　　　　　　　　　　　　　　　填表日期：　年　月　日

姓名	性别	文化程度（学历）	岗位	从事财务工作年限	接受项目财务培训次数	专兼职情况	是否会使用项目财务软件	全球基金项目管理任务占总工作量的比重

表 8 财务督导情况调查表

填表单位：

年份	接受本级以上财务督导次数	对本级以下财务督导次数
2003		
2004		
2005		
2006		
2007		
合计		

表 9　设备物资情况调查表

填表单位：　　　　　　　　　　　　　　　　　　　　　　　　　　　　填表日期：

设备物资名称	数量	总金额（人民币 元）	获得途径	下拨时间	运行情况	是否为项目专用	备注
显微镜							
计算机							
打印机							
传真机							
4 轮驱动皮卡车							
125C 摩托车							
越野车 / 面包车							
商务车							
…							
设备小计	–		–	–	–	–	–
磷酸氯 / 伯喹片剂							
双氢青蒿素片剂							
蒿甲醚针剂							
青蒿琥酯片剂							
磷酸伯氨喹片剂							
一次性注射器							
长效蚊帐							
快速诊断试纸条（RDT）							
…							
物资小计	–		–	–	–	–	–
设备物资合计	–		–	–	–	–	–

注：1 设备物资栏可根据各项目单位实际情况增减；

2 运行情况分良好、报废、毁损、遗失四种情况填写；

3 获得途径栏填写项目拨入或自购。

表 10 财务及物资管理评分表

评估单位		评估组长	
评估时间		总 分	
评估项目	内 容	100 分	实得分
一、财务人员队伍建设	1．各级项目办财务人员配置是否齐全	5	
	2．各级项目办财务人员不相容职务是否分人担任	2	
	3．财务人员与项目人员沟通是否经常沟通	3	
二、预算制订与预算执行	1．财务人员是否参与、了解项目预算	2	
	2．项目支出标准是否符合预算标准	2	
	3．项目资金的使用是否与工作计划相对应	2	
	4．预算调整是否有批准	4	
三、项目资金管理	1．银行账号是否独立设置	2	
	2．是否严格遵守中国人民银行颁布的《现金管理暂行条例》和《银行存款支付结算办法》	3	
	3．现金日记账和银行存款日记账是否账实相符	3	
	4．是否使用“全球基金项目空白票据购置、领用登记簿”，及时登记空白票据的购入、使用和结存	2	
四、项目财务管理	1．是否有相关的项目财务管理、物资管理制度及实施情况	2	
	2．项目资金支出是否严格执行授权批准制度，是否使用全球基金专用凭证	2	
	3．项目资金使用是否合规，是否存在挤占挪用项目资金的情况	2	
	4.是否将全球基金资金按照病种建账管理、是否分工作目标进行财务核算	2	
	5．是否使用《全球基金财务管理手册》规定的会计科目进行财务核算，科目使用是否合理	2	
五、报表及审计	1．调阅财务季报、半年报和年报，是否账表相符	5	
	2．省、市、县级项目每年是否进行了审计，是否有审计报告	5	

续表

评估单位		评估组长	
评估时间		总　分	
评估项目	内　容	100分	实得分
六、会计档案管理	调阅项目会计资料，检查财务票据、账簿、报表的装订和保管情况	10	
七、项目物资管理	1. 项目固定资产和药品的采购是否按工作计划完成，是否及时下拨给省、县级项目点	2	
	2. 项目固定资产和药品的调拨、领用手续是否健全	2	
	3. 是否按照《全球基金财务管理手册》的要求，建立相应的固定资产和项目物品辅助账	4	
	4. 清点全球基金项目固定资产和药品，检查账实是否相符	2	
八、培训及督导	1. 各级项目点是否按照工作计划对下一级项目点财务人员进行了培训和督导	5	
	2. 各级项目点是否有督导、培训资料	5	
九、内部控制制度	1. 是否有项目的内部控制制度	1	
	2. 是否有授权批准控制	1	
	3. 财产保全控制	2	
	4. 内部报告控制	3	
	5. 财务电子信息系统的数据输入与输出、文件储存与保管、网络安全等方面的控制	3	
十、其他	根据项目点具体情况，提出评估要求和内容	10	

表 11　项目地区疟防投入调查表

调查项目	调查内容	印象描述	备注
卫生行政部门组织和支持项目活动	卫生行政部门将本项目作为疟疾防治规划的重要部分		
	卫生行政部门对项目的支持和参与程度		
疟疾防治资金投入		项目执行五年内,项目地区疟防资金投入 总额为　　　元; 其中全球基金项目资金投入占　　% 政府资金投入占　% 其他资金来源占　% 评价:	

注:本表请根据座谈、实地调查后主观印象填写,请在“印象描述一栏”填写您对该项目地区各项调查内容现状的评价。

表 12　疟疾防治资金投入情况表

单位：万元

年度	政府支持	全球基金			其他	合计
		第一轮	第五轮	第六轮		
2003						
2004						
2005						
2006						
2007						
合计						
所占比例(%)						—

填表单位：　　　　填表日期：　年　月　日

附录3：管理方案附表

表1　全球基金疟疾项目单位基本情况表

分级	数据管理流程说明		负责人	时限要求
村级	涂制血片，填写送检单，及时送乡卫生院血检。		村医	每月
	填写“疟疾项目病人诊治月登记表”一式两份并保存其中一份			
	上报“疟疾项目病人诊治月登记表”一份			
乡级	村级送检资料	保存其送检资料，及时血检和记录，并核定其“疟疾项目病人诊治月登记表”。	乡卫生院防保组	每月
	乡个体医送检资料	涂制血片，填写送检单，及时送乡卫生院血检。	乡个体医生	
		填写“疟疾项目病人诊治月登记表”一式两份并保存其中一份		
		上报“疟疾项目病人诊治月登记表”一份		
		保存其送检资料，及时血检和记录，并核定其“疟疾项目病人诊治月登记表”。	乡卫生院防保组	
	乡卫生院本级血检资料	血检门诊病人，根据血检记录核定其“疟疾项目病人诊治月登记表”。	乡卫生院防保组	
	编制和上报乡级月汇总表			

续表

分级	数据管理流程说明		负责人	时限要求
县级	乡级上报资料	核实和保存乡级上报资料	县项目办	每月
	县级医院血检资料	血检门诊病人，根据血检记录填写“疟疾项目病人诊治月登记表”。	县级医院	
		收集、核实其“疟疾项目病人诊治月登记表”相关数据。	县项目办	
	县 CDC 血检资料	血检门诊病人，根据血检记录填写“疟疾项目病人诊治月登记表”。	县 CDC	
		收集、核实其“疟疾项目病人诊治月登记表”相关数据。	县项目办	
	编制和上报县级月汇总表		县项目办	
	编制和上报县级季度报表		县项目办	季度结束15日内
省级	核实和保存县级上报表		省项目办	季度结束30日内
	编制省级季度汇总表			
	编制和上报省级季度报表			
国家级	核实和保存省级季度上报表		国家项目办	季度结束45日内
	编制国家级季度汇总表			
	编制和上报国家级季度报表			

表2 第____轮 流动人口发热病人血检的人数和比例乡级汇总表

___乡 __年 __季度　　　　填表人：　　　　填表日期：　　　　上报单位盖章：

行政村		____月份		____月份		____月份		合计	
		发热病人数	血检人数	发热病人数	血检人数	发热病人数	血检人数	发热病人数	血检人数
	村医送检								
	乡个体医送检								
	乡卫生院本级血检								
	小计								
	村医送检								
	乡个体医送检								
	乡卫生院本级血检								
	小计								
	村医送检								
	乡个体医送检								
	乡卫生院本级血检								
	小计								
	村医送检								
	乡个体医送检								
	乡卫生院本级血检								
	小计								
	村医送检								
	乡个体医送检								
	乡卫生院本级血检								
	小计								
	村医送检								
	乡个体医送检								
	乡卫生院本级血检								
	小计								
	村医送检								
	乡个体医送检								
	乡卫生院本级血检								
	小计								
	村医送检								

续表

	乡个体医送检
	乡卫生院本级血检
	小计
	村医送检
	乡个体医送检
	乡卫生院本级血检
	小计
	村医送检
	乡个体医送检
	乡卫生院本级血检
	小计
合计	村医送检
	乡个体医送检
	乡卫生院本级血检
	小计

表3 第____轮 流动人口发热病人血检的人数和比例县级汇总表

___乡__年__季度　　　　填表人：　　　　填表日期：　　　　上报单位盖章：

项目乡镇		____月份			____月份			____月份			合计		
		发热病人数	血检人数	血检率(%)	发热病人数	血检人数	血检率(%)	发热病人数	血检人数	血检率(%)	发热病人数	血检人数	血检率(%)
	乡级上报												
	县 CDC 血检												
	县级医院血检												
	小计												
	乡级上报												
	县 CDC 血检												
	县级医院血检												
	小计												
	乡级上报												
	县 CDC 血检												
	县级医院血检												
	小计												
	乡级上报												
	县 CDC 血检												
	县级医院血检												
	小计												
	乡级上报												
	县 CDC 血检												
	县级医院血检												
	小计												

续表

___乡__年__季度　　填表人：　　填表日期：　　上报单位盖章：

项目乡镇		___月份			___月份			___月份			合计		
		发热病人数	血检人数	血检率（%）	发热病人数	血检人数	血检率（%）	发热病人数	血检人数	血检率（%）	发热病人数	血检人数	血检率（%）
	乡级上报												
	县 CDC 血检												
	县级医院血检												
	小计												
	乡级上报												
	县 CDC 血检												
	县级医院血检												
	小计												
	乡级上报												
	县 CDC 血检												
	县级医院血检												
	小计												
	乡级上报												
	县 CDC 血检												
	县级医院血检												
	小计												
合计	乡级上报												
	县 CDC 血检												
	县级医院血检												
	小计												

表 4　第 ___ 轮流动人口发热病人血检的人数和比例省级汇总表

___ 乡 __ 年 __ 季度　　填表人：　　填表日期：　　上报单位盖章：

项目县	第 1 季度			第 2 季度			第 3 季度			第 4 季度			合计		
	发热病人数	血检人数	血检率（%）	发热病人数	血检人数	血检率（%）	发热病人数	血检人数	血检率（%）	发热病人数	血检人数	血检率（%）	发热病人数	血检人数	血检率（%）
合计															

表 5 第 ___ 轮流动人口发热病人血检的人数和比例国家级汇总表

__ 年　　填表人：　　填表日期：　　上报单位盖章：

项目省	第 1 季度			第 2 季度			第 3 季度			第 4 季度			合计		
	发热病人数	血检人数	血检率(%)	发热病人数	血检人数	血检率(%)	发热病人数	血检人数	血检率(%)	发热病人数	血检人数	血检率(%)	发热病人数	血检人数	血检率(%)
合计															

表6 第 ___ 轮接受规范治疗的当地居民疟疾病人通过显微镜确诊的人数和比例乡级汇总表

___ 乡 __ 年 __ 季度　　　填表人：　　　填表日期：　　　上报单位盖章：

行政村		___月份		___月份		___月份		合计	
		规范治疗数	血检确诊数	规范治疗数	血检确诊数	规范治疗数	血检确诊数	规范治疗数	血检确诊数
	村医诊治								
	乡个体医诊治								
	乡卫生院诊治								
	小计								
	村医诊治								
	乡个体医诊治								
	乡卫生院诊治								
	小计								
	村医诊治								
	乡个体医诊治								
	乡卫生院诊治								
	小计								
	村医诊治								
	乡个体医诊治								
	乡卫生院诊治								
	小计								
	村医诊治								
	乡个体医诊治								
	乡卫生院诊治								
	小计								
	村医诊治								
	乡个体医诊治								
	乡卫生院诊治								
	小计								
	村医诊治								
	乡个体医诊治								
	乡卫生院诊治								
	小计								
	村医诊治								
	乡个体医诊治								
	乡卫生院诊治								
	小计								
	村医诊治								
	乡个体医诊治								
	乡卫生院诊治								
	小计								
	村医诊治								
	乡个体医诊治								
	乡卫生院诊治								
	小计								
合计	村医诊治								
	乡个体医诊治								
	乡卫生院诊治								
	小计								

表 7　第 ___ 轮接受规范治疗的当地居民疟疾病人通过显微镜确诊的人数和比例县级汇总表

___ 乡 __ 年 __ 季度　　　填表人：　　　填表日期：　　　上报单位盖章：

项目乡镇		____月份			____月份			____月份			合计		
		规范治疗数	血检确诊数	确诊率(%)	规范治疗数	血检确诊数	确诊率(%)	规范治疗数	血检确诊数	确诊率(%)	规范治疗数	血检确诊数	确诊率(%)
	乡级上报												
	县 CDC 诊治												
	县级医院诊治												
	小计												
	乡级上报												
	县 CDC 诊治												
	县级医院诊治												
	小计												
	乡级上报												
	县 CDC 诊治												
	县级医院诊治												
	小计												
	乡级上报												
	县 CDC 诊治												
	县级医院诊治												
	小计												
	乡级上报												
	县 CDC 诊治												
	县级医院诊治												
	小计												
	乡级上报												
	县 CDC 诊治												

___乡__年__季度　　　填表人：　　填表日期：　　上报单位盖章：

项目乡镇		___月份			___月份			___月份			合计		
		规范治疗数	血检确诊数	确诊率（%）	规范治疗数	血检确诊数	确诊率（%）	规范治疗数	血检确诊数	确诊率（%）	规范治疗数	血检确诊数	确诊率（%）
	县级医院诊治												
	小计												
	乡级上报												
	县 CDC 诊治												
	县级医院诊治												
	小计												
	乡级上报												
	县 CDC 诊治												
	县级医院诊治												
	小计												
	乡级上报												
	县 CDC 诊治												
	县级医院诊治												
	小计												
	乡级上报												
	县 CDC 诊治												
	县级医院诊治												
	小计												
合计	乡级上报												
	县 CDC 诊治												
	县级医院诊治												
	小计												

表 8　第　轮 ___ 接受规范治疗的当地居民疟疾病人通过显微镜确诊的人数和比例省级汇总表

___ 省 __ 年　　　　填表人：　　　　填表日期：

项目县	第 1 季度			第 2 季度			第 3 季度			第 4 季度			合计		
	规范治疗数	血检确诊数	确诊率(%)	规范治疗数	血检确诊数	确诊率(%)	规范治疗数	血检确诊数	确诊率(%)	规范治疗数	血检确诊数	确诊率(%)	规范治疗数	血检确诊数	确诊率(%)
合计															

表 9　第 ___ 轮接受规范治疗的当地居民疟疾病人通过显微镜确诊的人数和比例国家级汇总表

___ 年　　　　填表人：　　　　填表日期：

项目省	第 1 季度			第 2 季度			第 3 季度			第 4 季度			合计		
	规范治疗数	血检确诊数	确诊率（%）	规范治疗数	血检确诊数	确诊率（%）	规范治疗数	血检确诊数	确诊率（%）	规范治疗数	血检确诊数	确诊率（%）	规范治疗数	血检确诊数	确诊率（%）
合计															

表 10　接受规范治疗的疟疾病人数据管理流程表

分级	数据管理流程说明		负责人	时限要求
村级	开具双联疟疾病人处方并保存其中一联		村医	每月
	填写“疟疾项目病人诊治月登记表”一式两份并保存其中一份			
	上报“疟疾项目病人诊治月登记表”一份和另一联处方			
乡级	村级上报资料	收集村级上报资料	乡卫生院防保组	每月
		核对其上报资料，在处方上标明“流动人口”或“当地居民”，“规范治疗”或“不规范治疗”，并核定其“疟疾项目病人诊治月登记表”相应数据。		
		将其上报处方按人口类型和规范治疗与否分类，与其“疟疾项目病人诊治月登记表”一起存档。		
	乡个体医诊治资料	开具双联疟疾病人处方并保存其中一联	乡个体医生	
		填写“疟疾项目病人诊治月登记表”一式两份并保存其中一份		
		收集其“疟疾项目病人诊治月登记表”一份和另一联处方	乡卫生院防保组	
		核对其上报资料，在处方上标明“流动人口”或“当地居民”，“规范治疗”或“不规范治疗”，并核定其“疟疾项目病人诊治月登记表”相应数据。		
		将其上报处方按人口类型和规范治疗与否分类，与其“疟疾项目病人诊治月登记表”一起存档。		
	乡卫生院诊治资料	开具双联疟疾病人处方并保存其中一联	乡卫生院门诊	
		填写“疟疾项目病人诊治月登记表”一式两份并保存其中一份		
		收集其“疟疾项目病人诊治月登记表”一份和另一联处方	乡卫生院防保组	
		核对其上报资料，在处方上标明“流动人口”或“当地居民”，“规范治疗”或“不规范治疗”，并核定其“疟疾项目病人诊治月登记表”相应数据。		
		将其上报处方按人口类型和规范治疗与否分类，与其“疟疾项目病人诊治月登记表”一起存档。		
	编制和上报乡级月汇总表		乡卫生院防保组	

续表

分级	数据管理流程说明		负责人	时限要求
县级	乡级上报资料	核实和保存乡级上报资料	县项目办	每月
	县级医院诊治资料	开具双联疟疾病人处方并保存其中一联	县级医院门诊	
		填写“疟疾项目病人诊治月登记表”一式两份并保存其中一份		
		收集其“疟疾项目病人诊治月登记表”一份和另一联处方	县项目办	
		核对其上报资料,在处方上标明“流动人口”或“当地居民”,“规范治疗”或“不规范治疗”,并核定其“疟疾项目病人诊治月登记表”相应数据。		
		将其上报处方按人口类型和规范治疗与否分类,与其“疟疾项目病人诊治月登记表”一起存档。		
	县 CDC 诊治资料	开具双联疟疾病人处方并保存其中一联	县 CDC 门诊	
		填写“疟疾项目病人诊治月登记表”一式两份并保存其中一份		
		收集其“疟疾项目病人诊治月登记表”一份和另一联处方	县项目办	
		核对其上报资料,在处方上标明“流动人口”或“当地居民”,“规范治疗”或“不规范治疗”,并核定其“疟疾项目病人诊治月登记表”相应数据。		
		将其上报处方按人口类型和规范治疗与否分类,与其“疟疾项目病人诊治月登记表”一起存档。		
	编制和上报县级月汇总表		县项目办	
	编制和上报县级季度报表		县项目办	季度结束 15 日内
省级	核实和保存县级上报表		省项目办	季度结束 30 日内
	编制省级季度汇总表			
	编制和上报省级季度报表			
国家级	核实和保存省级季度上报表		国家项目办	季度结束 45 日内
	编制国家级季度汇总表			
	编制和上报国家级季度报表			

表 11　第 ___ 轮规范治疗的疟疾病人数和比例乡级汇总表

□流动人口:□当地居民

___ 乡 __ 年 __ 季度　　填表人:　　填表日期:　　上报单位盖章:

行政村	______月份				______月份				______月份				合计			
	疟疾病人数	规范治疗数	不规范治疗数	规范治疗率(%)	疟疾病人数	规范治疗数	不规范治疗数	规范治疗率(%)	疟疾病人数	规范治疗数	不规范治疗数	规范治疗率(%)	疟疾病人数	规范治疗数	不规范治疗数	规范治疗率(%)
村医诊治																
乡个体医诊治																
乡卫生院诊治																
小计																
村医诊治																
乡个体医诊治																
乡卫生院诊治																
小计																
村医诊治																
乡个体医诊治																
乡卫生院诊治																
小计																
村医诊治																
乡个体医诊治																
乡卫生院诊治																
小计																
村医诊治																
乡个体医诊治																
乡卫生院诊治																
小计																
村医诊治																
乡个体医诊治																
乡卫生院诊治																
小计																
村医诊治																
乡个体医诊治																

___乡__年__季度　　　　填表人：　　　　填表日期：　　　　上报单位盖章：

行政村		____月份				____月份				____月份				合计			
		疟疾病人数	规范治疗数	不规范治疗数	规范治疗率(%)	疟疾病人数	规范治疗数	不规范治疗数	规范治疗率(%)	疟疾病人数	规范治疗数	不规范治疗数	规范治疗率(%)	疟疾病人数	规范治疗数	不规范治疗数	规范治疗率(%)
	乡卫生院诊治																
	小计																
	村医诊治																
	乡个体医诊治																
	乡卫生院诊治																
	小计																
	村医诊治																
	乡个体医诊治																
	乡卫生院诊治																
	小计																
	村医诊治																
	乡个体医诊治																
	乡卫生院诊治																
	小计																
合计	村医诊治																
	乡个体医诊治																
	乡卫生院诊治																
	小计																

表 12　第 ___ 轮规范治疗的疟疾病人数和比例县级汇总表

□流动人口：□当地居民

___ 乡 __ 年 __ 季度　　　　填表人：　　　　填表日期：　　　　上报单位盖章：

项目乡镇	____月份				____月份				____月份				合计			
	疟疾病人数	规范治疗数	不规范治疗数	规范治疗率(%)	疟疾病人数	规范治疗数	不规范治疗数	规范治疗率(%)	疟疾病人数	规范治疗数	不规范治疗数	规范治疗率(%)	疟疾病人数	规范治疗数	不规范治疗数	规范治疗率(%)
乡级上报																
县 CDC 诊治																
县级医院诊治																
小计																
乡级上报																
县 CDC 诊治																
县级医院诊治																
小计																
乡级上报																
县 CDC 诊治																
县级医院诊治																
小计																
乡级上报																
县 CDC 诊治																
县级医院诊治																
小计																
乡级上报																
县 CDC 诊治																
县级医院诊治																
小计																
乡级上报																
县 CDC 诊治																
县级医院诊治																
小计																

___乡___年___季度　　填表人：　　填表日期：　　上报单位盖章：

项目乡镇		___月份				___月份				___月份				合计			
		疟疾病人数	规范治疗数	不规范治疗数	规范治疗率(%)	疟疾病人数	规范治疗数	不规范治疗数	规范治疗率(%)	疟疾病人数	规范治疗数	不规范治疗数	规范治疗率(%)	疟疾病人数	规范治疗数	不规范治疗数	规范治疗率(%)
	乡级上报																
	县 CDC 诊治																
	县级医院诊治																
	小计																
	乡级上报																
	县 CDC 诊治																
	县级医院诊治																
	小计																
	乡级上报																
	县 CDC 诊治																
	县级医院诊治																
	小计																
	乡级上报																
	县 CDC 诊治																
	县级医院诊治																
	小计																
合计	乡级上报																
	县 CDC 诊治																
	县级医院诊治																
	小计																

表 13　第 ___ 轮规范治疗的疟疾病人数和比例省级汇总表

□流动人口：□当地居民

___ 乡 __ 年 __ 季度　　　填表人：　　　填表日期：　　　上报单位盖章：

项目县	第 1 季度				第 2 季度				第 3 季度				第 4 季度				合计			
	疟疾病人数	规范治疗数	不规范治疗数	规范治疗率(%)	疟疾病人数	规范治疗数	不规范治疗数	规范治疗率(%)	疟疾病人数	规范治疗数	不规范治疗数	规范治疗率(%)	疟疾病人数	规范治疗数	不规范治疗数	规范治疗率(%)	疟疾病人数	规范治疗数	不规范治疗数	规范治疗率(%)
合计																				

表 14 第 ___ 轮规范治疗的疟疾病人数和比例省级汇总表

□流动人口：□当地居民

___ 年　　　　填表人：　　　　填表日期：

项目省	第 1 季度				第 2 季度				第 3 季度				第 4 季度				合计			
	疟疾病人数	规范治疗数	不规范治疗数	规范治疗率（%）	疟疾病人数	规范治疗数	不规范治疗数	规范治疗率（%）	疟疾病人数	规范治疗数	不规范治疗数	规范治疗率（%）	疟疾病人数	规范治疗数	不规范治疗数	规范治疗率（%）	疟疾病人数	规范治疗数	不规范治疗数	规范治疗率（%）
合计																				

表 15　第 ___ 轮疟疾项目病人诊治月登记表

□流动人口：□当地居民

__ 年 __ 月　　上服单位及填表人：　　上报日期：　　核定单位及核定人：　　核定日期：

姓名	性别	年龄	住址	发病时间	就诊时间	送检时间	治疗时间	诊断结果				血检情况						治疗情况			人口类型	
								疟疾病例			其他	未血检	血检					未抗疟治疗	抗疟治疗		流动人口	当地居民
								血检阳性	典型临床症状	药物试治有效			Pv	Pf	混合感染	阴性			规范	不规范		

1、流动人口：指在当地居住时间小于3个月的外国、外省、外县人口。2、规范治疗：符合全球基金管理与技术规范中治疗方案的即为规范治疗。

人口类型	发病人数	血检人数	疟疾病人数	疟疾病人规范治疗数		
				总数	确诊病例数	%
流动人口						
当地居民						
合计						

表 16　杀虫剂浸泡蚊帐数据管理流程表

分级	数据管理流程说明	负责人	时限要求
乡级	制订实施方案，开展杀虫剂浸泡蚊帐工作，保存工作记录表	乡卫生院防保组	每次
	编制和上报乡级月汇总表	乡卫生院防保组	每月
县级	核实和保存乡级上报资料	县项目办	每月
	编制和上报县级月汇总表		
	编制和上报县级季度报表	县项目办	季度结束 15 日内
省级	核实和保存县级上报表	省项目办	季度结束 30 日内
	编制省级季度汇总表		
	编制和上报省级季度报表		
国家级	核实和保存省级季度上报表	国家项目办	季度结束 45 日内
	编制国家级季度汇总表		
	编制和上报国家级季度报表		

表 17　第____轮　____县___乡___村___自然村　杀虫剂浸泡蚊帐工作记录表

编号	户主姓名	户内人数	拥有蚊帐数	浸泡蚊帐数	受益人签名
合计					

实施单位________________　　浸帐人员________________　　浸帐时间____________

表 18 第 ____ 轮 杀虫剂浸泡蚊帐数量乡级汇总表

____ 乡 ___ 年 ___ 季度　　填表人：　　填表日期：　　上报单位盖章：

行政村	____ 月份	____ 月份	____ 月份	合计
合计				

表 19 第 ____ 轮 杀虫剂浸泡蚊帐数量县级汇总表

____ 县 ___ 年 ___ 季度　　填表人：　　填表日期：　　上报单位盖章：

项目乡镇	____ 月份	____ 月份	____ 月份	合计
合计				

表 20 第____轮 杀虫剂浸泡蚊帐数量省级汇总表

____省___年　　　　填表人：　　　　填表日期：

项目县	第1季度	第2季度	第3季度	第4季度	合计
合计					

表 21 第____轮 杀虫剂浸泡蚊帐数量国家级汇总表

___年　　　　填表人：　　　　填表日期：

项目县	第1季度	第2季度	第3季度	第4季度	合计
合计					

表 22　乡、村医生和镜检员培训数据管理流程表

分级	数据管理流程说明	负责人	时限要求
县级	按工作计划组织实施培训	县项目办	每次
	保存培训通知、日程、讲义、签到簿等		
	编制和上报县级月汇总表	县项目办	每月
	编制和上报县级季度报表	县项目办	季度结束 15 日内
省级	核实和保存县级上报表	省项目办	季度结束 30 日内
	编制省级季度汇总表		
	编制和上报省级季度报表		
国家级	核实和保存省级季度上报表	国家项目办	季度结束 45 日内
	编制国家级季度汇总表		
	编制和上报国家级季度报表		

表 23　第 ___ 轮　乡、村医生和镜检员培训人数和比例县级汇总表

项目乡镇	乡村医生和镜检员总数	接受早期诊断和规范治疗培训的人数			
		______月份	______月份	______月份	合计
合计					

表 24 第 ___ 轮乡、村医生和镜检员培训人数和比例省级汇总表

___ 省 ___ 年　　　　填表人：　　　　填表日期：

项目县	乡村医生和镜检员总数	第 1 季度		第 2 季度		第 3 季度		第 4 季度		合计	
		培训人数	%	培训人数	%	培训人数	%	培训人数	%	培训人数	%
合计											

表 25　第 ___ 轮规乡、村医生和镜检员培训人数和比例国家级汇总表

项目省	乡村医生和镜检员总数	第 1 季度		第 2 季度		第 3 季度		第 4 季度		合计	
		培训人数	%	培训人数	%	培训人数	%	培训人数	%	培训人数	%
合计											

表 26　收到健康教育材料的户数和比例数据管理流程表

分级	数据管理流程说明	负责人	时限要求
县级	按计划开展疟疾健康教育活动，并统计受益户数	县项目办	每次
	保存工作记录和健康教育材料		
	编制和上报县级月汇总表	县项目办	每月
	编制和上报县级季度报表	县项目办	季度结束 15 日内
省级	核实和保存县级上报表	省项目办	季度结束 30 日内
	编制省级季度汇总表		
	编制和上报省级季度报表		
国家级	核实和保存省级季度上报表	国家项目办	季度结束 45 日内
	编制国家级季度汇总表		
	编制和上报国家级季度报表		

表 27 第 ____ 轮 收到健康教育材料的户数和比例县级汇总表

____ 县 ___ 年 ___ 季度　　填表人：　　填表日期：　　上报单位盖章：

项目乡镇	总户数	接受疟疾健康教育材料的户数			
		_____ 月份	_____ 月份	_____ 月份	合计
合计					

表 28 第 ___ 轮收到健康教育材料的户数和比例省级汇总表

___ 省 ___ 年　　　　填表人：　　　　填表日期：

项目县	总户数	第 1 季度		第 2 季度		第 3 季度		第 4 季度		合计	
		受益户数	%	受益户数	%	受益户数	%	受益户数	%	受益户数	%
合计											

表 29 第 ___ 轮收到健康教育材料的户数和比例国家级级汇总表

___ 年　　　　填表人：　　　　填表日期：

项目县	总户数	第 1 季度		第 2 季度		第 3 季度		第 4 季度		合计	
		受益户数	%	受益户数	%	受益户数	%	受益户数	%	受益户数	%
合计											

表 30 M&E 指标县级季度报表

项目县：　　季度时段：　　上报日期：　　签字盖章：

项目目标	考核指标	本期实际值			备注
		分子	分母	%	
目标 1：使云南省边境地区流动人口更好地获得疟疾诊断和合理治疗。	就诊的流动人口发热病人中得到镜检的人数和比例				
	就诊的流动人口疟疾病人得到规范治疗的人数和比例				
目标 2：使云南和海南流行区居民得到更好的早期诊断和个人防护。	目标地区乡、村医生和镜检员接受早期诊断和规范治疗（EDAT）培训的人数和比例				
	云南和海南当地居民疟疾病人中接受规范治疗的人数和比例				
	接受规范治疗的疟疾病人中通过镜检确诊的人数和比例				
	杀虫剂浸泡蚊帐的数量				
目标 3：使云南和海南目标地区居民更有效地采取疟疾预防措施，及时治疗。	目标地区家庭收到“信息、教育和交流（IEC）”和健康教育（HE）材料的户数和比例				

其他说明：

表 31 M&E 指标省级季度报表

项目县：　　季度时段：　　上报日期：　　签字盖章：

项目目标	考核指标	基线		累计	累计	差异的原因	本期	本期	差异的原因
		值	年月	目标	结果	及改进计划	目标	结果	及改进计划
总目标：遏制项目省疟疾流行，控制多重抗性恶性疟扩散。	云南 25 个项目县和海南 10 个项目县的疟疾发病率								
	海南 10 个项目县的恶性疟发病率								
	云南和海南疟疾报告死亡人数								
	拥有杀虫剂浸泡蚊帐的家庭比例								
	目标地区中小学生能够正确回答至少 3 个与疟疾相关问题的比例								
	发热病人在症状出现 2 天内求诊的比例								
目标 1：使云南省边境地区流动人口更好地获得疟疾诊断和合理治疗。	就诊的流动人口发热病人中得到镜检的人数和比例								
	就诊的流动人口疟疾病人得到规范治疗的人数和比例								
目标 2：使云南和海南流行区居民得到更好的早期诊断和个人防护。	目标地区乡、村医生和镜检员接受早期诊断和规范治疗（EDAT）培训的人数和比例								
	云南和海南当地居民疟疾病人中接受规范治疗的人数和比例								

续表

项目县：　　季度时段：　　上报日期：　　签字盖章：

项目目标	考核指标	基线		累计目标	累计结果	差异的原因及改进计划	本期目标	本期结果	差异的原因及改进计划
		值	年月						
	接受规范治疗的疟疾病人中通过镜检确诊的人数和比例								
	杀虫剂浸泡蚊帐的数量								
目标3：使云南和海南目标地区居民更有效地采取疟疾预防措施，及时治疗。	目标地区家庭收到“信息、教育和交流(IEC)”和健康教育(HE)材料的户数和比例								
目标4：优化云南、海南及其他八个项目省疟疾控制项目管理。	疟疾病例通过信息网络报告的比例								

其他说明：

附录 4：技术规范附表

表 1 ______ 省 ______ 县县级基线调查汇总表

疟疾疫情 *				血检能力		县发热病人血检		
人口数	病例数	Pf 数	死亡数	乡卫生院总数	开展血检的乡卫生院数	血检数	血检阳性数	恶性疟阳性数

注：* 按上年度县统计局公布的人口数和县疾控中心上报的疟疾疫情数统计。

调 查 者 __________

调查时间 __________

表 2 ______ 省 ______ 县调查乡基线调查汇总表

乡镇名	人口数	疟疾疫情 *			镜检员培训		发热病人血检			规范治疗	
		病例数	恶性疟数	死亡数	乡院镜检员数	经培训镜检员数	血检数	阳性数	恶性疟数	检查处方数	规范处方数
合计											

注：* 按上年度县统计局公布的人口数和县疾控中心上报的疟疾疫情数统计。

调 查 者 __________

调查时间 __________

表 3 ______ 省 ______ 县调查村基线调查汇总表

调查乡	调查村	人口数	报告疟疾疫情			村/个体医		规范疟疾治疗情况		走访调查							
			病例数	Pf数	死亡数	村/个体医数	经培训人数	检查处方数	规范处方数	户数	调查人数	疟史人数	治疗人数	规范治疗人数	休治人数	使用蚊帐人数	使用药帐人数
	合计																
	合计																
	合计																
合计																	

调 查 者 ____________

调查时间 ____________

表 4 ______ 省 ______ 县基线调查疫情核查表

乡名	报告疫情			血检登记				抗疟处方		村走访				
	县病例报告数	乡病例报告数	名单符合例数	县报告血检阳性数	乡血检阳性登记数	名单符合例数	乡报告病例数	乡抗疟药处方登记数	名单符合例数	村名	走访人数	乡报告病例数	村走访病例数	名单符合例数

调 查 者 __________

调查时间 __________

表 5 ______ 云南省 ______ 县边境口岸流动人口疟疾监测情况基线调查表

口岸名称	出入境人口数	有医疗诊所的口岸数	有镜检条件口岸诊所数	有发热病人血检的诊所数	发热病人血检数	疟原虫阳性数	恶性疟数	疟疾病人治疗数	使用抗疟药处方数	规范使用抗疟药处方数

注：请注明正规与非正规口岸

调 查 者 __________

调查时间 __________

表 6 ______ 县 ______ 乡镇上山住宿人群疟疾监测情况基线调查表

行政村名	总人口数	本村病例报告数	上山住宿人数	其中使用蚊帐人数	其中服预防药人数	其中有疟史者人数	其中血检人数	其中血检阳性人数	其中恶性疟数	其中因疟疾死亡数	其中接受治疗人数	其中接受规范治疗人数

调 查 者 ____________

调查时间 ____________

表 7 流动人口集中地区的疟疾监测情况基线调查表

行政村名	总人口数	流动人口		其中报告疟疾病例数	其中血检人数	其中血检阳性人数	其中恶性疟数	其中因疟疾死亡数	其中接受治疗人数	其中接受规范治疗人数
		总数	来往海南云南人数							

调 查 者 ____________

调查时间 ____________

表 8 ______ 省 ______ 县居民家庭走访调查表 编号

1．乡(镇) ________，行政村 ________，居民组或自然村 ________；
2．户主姓名 ________，家庭人口数： □□
3．家中疟疾发病情况：者：无，有 □
有疟疾发病人数 □□；
4．家中疟疾病人就诊情况：无，有 □(□□ 人)；
5．家中疟疾病人治疗情况：未治，有治 □
(治疗□□人 ，其中规范 □□人 ，不规范 □□人)；
6．家中疟疾病人休止期根治情况：无，有 □ (接受休止期根治人数□□)；
7．防蚊情况：夏季露宿(有，无)；□ 使用蚊帐人数□□，使用药浸蚊帐人数 □□；
8．疫情报告：①已报，②未报，③不知；(与县疫情报告名单：相符，不相符) □
9．村民疟防知识调查：
⑴ 被访者文化水平：1. 文盲，2. 小学，3. 初中，4. 高中以上； □
⑵ 疟疾是通过什么途径传染的？ (① 接触，② 食物，③ 蚊子，
④ 空气，⑤ 不知道)； □
⑶ 用什么方法可预防疟疾？ ①不接触病人，② 不吃不清洁食物，
③ 用蚊帐，④戴口罩，⑤不知道； □□□
⑷ 疟疾发病有什么主要的症状或不舒服？ ① 流鼻涕，② 发高热，
③ 拉肚子，④皮肤红肿，⑤不知道；(可选择一项或多项。) □□□□□
⑸ 你或你家人得了疟疾怎么办？ ①找医生看病，②不看病，③自己买药，
④外出躲病，⑤不知道； □
⑹ 得了疟疾要吃几天药？ ① 1 天，② 2 天，③ 3 天，④ 4 天以上，⑤不知道)； □

调 查 者 __________

调查时间 __________

表 9 中小学生疟防知识调查问卷

学校名称 ________ 1. 小学， 2. 中学 □
学生姓名：________ 年级 ________，班级 ________；
(1) 疟疾是通过什么途径传染的？ (①接触，②食物，③蚊子，
④空气，⑤ 不知道)； □
(2) 用什么方法可预防疟疾？ ①不接触病人，②不吃不清洁食物，③用蚊帐，
④戴口罩，⑤不知道；(可选择一项或多项。) □□□
(3) 疟疾发病有什么主要的症状或不舒服？ ① 流鼻涕，② 发高热，
③ 拉肚子，④ 皮肤红肿，⑤ 不知道；(可选择一项或多项。) □□□
(4) 你或你家人得了疟疾怎么办？ ① 找医生看病，② 不看病，自己买药，
③ 外出躲病，④不知道； □
(5) 得了疟疾要吃几天药？ ① 1 天，② 2 天，③ 3 天，
④ 4 天以上，⑤不知道)； □

调 查 者 __________

调查时间 __________

表 10 ________ 省 ________ 县基线调查疟防知识调查统计表

调查乡名	中小学生疟防知识调查		村民疟防知识调查		
	调查学生数	知晓疟防知识人数	调查村名	调查村民数	知晓疟防知识人数
			合计		
			合计		
			合计		
合计					

调 查 者 ____________

调查时间 ____________

表 11 专家对全球基金疟疾项目效果指标的了解程度调查表

（请在相应的栏中打√，了解程度指对指标含义的了解，不是对指标具体数值的了解）

效果指标	十分了解	比较了解	一般了解	不了解
疟疾总发病率下降幅度 (%)				
恶性疟发病率下降比例 (%)				
疟疾死亡减少的比例 (%)				
疟防知识普及率提高的比例 (%)				
输入性恶性疟下降的比例 (%)				
恶性疟抗药性降低程度 (%)				
乡村医生正确处方率提高的比例 (%)				
药浸蚊帐使用率提高的比例 (%)				
疟疾漏报率下降的比例 (%)				
血检覆盖率提高的比例 (%)				
血片抽查合格率提高的比例 (%)				
★★★				
★★★				

注：★★★ 您认为还应增加的指标及对其的了解程度。

表 12　各指标的重要性评价

（请根据您认为的重要程度在相应的分值栏中打√）

效果指标	很重要		重要		一般重要		较不重要		不重要	
	10	9	8	7	6	5	4	3	2	1
疟疾总发病率下降幅度 (%)										
恶性疟发病率下降比例 (%)										
疟疾死亡减少的比例 (%)										
疟防知识普及率提高的比例 (%)										
输入性恶性疟下降的比例 (%)										
恶性疟抗药性降低程度 (%)										
乡村医生正确处方率提高的比例 (%)										
药浸蚊帐使用率提高的比例 (%)										
疟疾漏报率下降的比例 (%)										
血检覆盖率提高的比例 (%)										
血片抽查合格率提高的比例 (%)										
★★★										
★★★										

注：★★★ 您认为还应增加的指标及对其的了解程度。

附录5：疟疾项目办组织结构

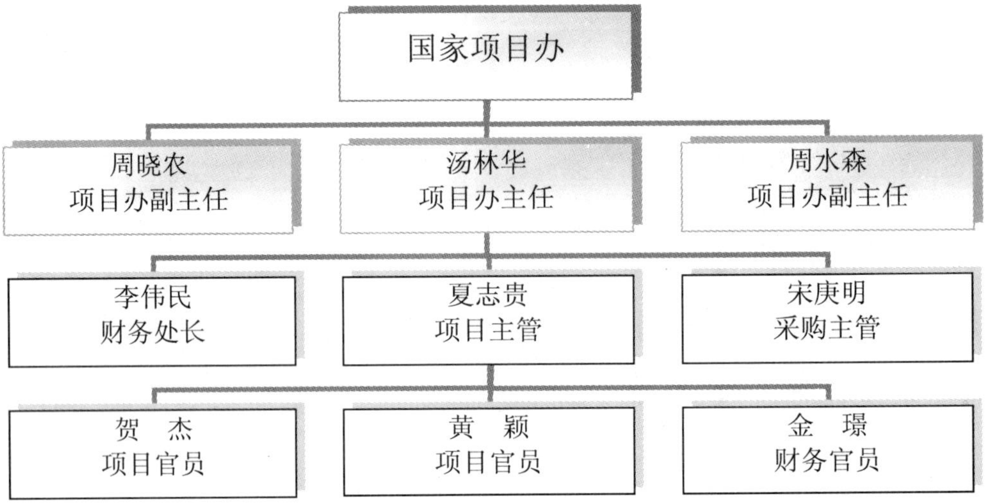

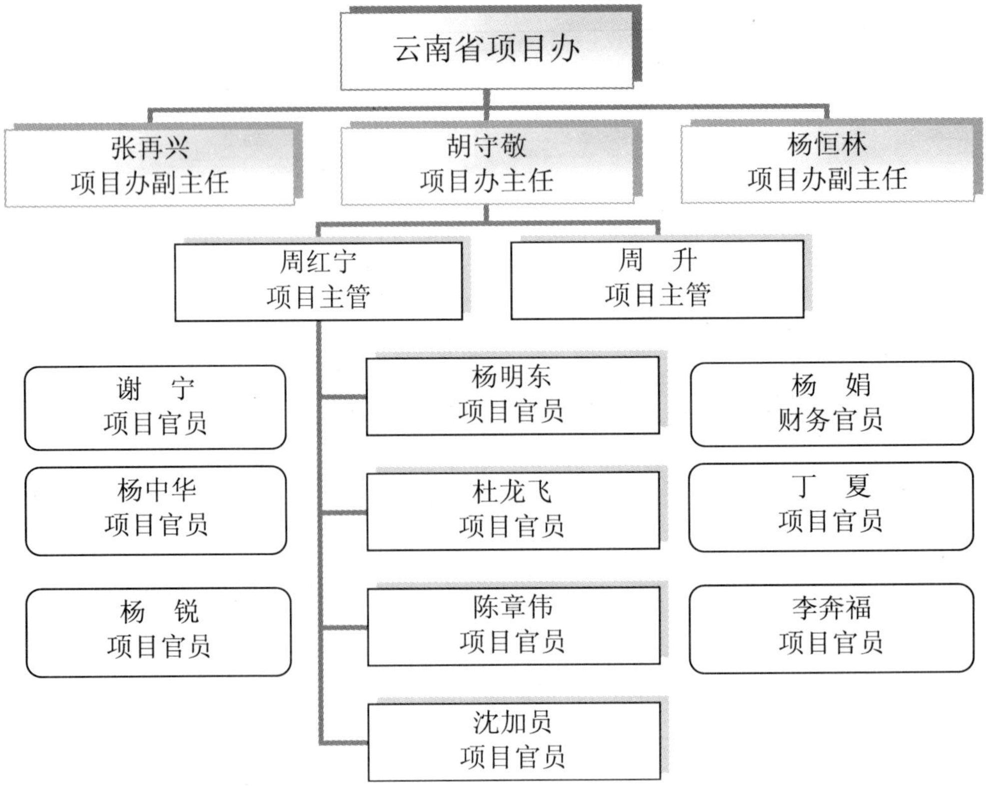

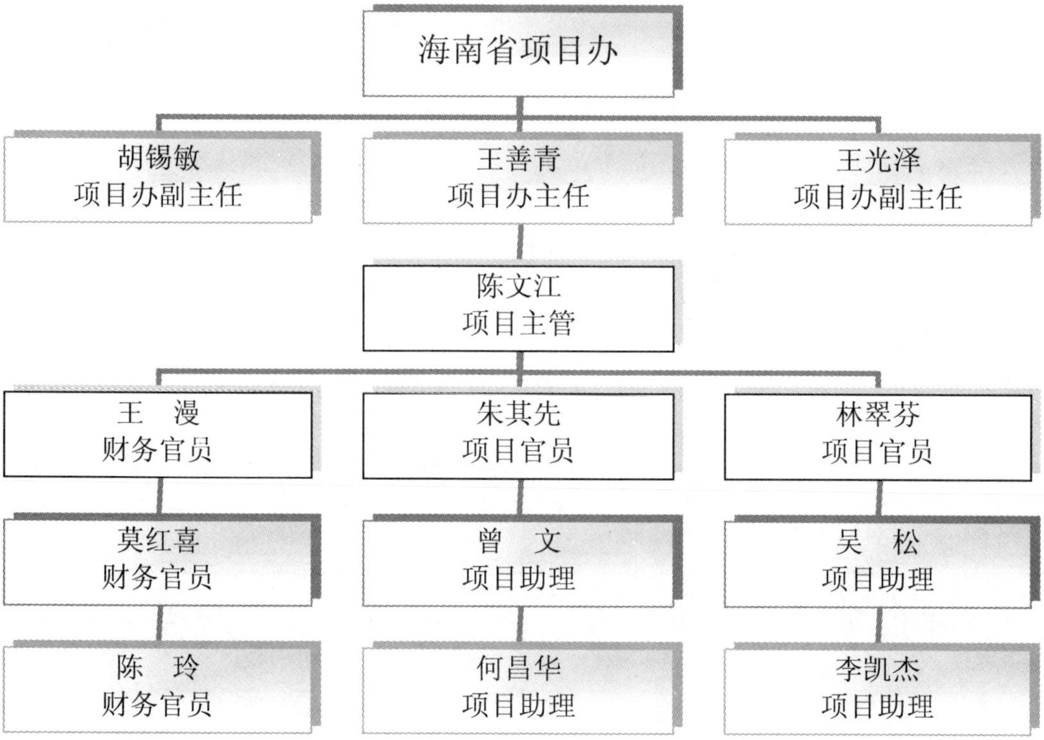
海南省项目办
胡锡敏
项目办副主任
王善青
项目办主任
王光泽
项目办副主任
陈文江
项目主管
王 漫
财务官员
朱其先
项目官员
林翠芬
项目官员
莫红喜
财务官员
曾 文
项目助理
吴 松
项目助理
陈 玲
财务官员
何昌华
项目助理
李凯杰
项目助理

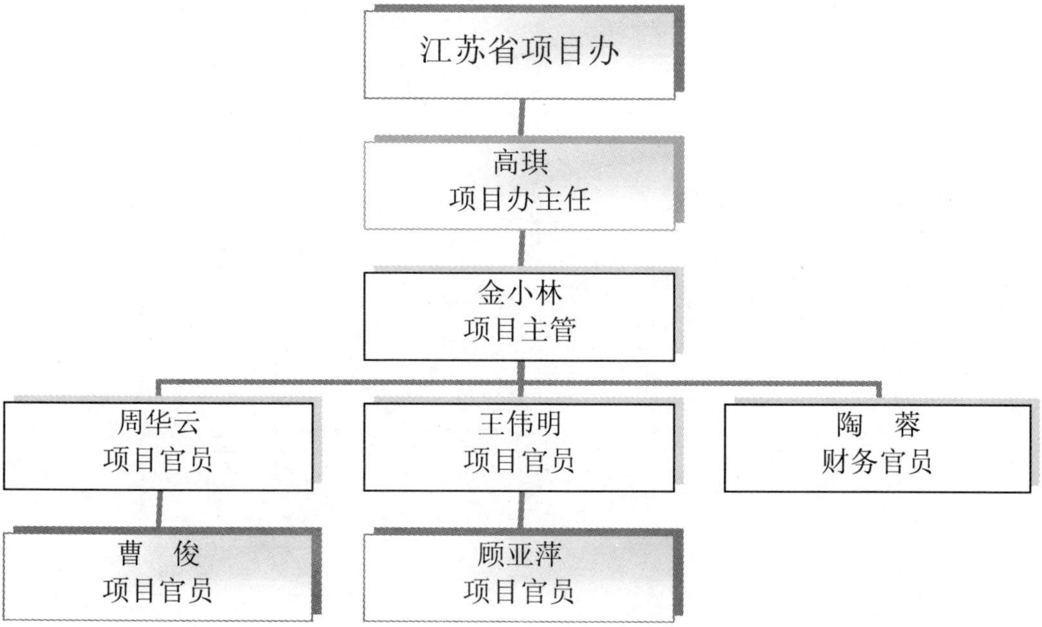
江苏省项目办
高琪
项目办主任
金小林
项目主管
周华云
项目官员
王伟明
项目官员
陶 蓉
财务官员
曹 俊
项目官员
顾亚萍
项目官员

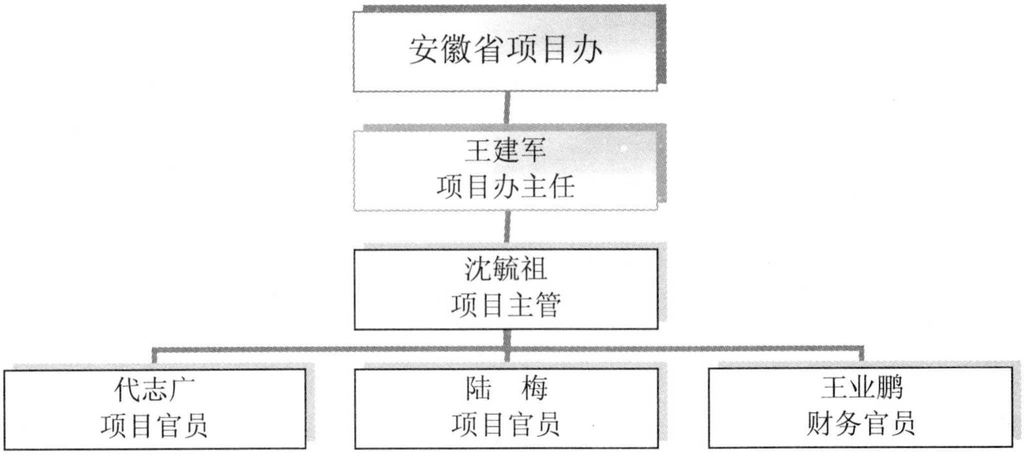
安徽省项目办
王建军
项目办主任
沈毓祖
项目主管
代志广
项目官员
陆 梅
项目官员
王业鹏
财务官员

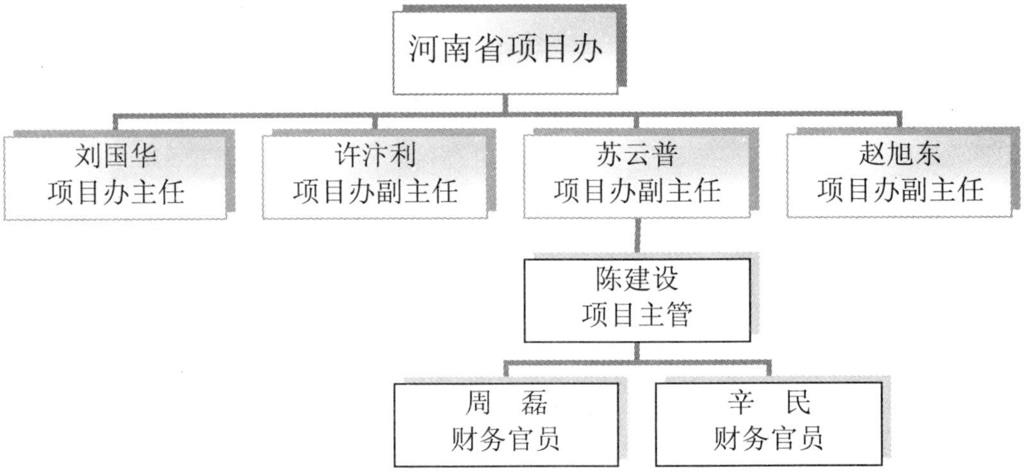
河南省项目办
刘国华
项目办主任
许汴利
项目办副主任
苏云普
项目办副主任
赵旭东
项目办副主任
陈建设
项目主管
周 磊
财务官员
辛 民
财务官员

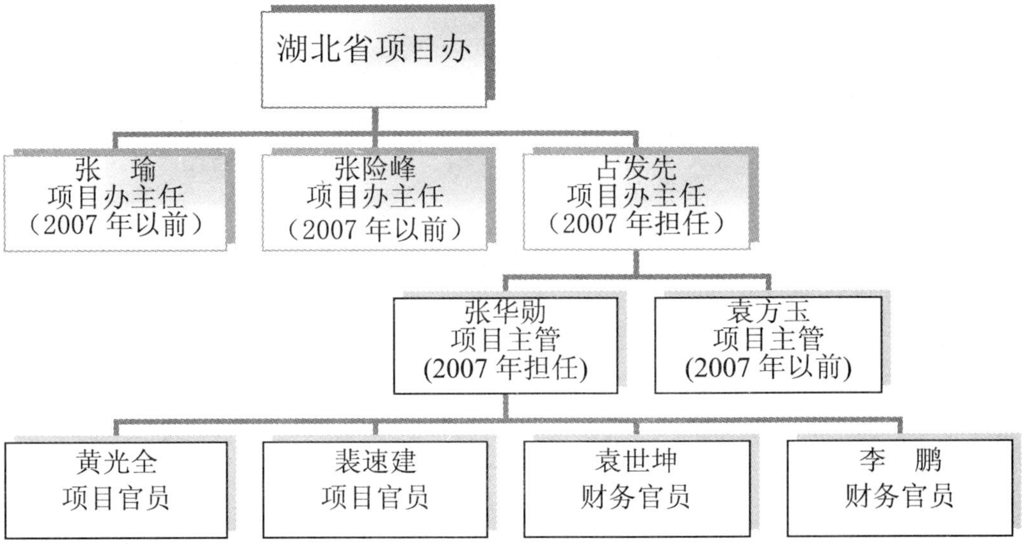
湖北省项目办
张 瑜
项目办主任
（2007 年以前）
张险峰
项目办主任
（2007 年以前）
占发先
项目办主任
（2007 年担任）
张华勋
项目主管
(2007 年担任)
袁方玉
项目主管
(2007 年以前)
黄光全
项目官员
裴速建
项目官员
袁世坤
财务官员
李 鹏
财务官员

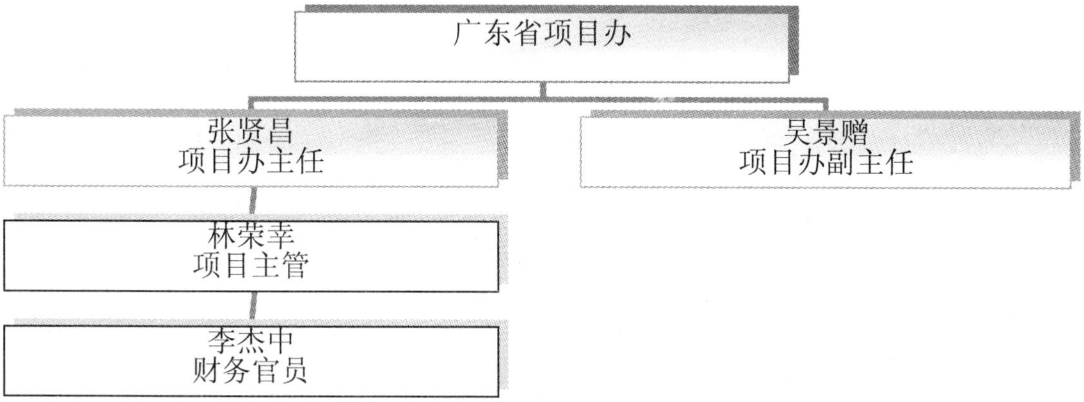
广东省项目办
张贤昌
项目办主任
吴景赠
项目办副主任
林荣幸
项目主管
李杰中
财务官员

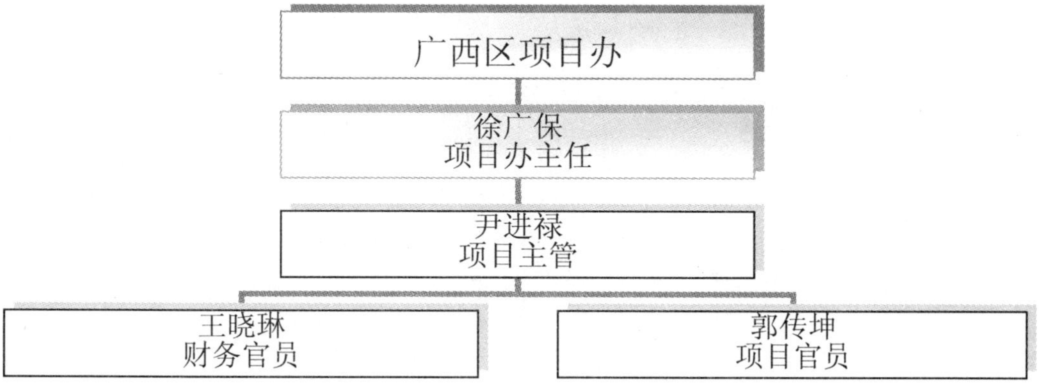
广西区项目办
徐广保
项目办主任
尹进禄
项目主管
王晓琳
财务官员
郭传坤
项目官员

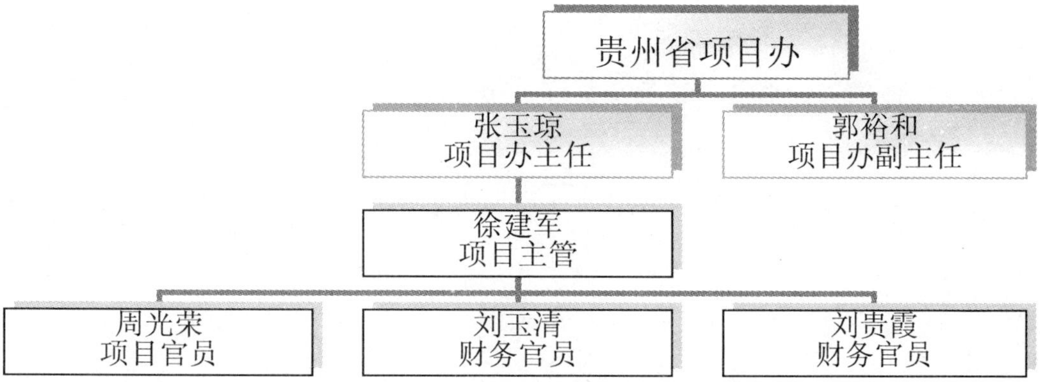
贵州省项目办
张玉琼
项目办主任
郭裕和
项目办副主任
徐建军
项目主管
周光荣
项目官员
刘玉清
财务官员
刘贵霞
财务官员

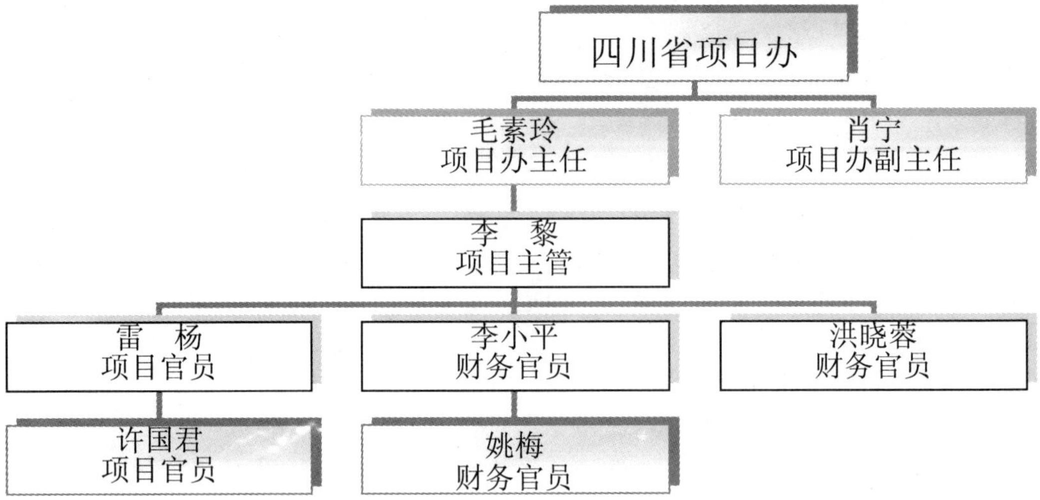
四川省项目办
毛素玲
项目办主任
肖宁
项目办副主任
李　黎
项目主管
雷　杨
项目官员
李小平
财务官员
洪晓蓉
财务官员
许国君
项目官员
姚梅
财务官员

附录 6：项目执行 5 年图片

一、项目会议

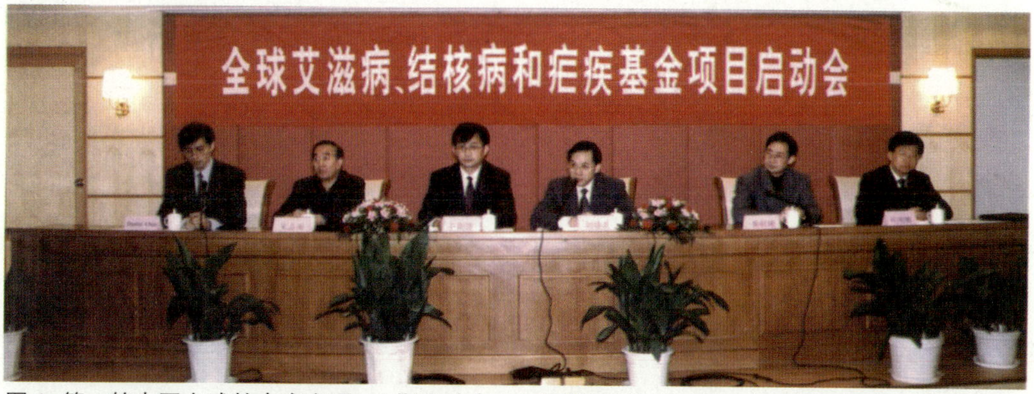

图 1 第一轮中国全球基金疟疾项目 I 期启动会在南京隆重召开（2003 年 3 月，江苏南京）

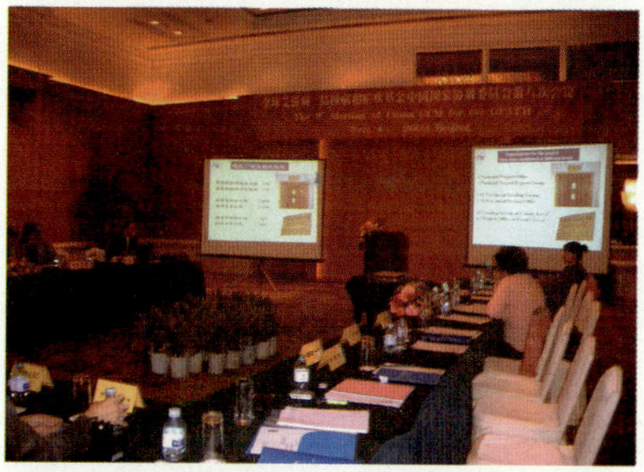

图 2 全球基金中国国家协调委员会（CCM）会议（2003 年 11 月，北京）

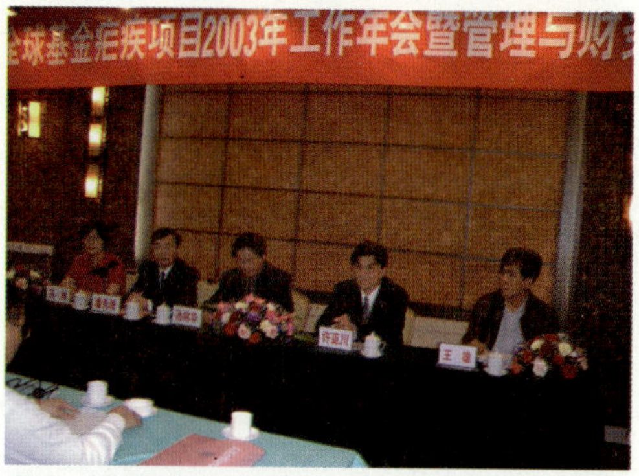

图 3 2003 年工作年会（2004 年 1 月，海南海口）

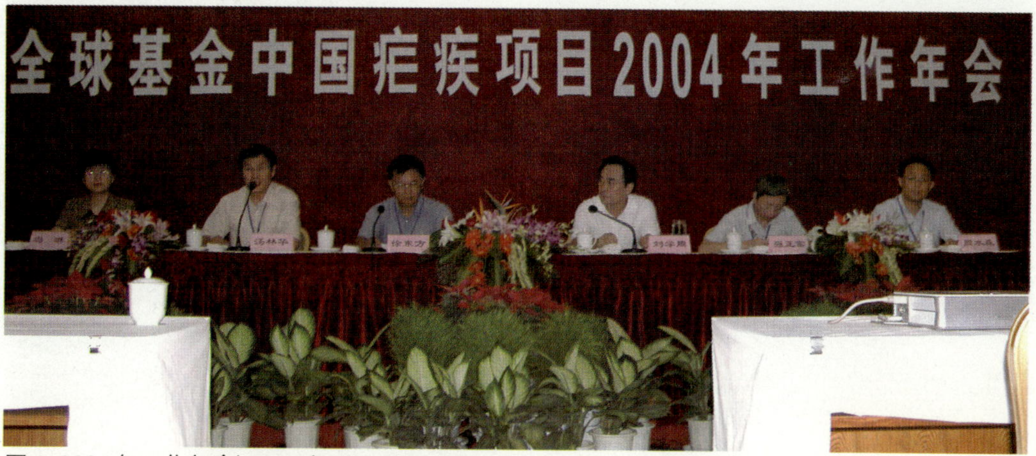

图4 2004年工作年会（2004年8月，河南郑州）

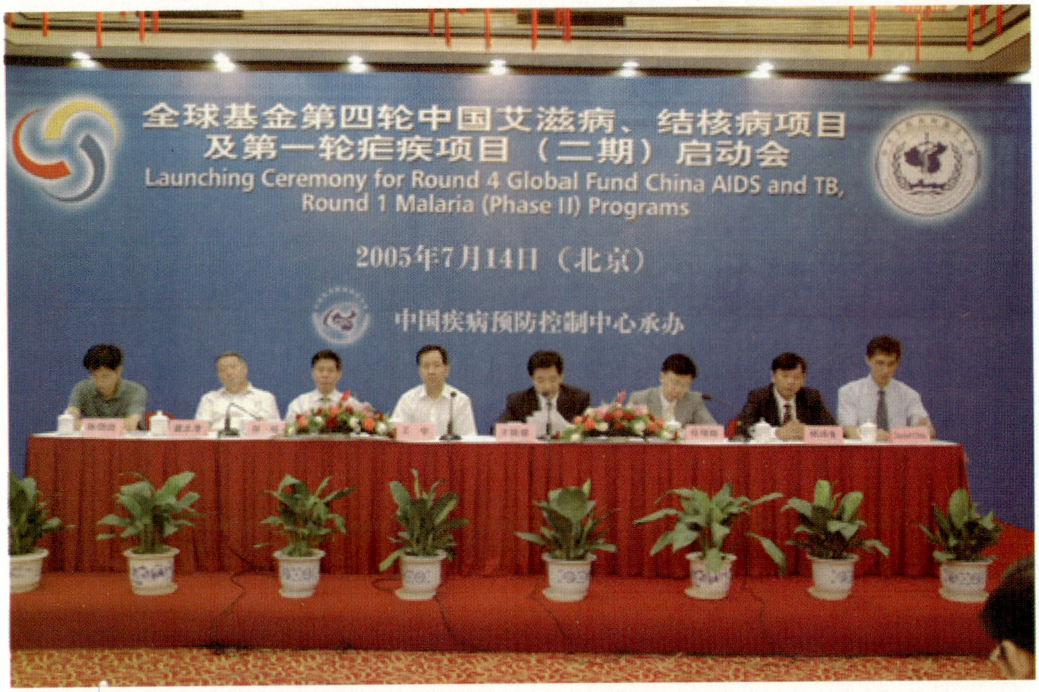

图5 第一轮中国全球基金疟疾项目 II 期启动会（2005 年 7 月，北京）

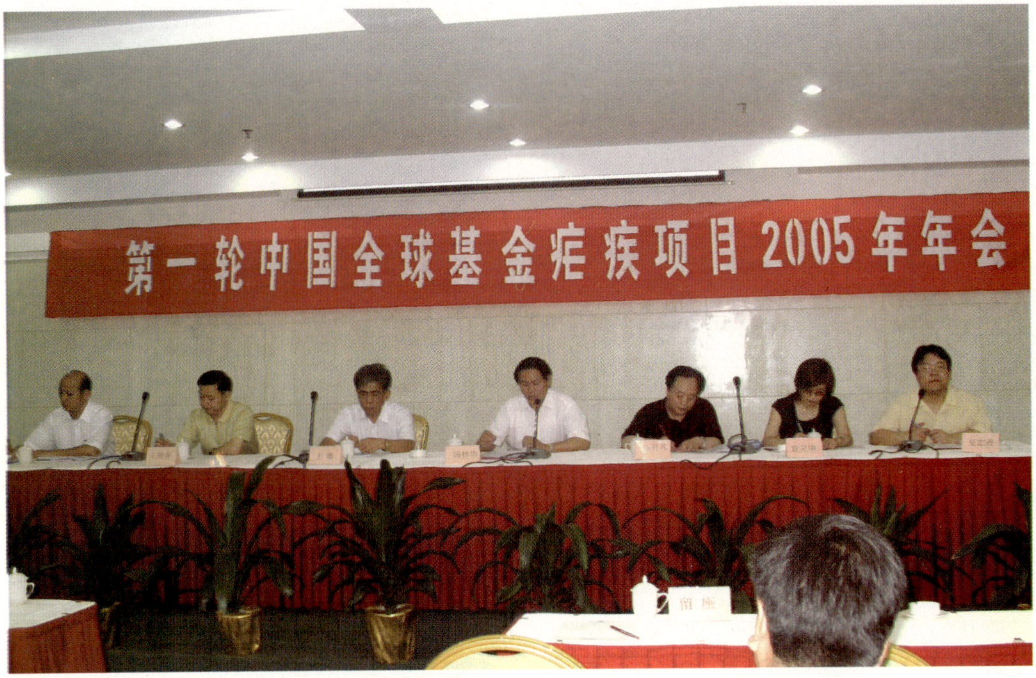

图6 2005 年年会（2006 年 6 月，海南三亚）

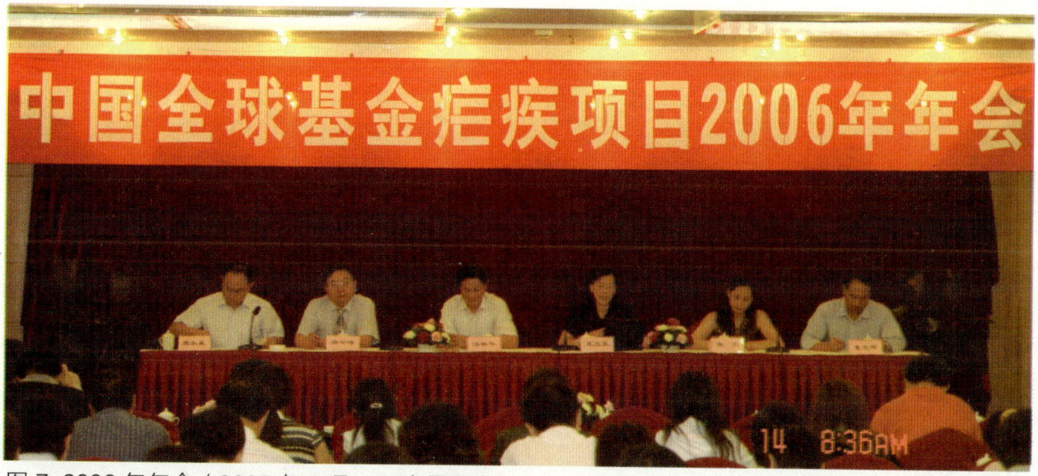

图 7 2006 年年会（2007 年 6 月，云南昆明）

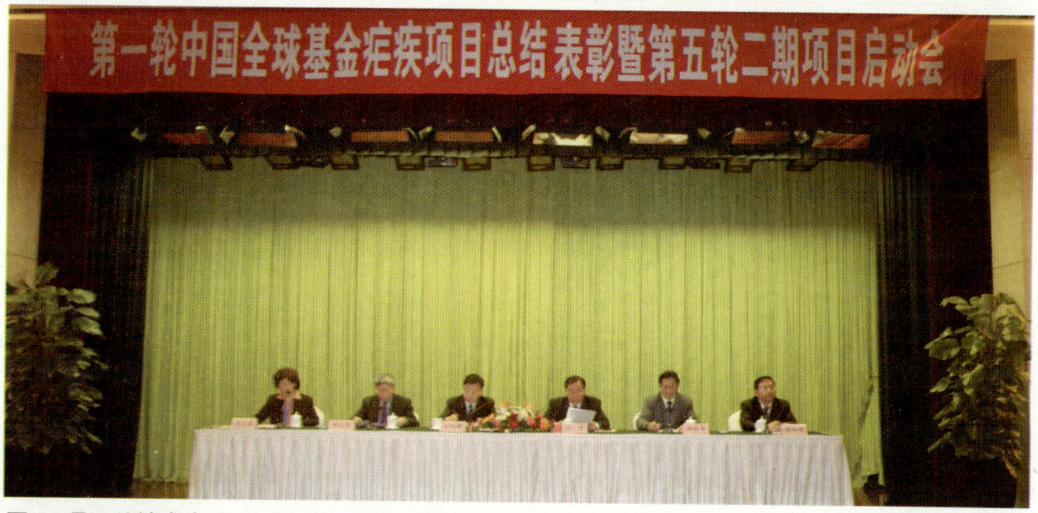

图 8 项目总结大会（2008 年 11 月，北京）

二、项目培训

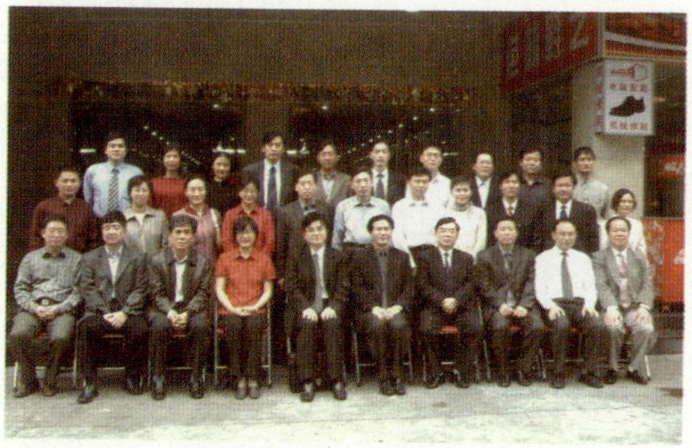

图 9 项目 I 期项目管理与财务培训（2003 年，海口）

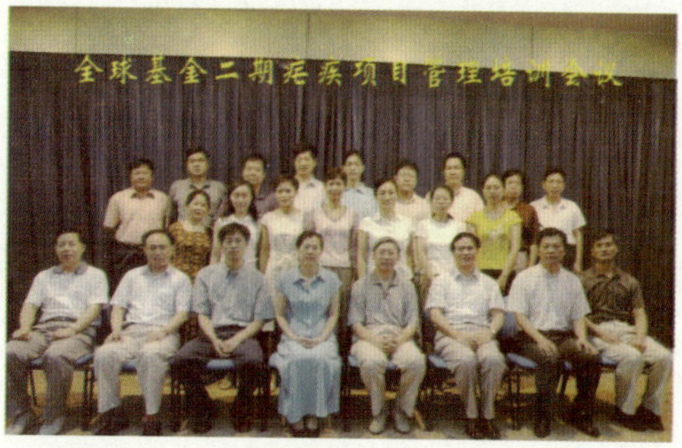

图 10 项目 II 期管理培训（2005 年，北京）

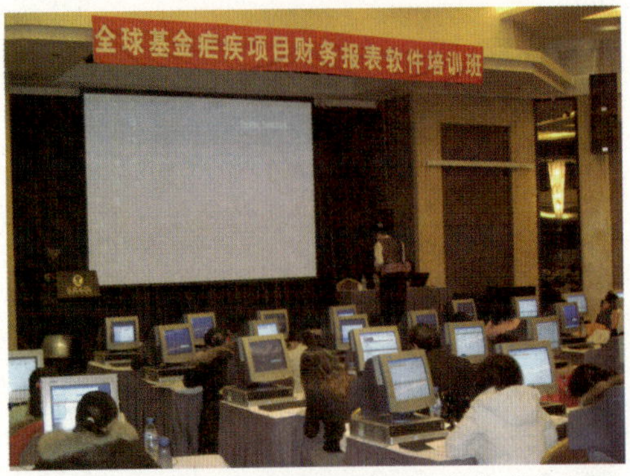

图 11　全球基金疟疾项目财务报表软件培训班（2007 年 11 月，上海）

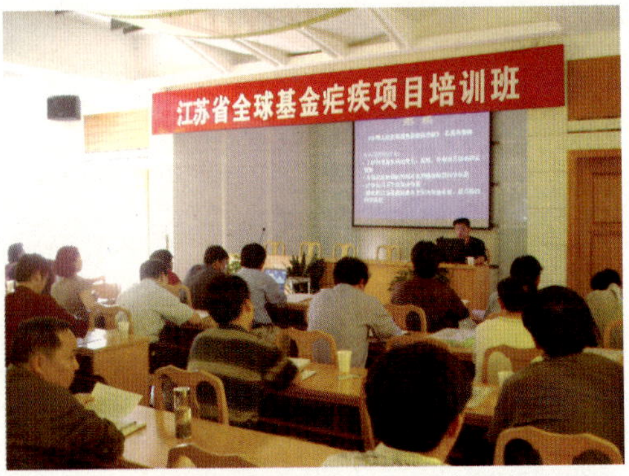

图 12　江苏省全球基金疟疾项目培训班（2003 年 4 月，江苏无锡）

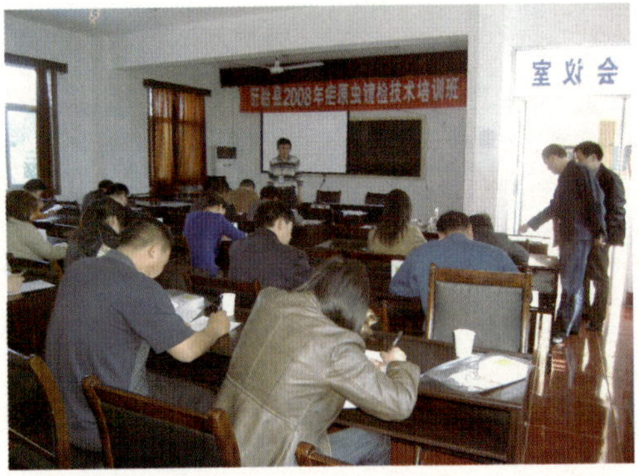

图 13　县级疟原虫镜检技术培训班（2004 年 8 月、江苏盱眙）

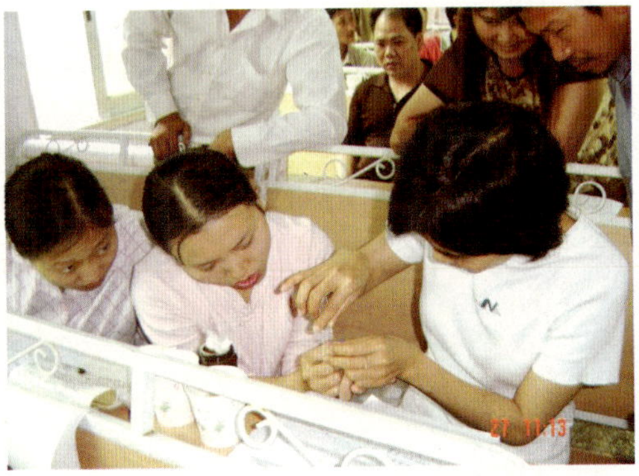

图 14　乡镇卫生院医务人员练习采血（2004 年，四川筠连）

三、项目实施现场活动

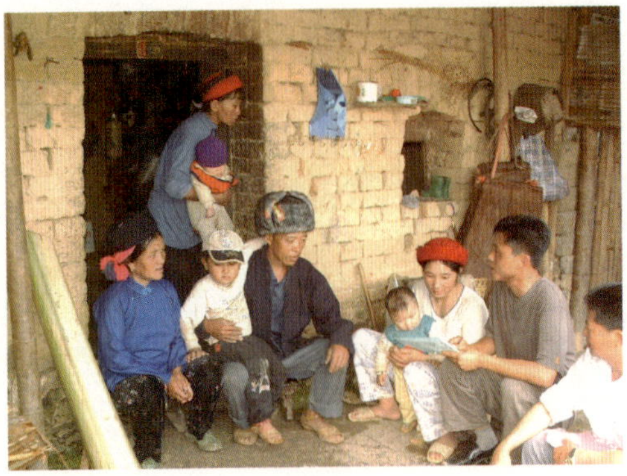

图 15　基线调查（2003 年 5 月，云南）

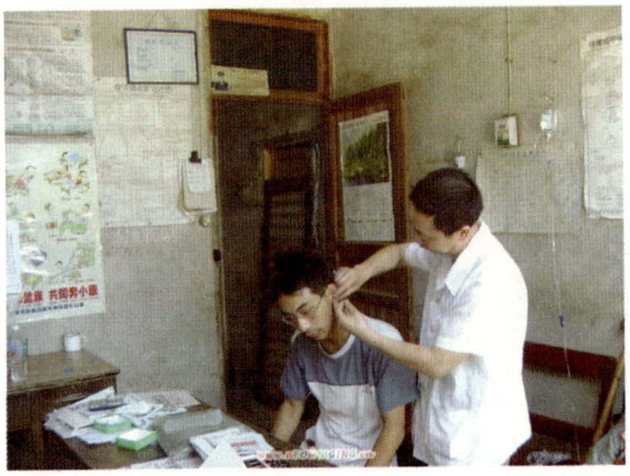

图 16　为发热病人采血

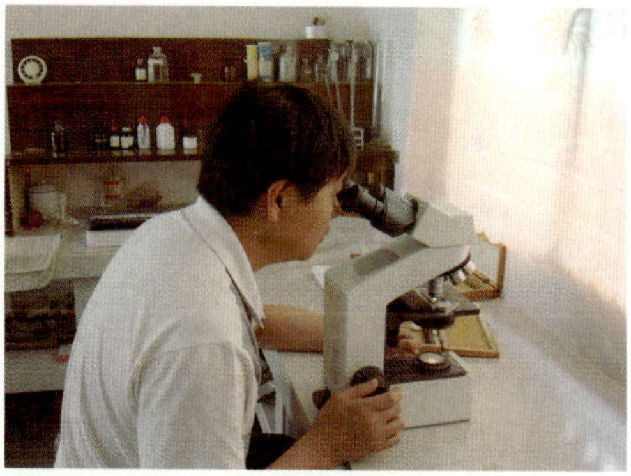
图 17 发热病人血片镜检诊断

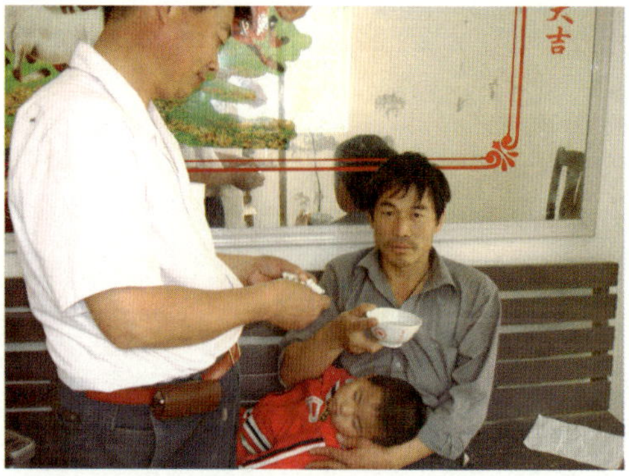
图 18 免费治疗病人

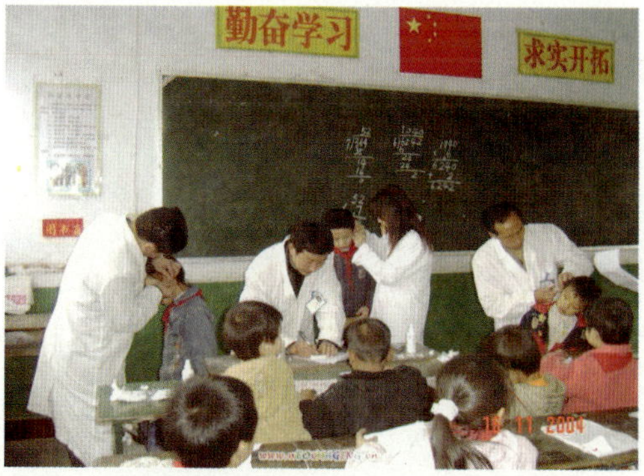

图 19 采集 IFA 血样

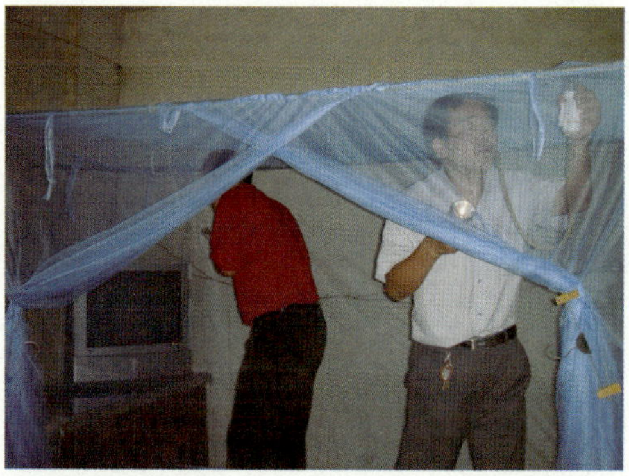
图 20 媒介监测

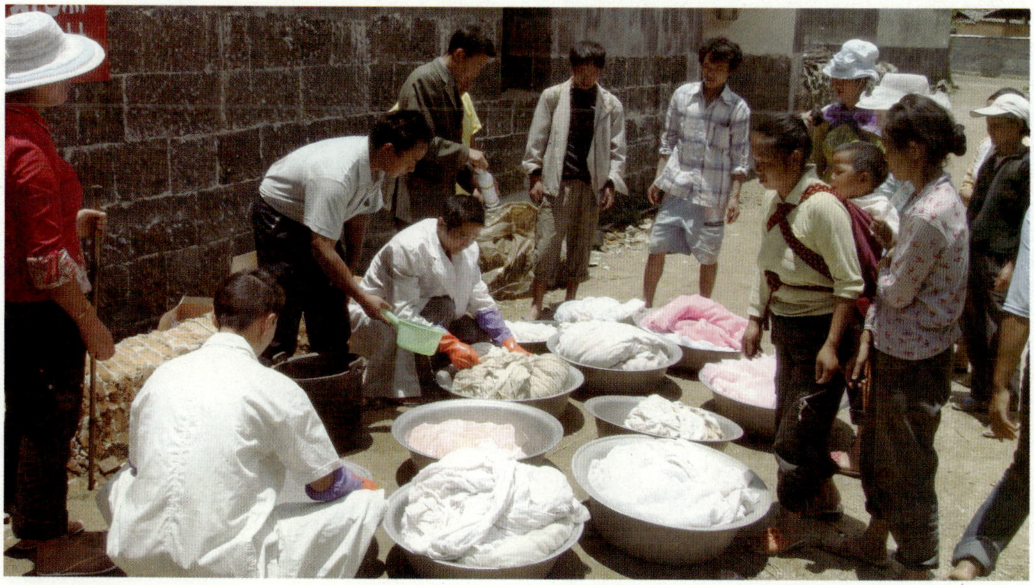
图 21 杀虫剂浸泡蚊帐

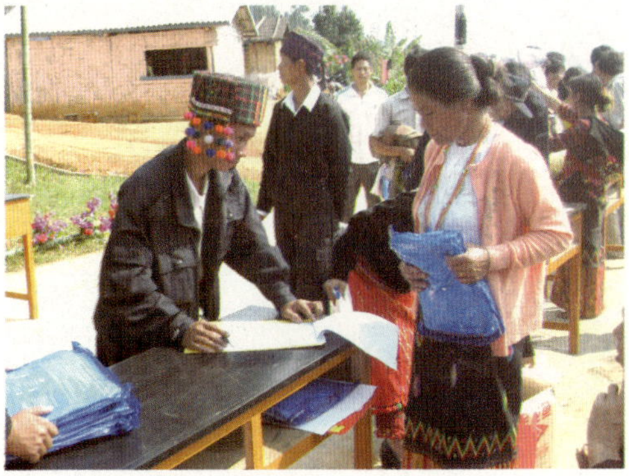

图 22 向村民发放免费的长效蚊帐

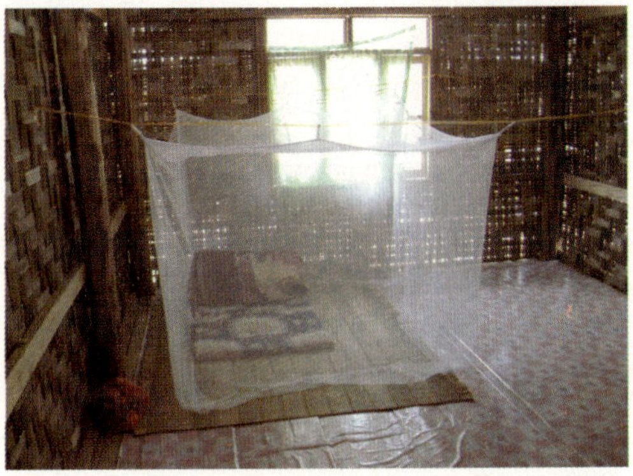

图 23 村民家里悬挂的项目免费提供的长效蚊帐

四、健教宣传活动

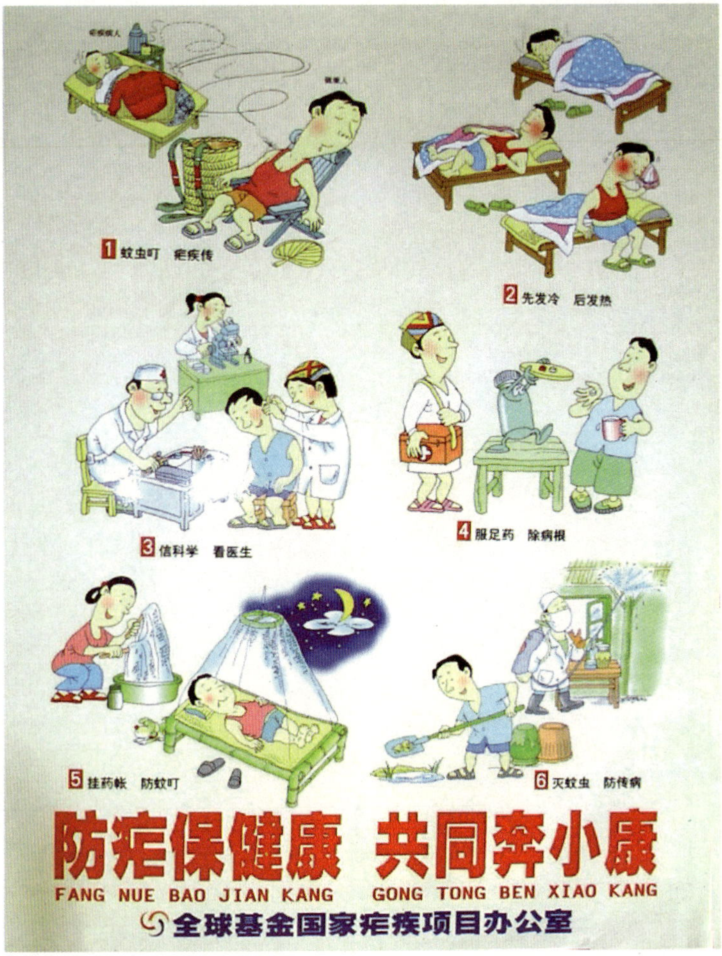

图 24 健康教育宣传画

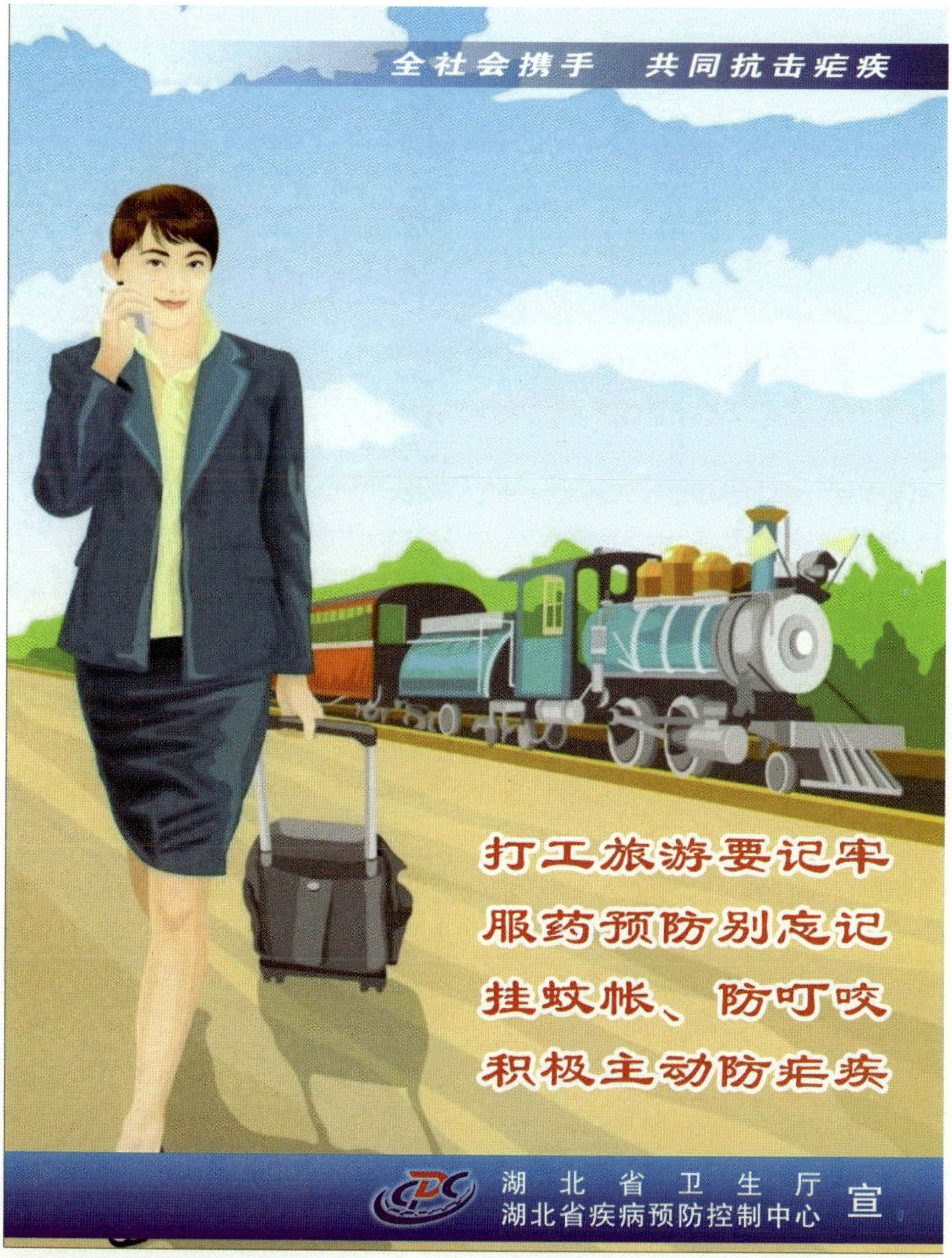
全社会携手　共同抗击疟疾
打工旅游要记牢
服药预防别忘记
挂蚊帐、防叮咬
积极主动防疟疾
湖　北　省　卫　生　厅
湖北省疾病预防控制中心
宣

图 25 健康教育宣传画

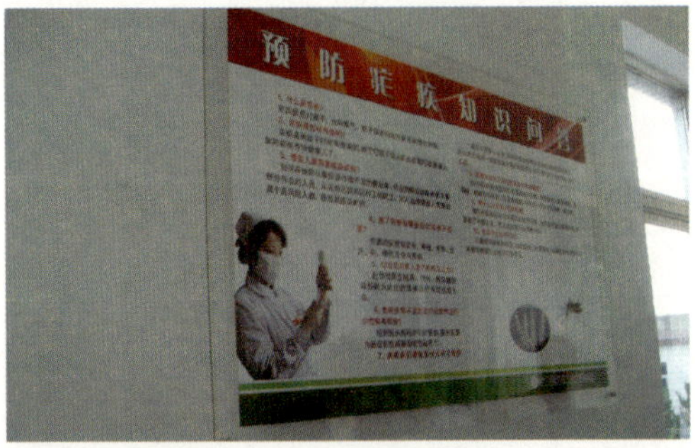

图 26 健教宣传知识问答墙体图片

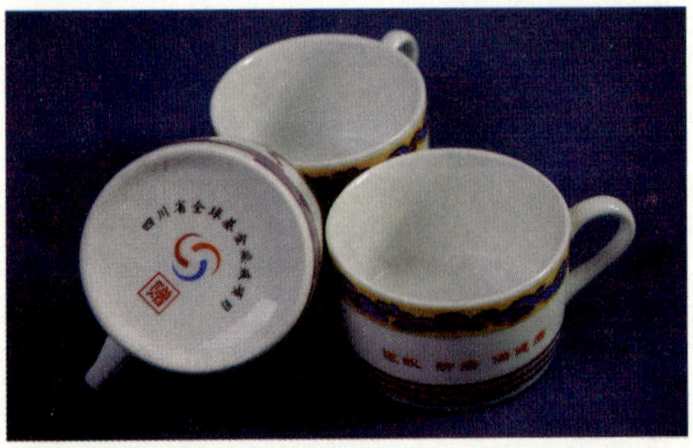

图 27 健康教育宣传茶杯

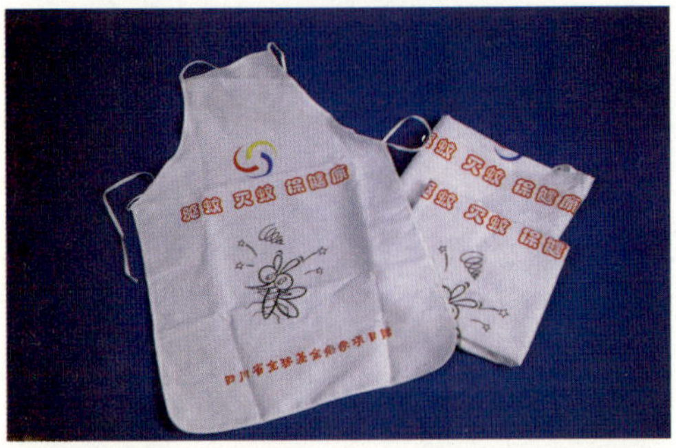

图 28 健教宣传围裙

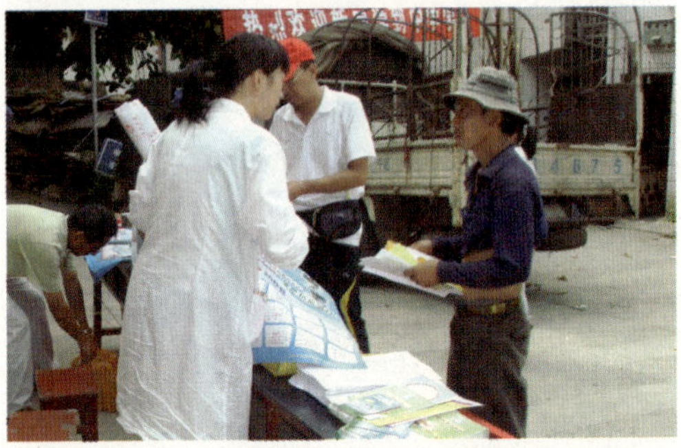

图 29 发放疟疾宣教材料

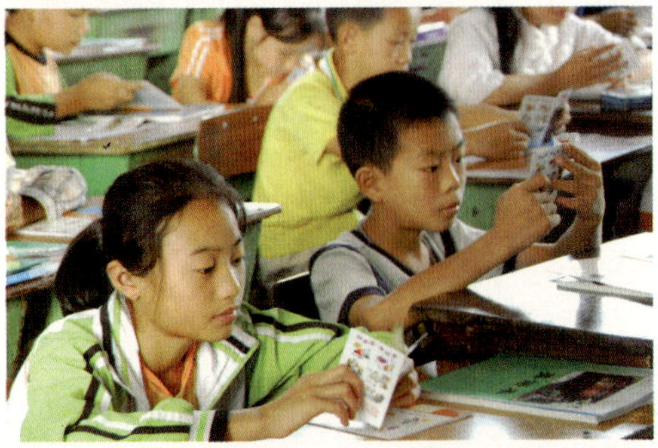

图 30 中小学生课堂疟防健康教育活动

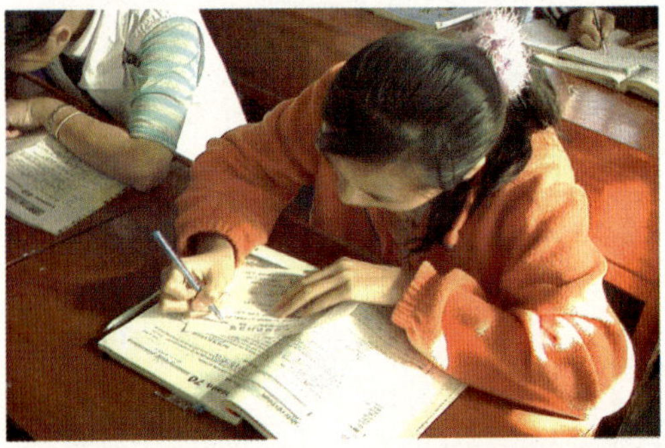

图 31 小学生在接受疟疾知识知晓情况问卷调查

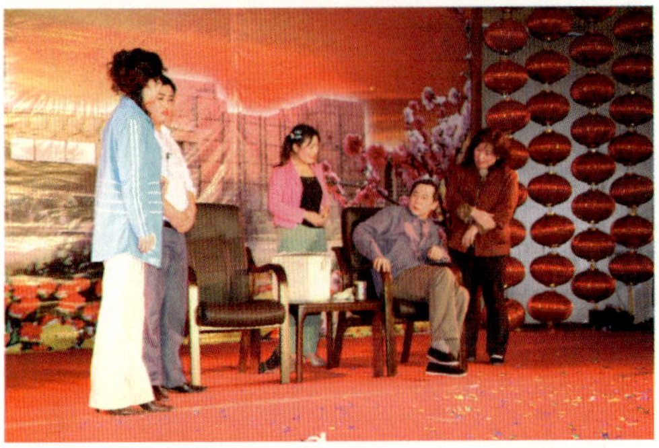

图 32 自编自演反映疟疾防治工作的小品“下乡”（2003 年 5 月，河南郑州）

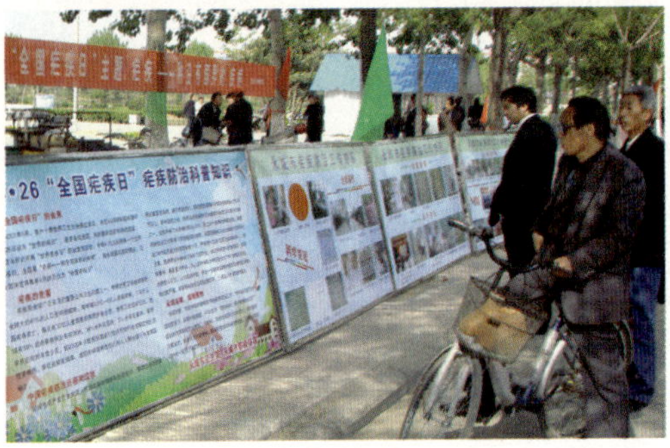

图 33 首届全国疟疾日宣传活动（2008 年 4 月，河南）

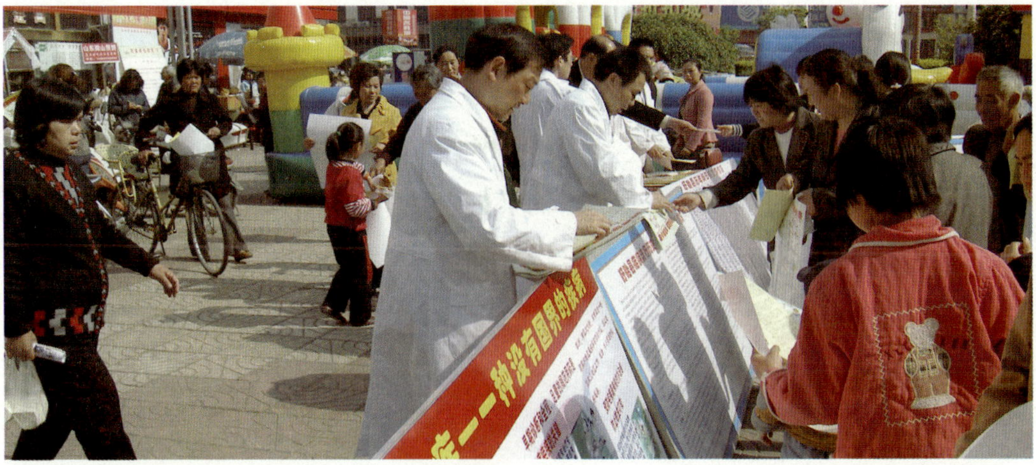

图 34 上街健教宣传（2008 年 4 月，江苏盱眙）

五、项目督导活动

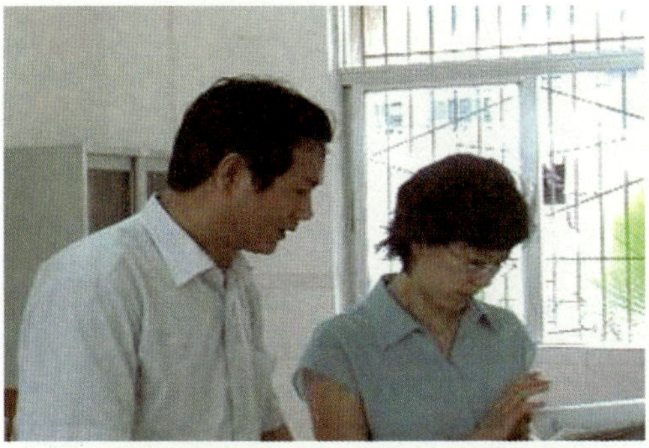

图 35 卫生部血防处王立英处长和国家疟疾项目办主任汤林华在海南省琼中县进行督导和调研（2004 年）

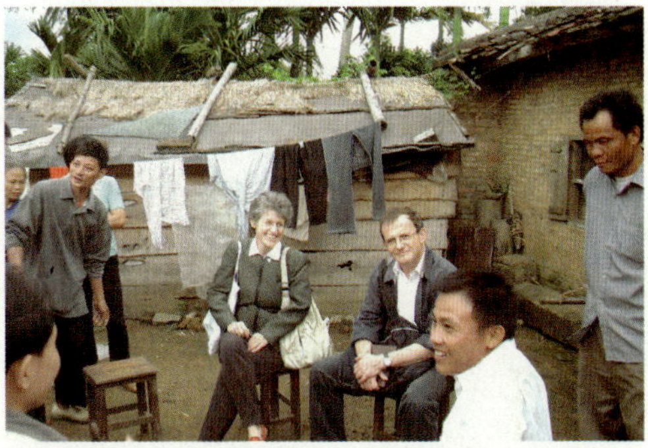

图 36 全球基金评估团赴海南进行项目 II 期实施前的能力评估（2004 年，海南白沙）

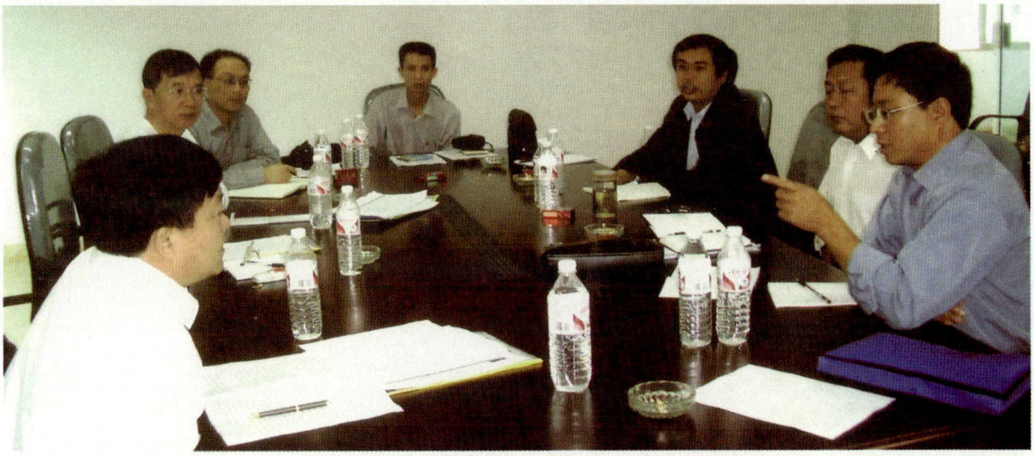

图 37 卫生部专家组到云南省全球基金项目县督导检查（2003 年 10 月）

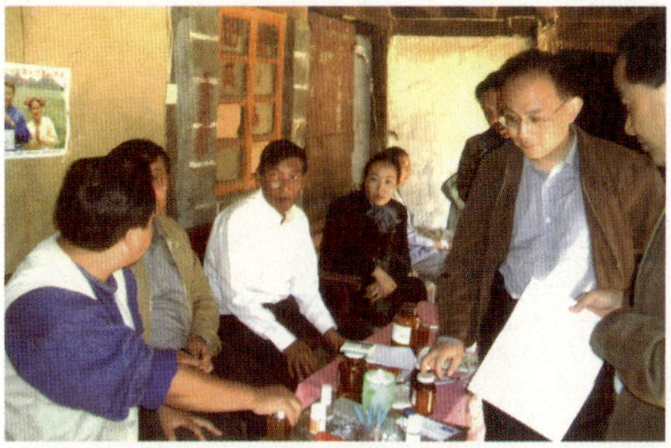

图 38　疟疾专家组赴云南处理中缅边境疟疾暴发（2003 年 11 月）

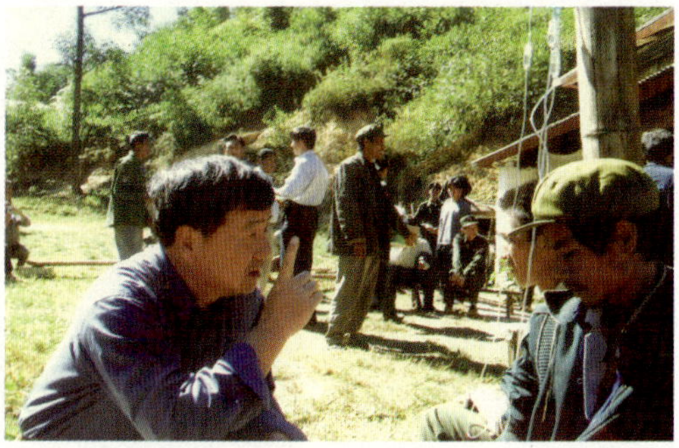

图 39　疟疾专家组在云南中缅边境进行现场流行病学调查（2003 年 11 月）

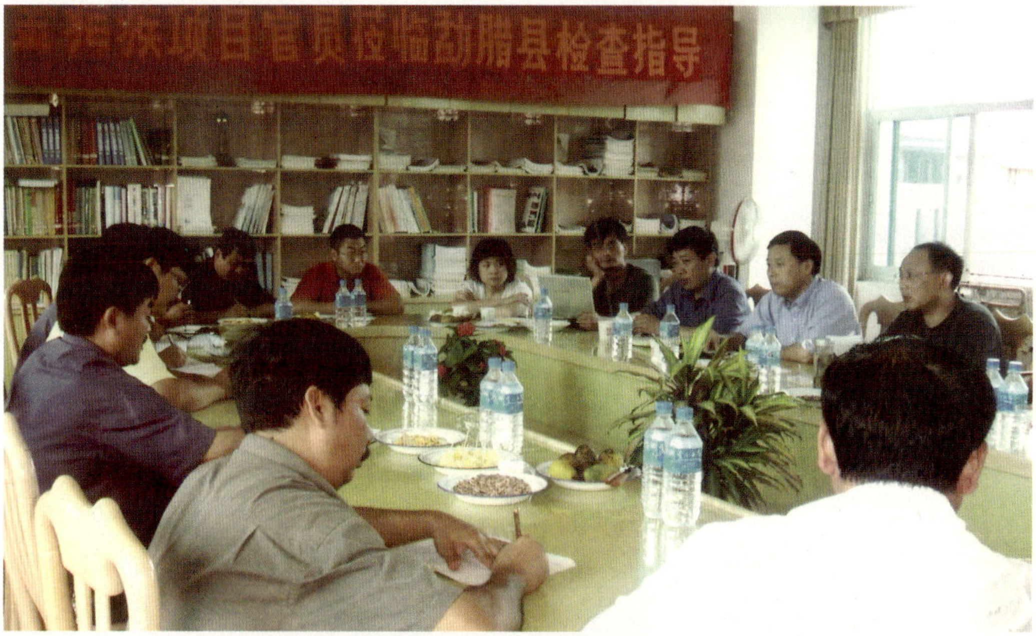

图 40　全球基金疟疾项目国家督导组对云南省项目现场督导（2004 年 7 月）

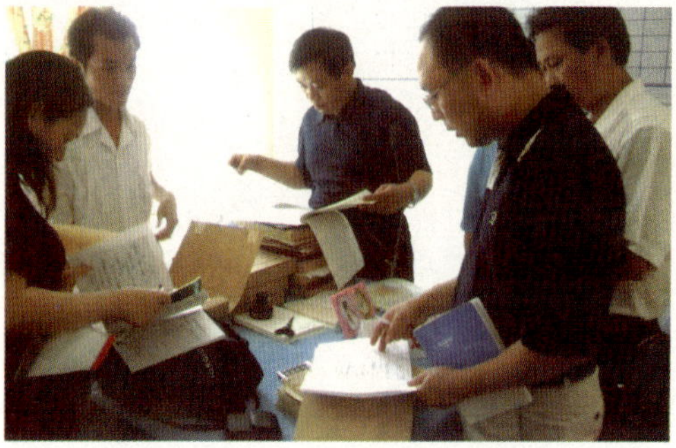

图 41　督导组检查项目办资料的可靠性、完整性

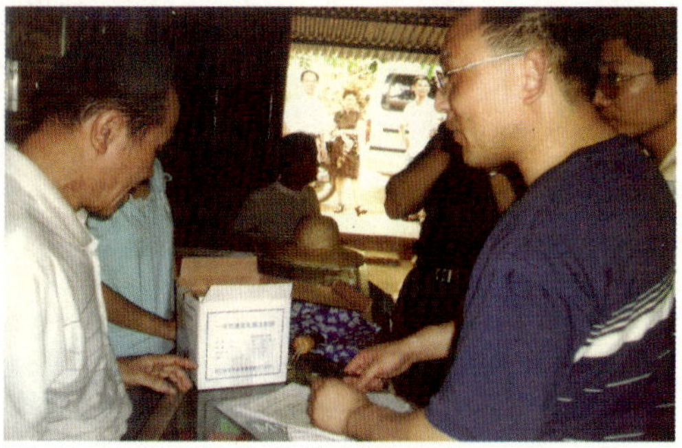

图 42　在村卫生室检查用药处方

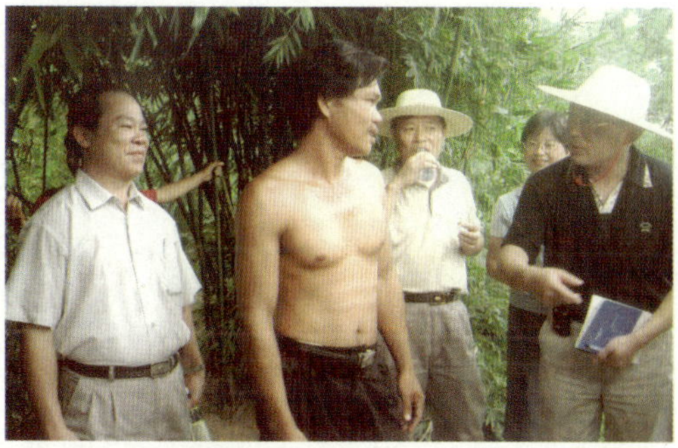

图 43 走访疟疾病人

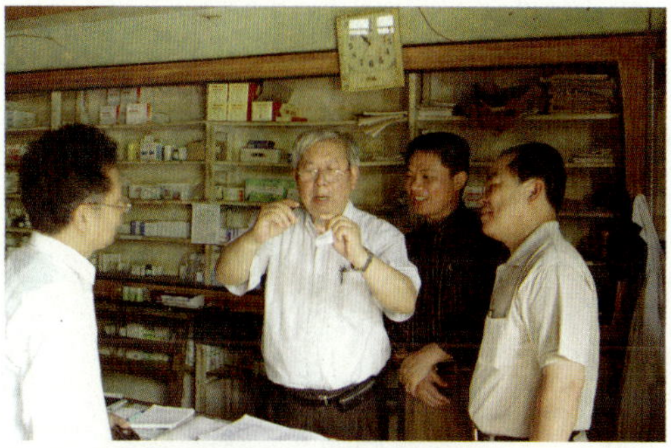

图 44 疟疾专家组在基层复查血片

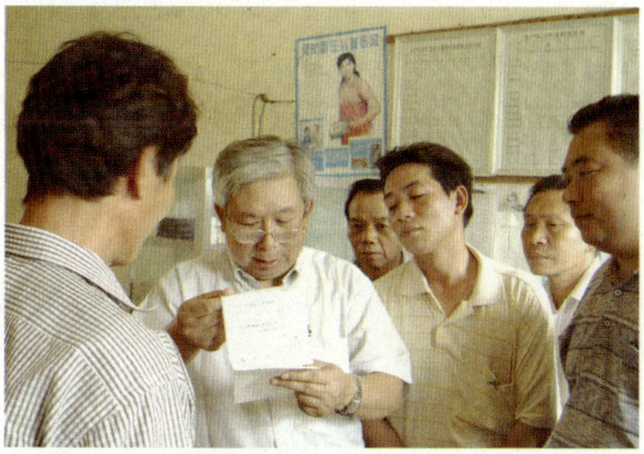

图 45 专家组在基层检查处方

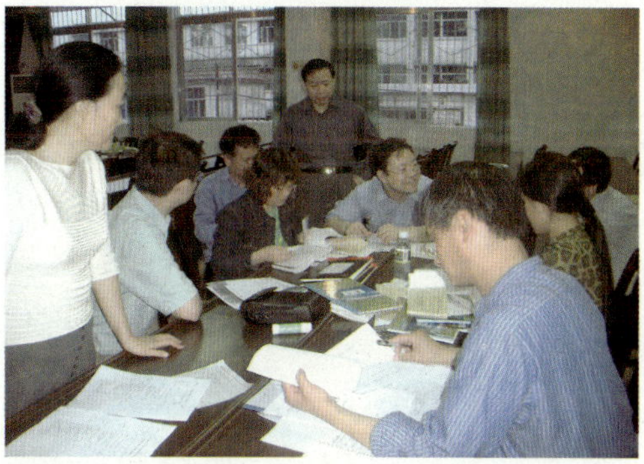

图 46 国家督导组在海南检查项目执行情况

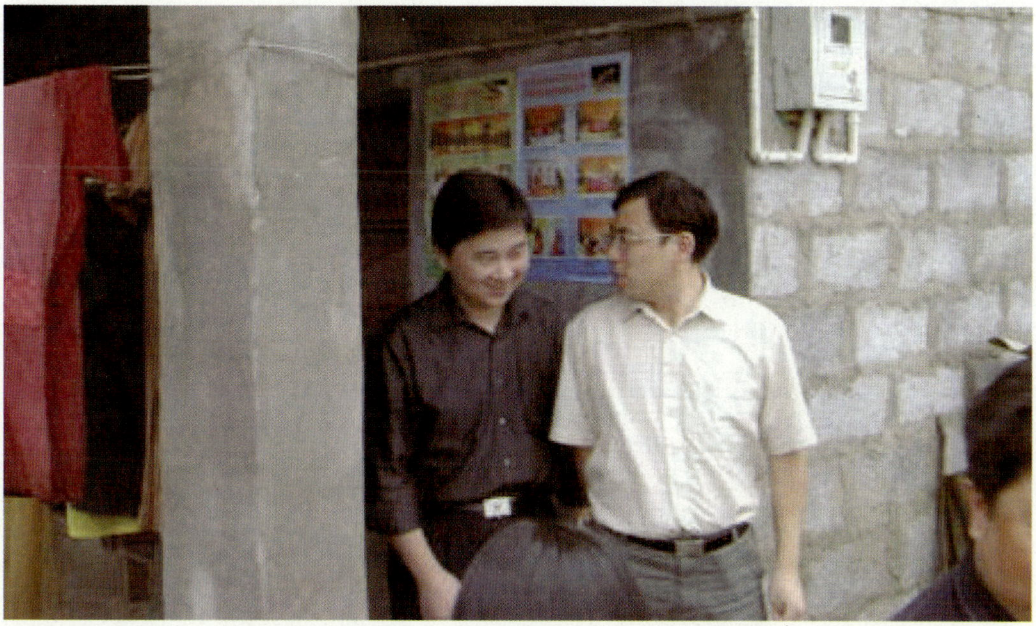

图 47 卫生部血防处夏刚副处长检查疟疾项目执行情况（2007 年 7 月，云南西盟）

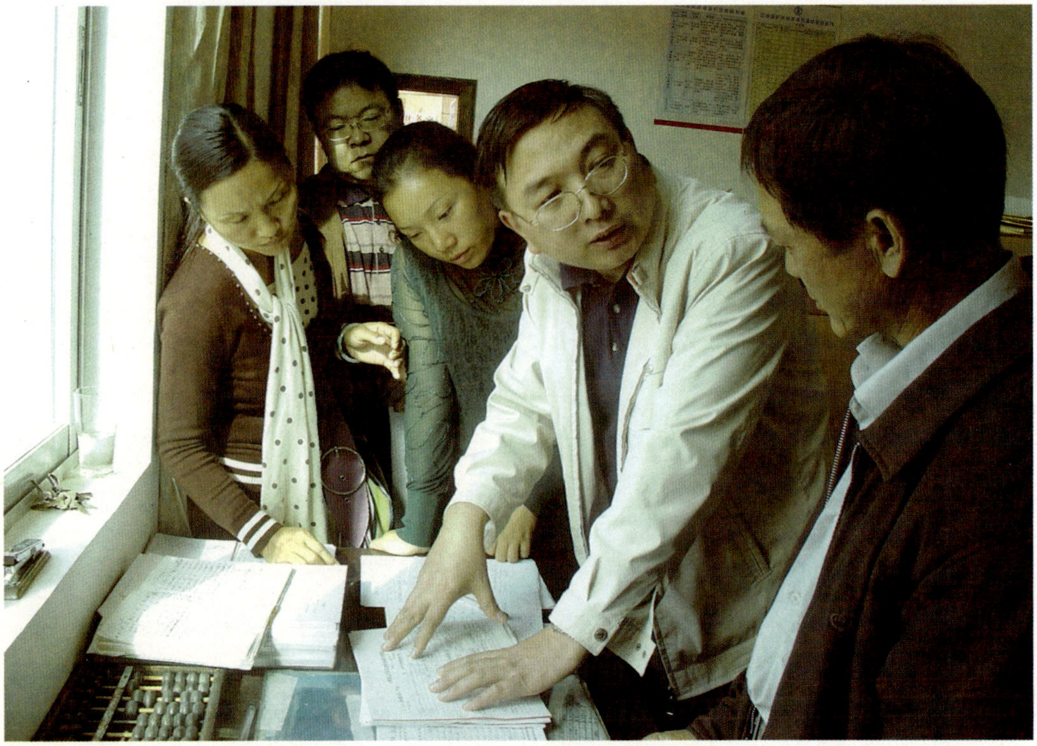

图 48 全球基金地方代理机构（LFA）徐岭峰主任现场核查数据（2005 年 11 月，云南孟连）

图 50 全球基金理事会专家现场检查疟疾项目（2007 年 11 月，海南琼中）

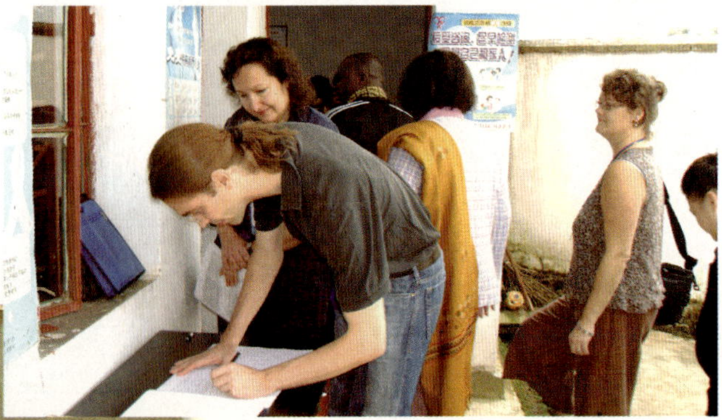

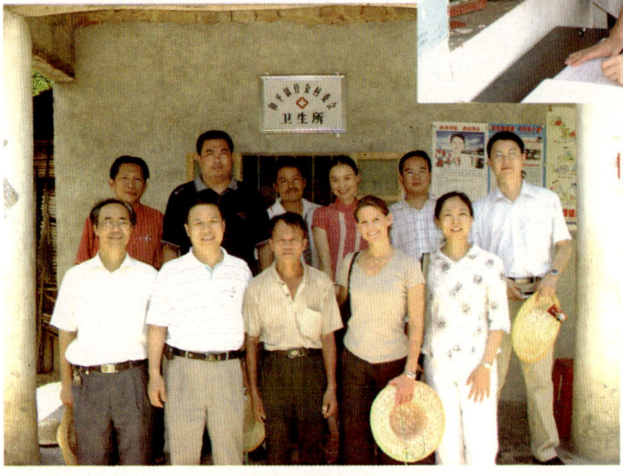

图 49 全球基金理事会专家在云南现场检查疟疾项目（2007 年 11 月，云南陇川）

六、终期评估

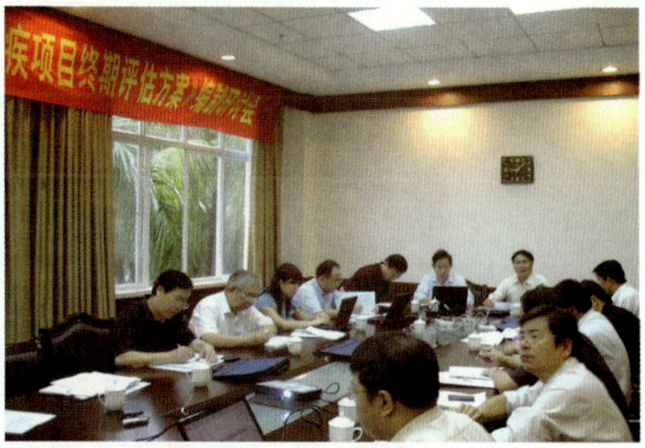

图 51《终期评估方案》编制研讨会（2007 年 11 月，海南琼海）

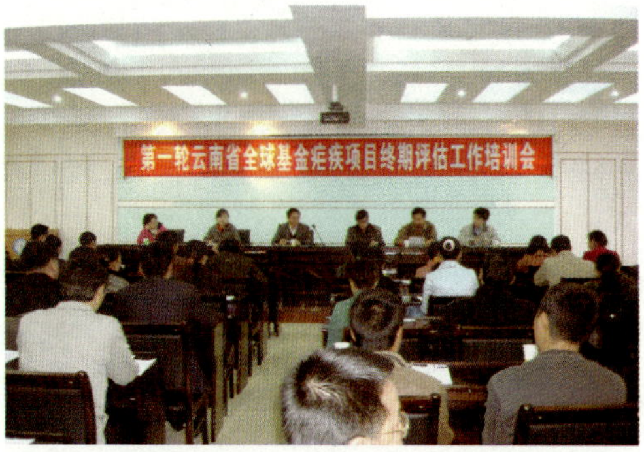

图 52 终期评估工作培训会（2008 年 3 月，云南思茅）

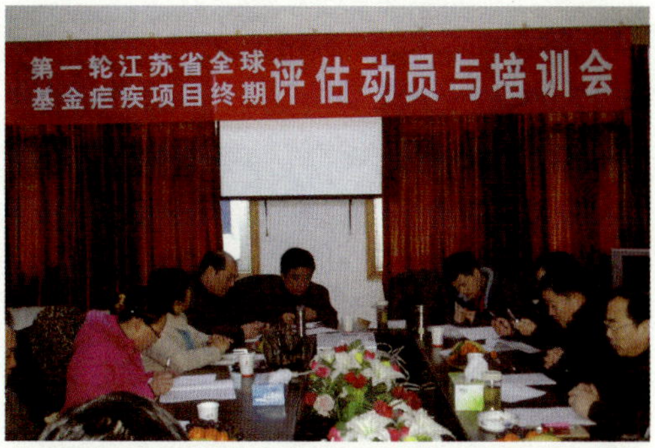

图 53 终期评估动员与培训（2008 年 2 月，江苏无锡）

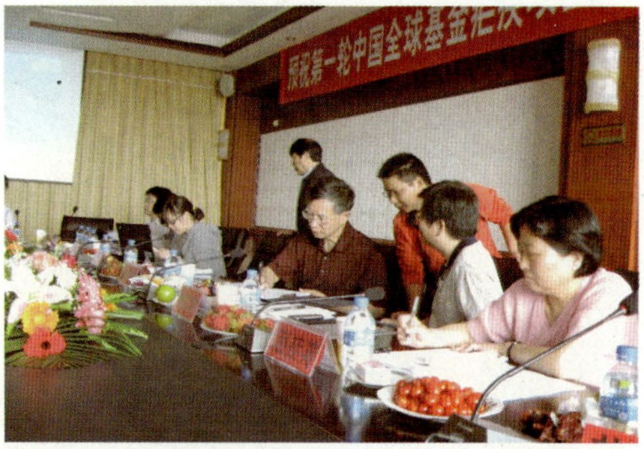

图 54 国家评估组对云南省项目实施情况进行评估（2008 年 5 月）

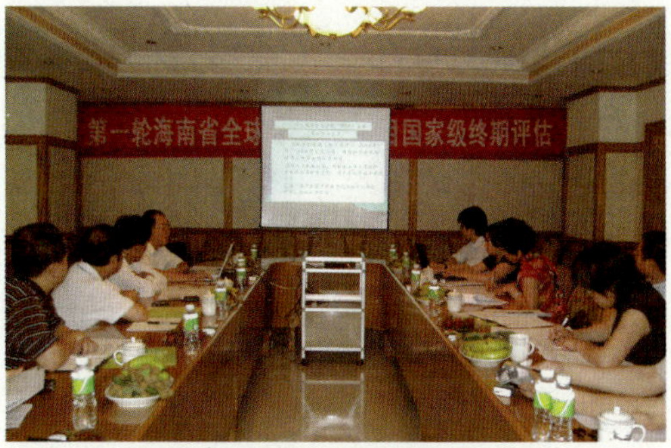

图 55 国家评估组对海南省项目实施情况进行评估（2008 年 5 月）

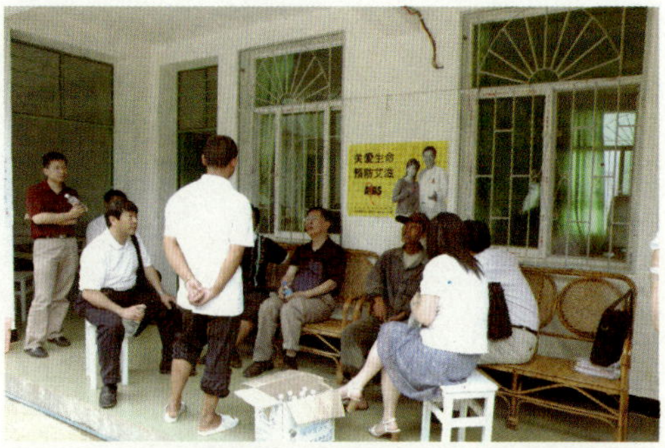

图 56 国家终期评估组在云南景洪与基层卫生人员交流（2008 年 5 月）

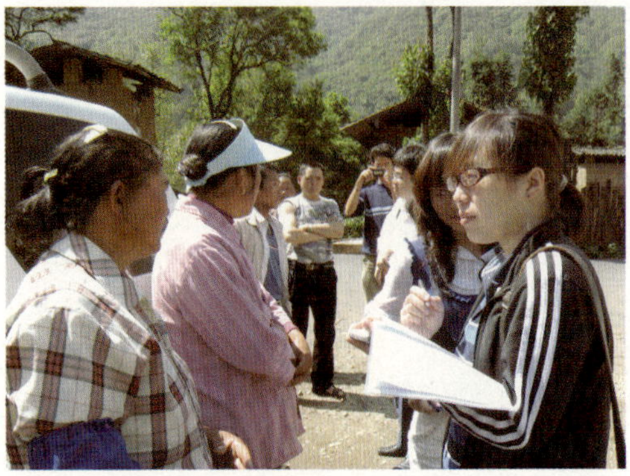

图 57　国家评估组走访杀虫剂浸泡蚊帐的受益人群（2008 年 5 月）

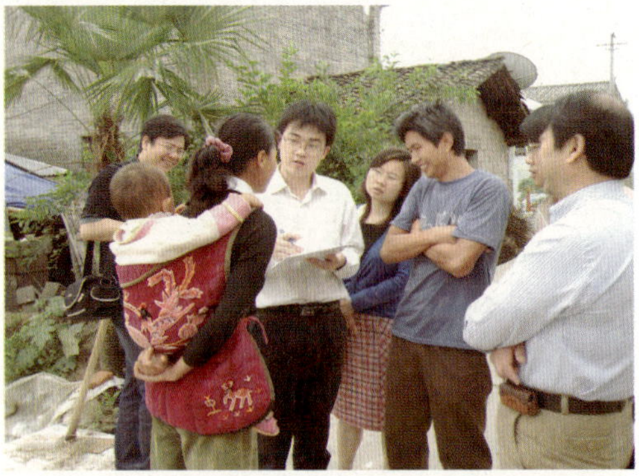

图 58　国家终期评估组在云南现场走访村民（2008 年 5 月）

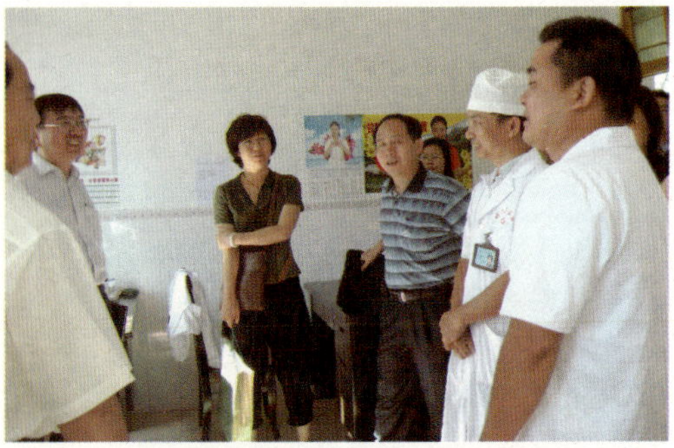

图 59　国家终期评估组在海南访谈村卫生室工作人员（2008 年 5 月）

七、项目交流

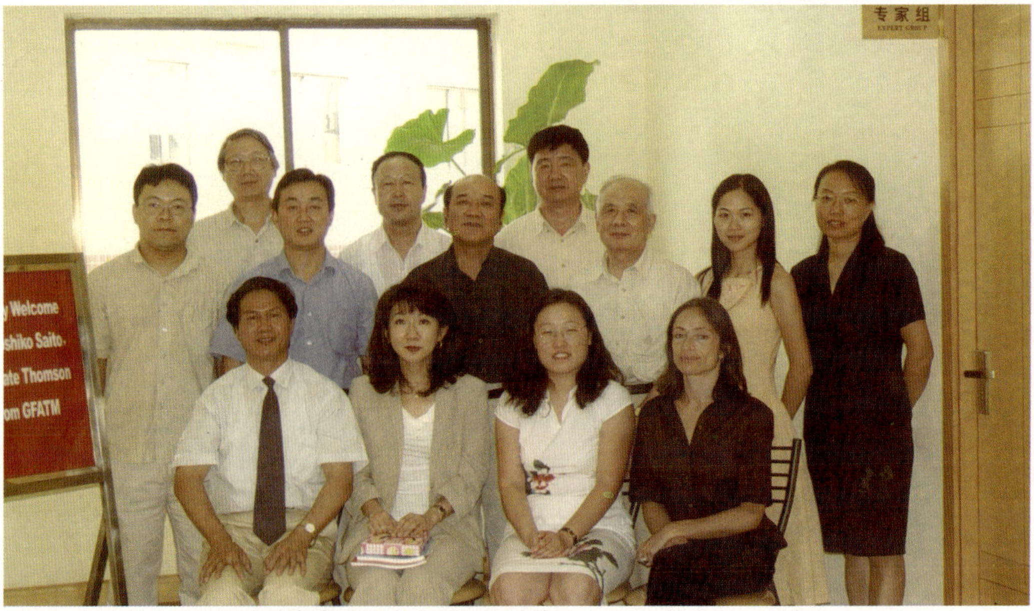

图 60　全球基金代表团来沪考察在华疟疾项目执行情况（2003 年 8 月，上海）

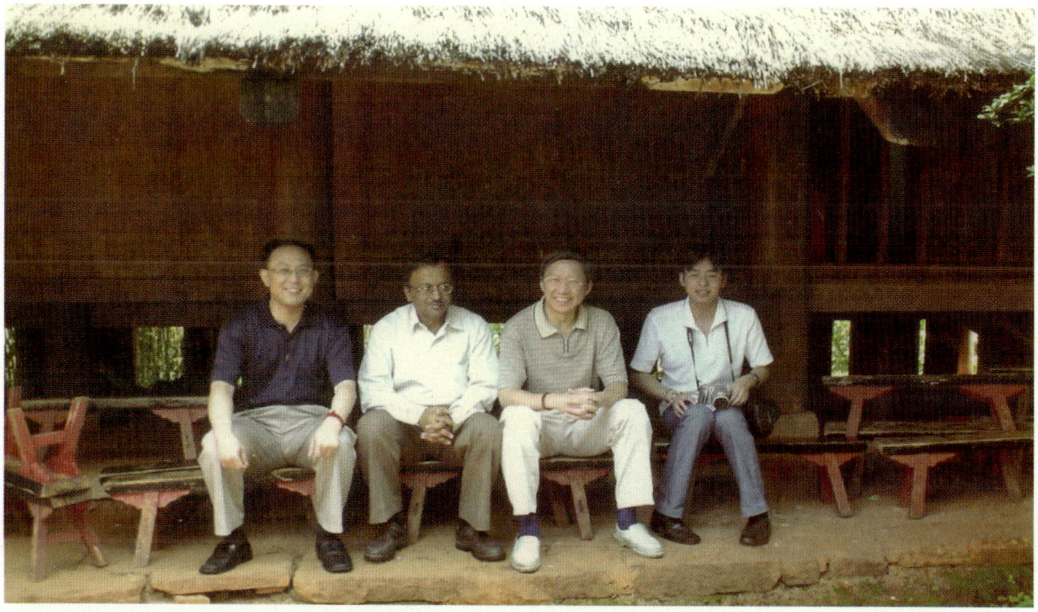

图 61 全球基金评估团对疟疾项目实地考察（2003 年 7 月，云南澜沧）

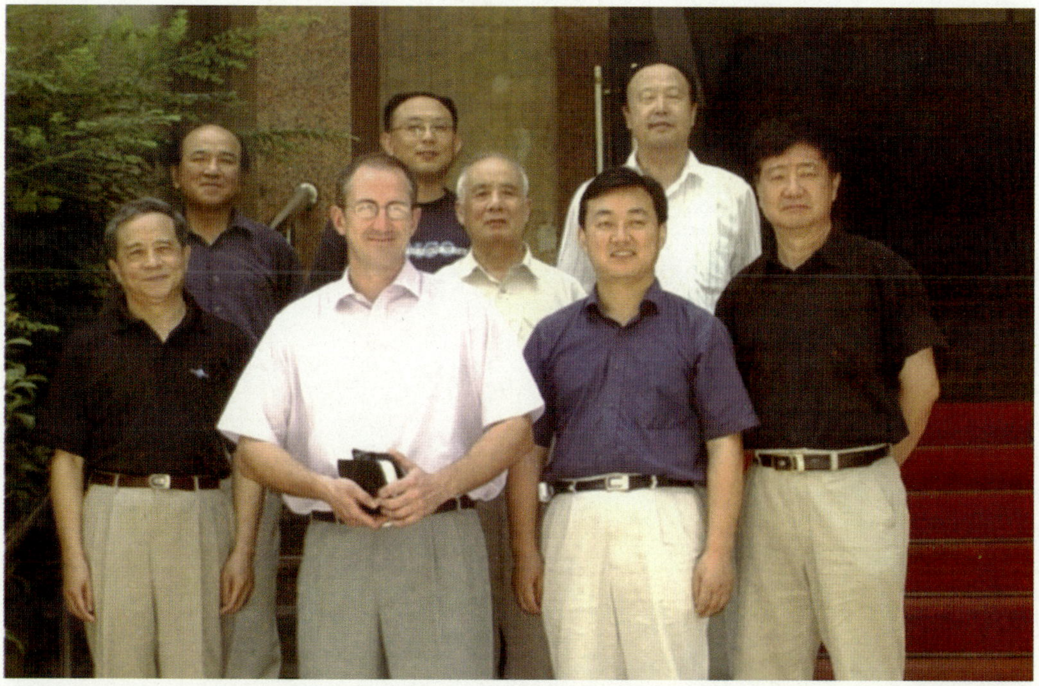

图 62 全球基金技术顾问 Hewitt Sean 博士为疟疾项目提供技术支持（2003 年 8 月，上海）

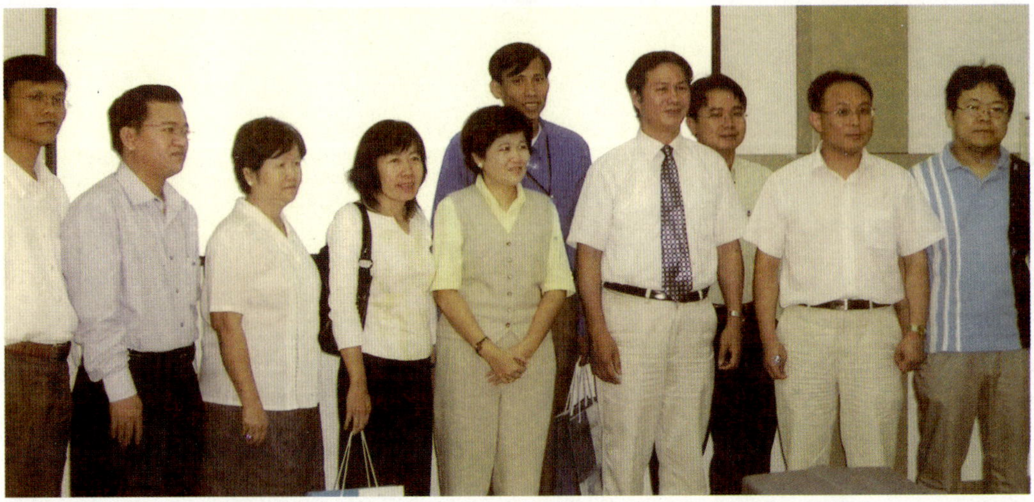

图 63 柬埔寨 PR 代表团访问中国全球基金疟疾国家项目办（2005 年 8 月，上海）

八、项目管理资料

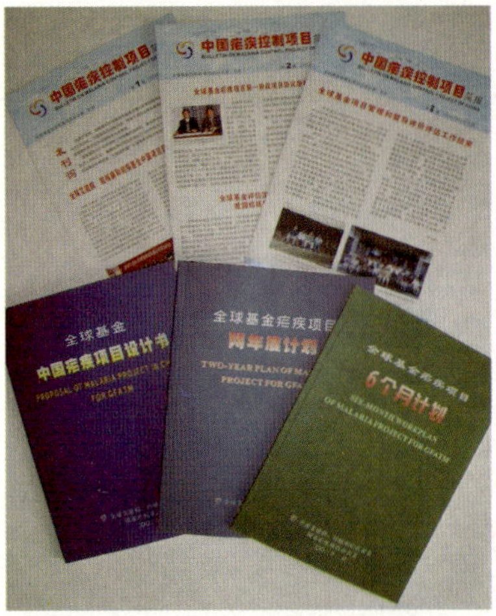

图 64 国家项目办编制的工作计划和项目通讯

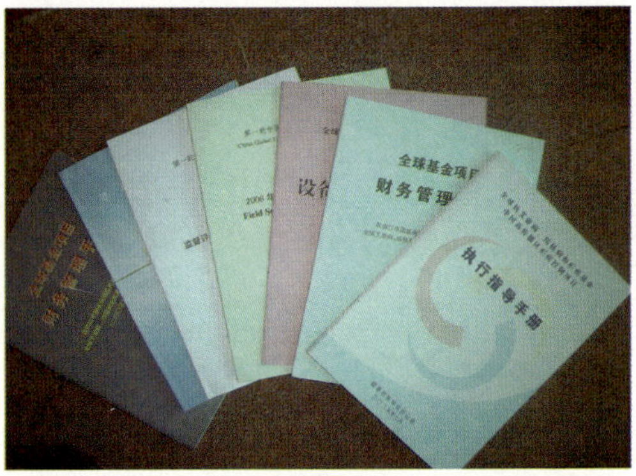

图 65 项目办编制的部分项目管理手册

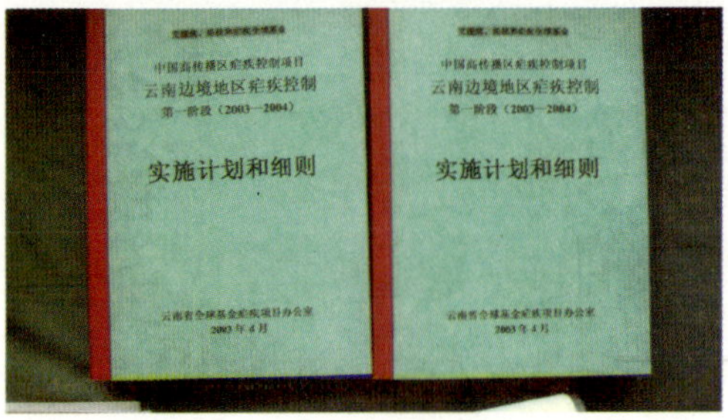

图 66 云南省第一阶段工作计划

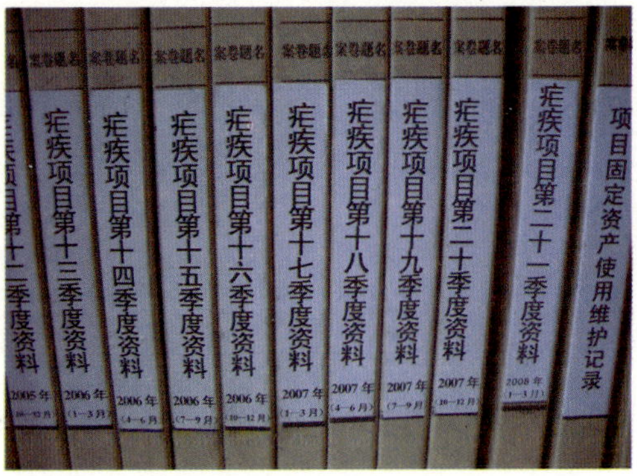

图 67 项目资料展示